# ADOLESCENTS' HEALTH

## A Developmental Perspective

# ADOLESCENTS' HEALTH
## A Developmental Perspective

**Inge Seiffge-Krenke**
*Universitat Mainz, Germany*

LEA LAWRENCE ERLBAUM ASSOCIATES, PUBLISHERS
1998 Mahwah, New Jersey London

Lawrence Erlbaum Associates, Inc., Publishers
10 Industrial Avenue
Mahwah, NJ 07430

Cover design by Kathryn Houghtaling Lacey

Library of Congress Cataloging-in-Publication Data

Seiffge-Krenke, Inge.
Adolescents' health : a developmental perspective / Inge Seiffge-Krenke.
p. cm.
Includes bibliographical references and index.
ISBN 0-8058-1839-1
1. Health behavior in adolescence. 2. Teenagers—Health and hygiene. I. Title.
RJ47.53.S44 1998
613'.0433—dc21 97-43413
CIP

Books published by Lawrence Erlbaum Associates are printed on acid-free paper, and their bindings are chosen for strength and durability.

Printed in the United States of America

10 9 8 7 6 5 4 3 2 1

*To Dirk, David, and Moritz Jakob*

# Contents


| | | |
|---|---|---|
| | Preface | **ix** |
| **1** | Theoretical Perspectives on Health and Illness | **1** |
| **2** | Problems in Assessing Health-Related Information | **18** |
| **3** | Epidemiological Findings on Health Problems, Diseases, and Health-Risk Behavior | **43** |
| **4** | Dealing With the Body | **70** |
| **5** | The Links Between Stress and Health | **99** |
| **6** | Social Support and Coping Style as Risk and Protective Factors | **124** |
| **7** | The Challenge of Coping With Chronic Illness | **151** |
| **8** | Health Care-Seeking Behavior in Adolescence | **181** |
| **9** | Some Implications for Prevention, Intervention, and Future Research | **209** |
| | References | **227** |
| | Author Index | **263** |
| | Subject Index | **275** |

# Preface

The primary aim of this volume is to integrate findings on health and illness in adolescence. To this end, I argue the value of following a developmental approach to the study of health or illness in general, and especially for adolescents. Throughout this book the importance of specific developmental processes and the contribution of these processes to understanding the reciprocity between health and illness is emphasized. This developmental perspective is also important because biological, social, and behavioral processes unique to the adolescent period have far-reaching consequences for health promotion, disease prevention, and disease recovery.

Compared to other age groups, adolescents enjoy a relatively good overall health status, yet report diffuse somatic complaints and are more likely to develop psychopathological symptoms. Thus, much attention is devoted to discussing the factors that may be responsible for this discrepancy. Special attention is given to adolescents who show cumulative deficits in their development due to their exposure to highly stressful events and lack of internal coping resources and social support in order to deal with these stressors. General data on both physical and emotional illness, health-related behaviors, and attitudes in adolescence are supplemented by findings obtained in the framework of my own longitudinal studies of adolescent health. It will be seen that studies of development in adolescence nearly invariably focus on the physical maturation process. Unfortunately, the effects of physical maturation on health-related behaviors shown by the adolescent in general and on interpersonal relationships with adults, including parents and health care professionals, have been largely overlooked. The chapters are organized according to several topics. Before embarking on a discussion of adolescent health and the factors that influence it, we need to give some consideration to a working definition of health. Chapter 1 summarizes the various theoretical models of health and illness and presents the development of the concepts of health and illness in lay persons. In chapter 2, the specific developmental barriers in obtaining diagnostic information in adolescent patients are outlined. In chapter 3, mortality and morbidity data from various adolescent populations offer rough estimates of adolescent health status. Chapter 4 presents an overview of the physical changes in adolescence and their effects on the interaction with health experts. Typical stressors for this age group and coping styles shown by normal and clinical samples of adolescents are described in chapters 5 and 6. Both chapters emphasize the adolescents' relationships with parents and friends as risk and protective factors. Chapter 7 is devoted to addressing these same issues in adolescents suffering from a chronic disease. The barriers in seeking health care or accepting offers of help are detailed in chapter 8. The book is concluded with a discussion of the major themes that emerge in the previous chapters in chapter 9. In addition, some considerations are made about the factors affecting adolescents' decisions to seek health care, and some suggestions are offered for prevention and intervention.

It is my hope that this book encourages others to assume a more integrated perspective toward the study of adolescence, a phase of development during which it is often difficult to distinguish between normal and disturbed developmental processes. I will be pleased if this book finds its way into the hands of many readers interested in the field of health psychology and hope that the discussion of the problems discussed herein proves useful in guiding those concerned with issues of adolescent health in their further research efforts.

## ACKNOWLEDGMENTS

In preparing this book, I profited from the stimulation, support, and assistance of many persons. I take this opportunity to thank all of those who have made it possible for me to complete the task. I would, however, like to specifically acknowledge the help of Judi Amsel and Nancy

Busch-Rossnagel who, by their interest and suggestions, encouraged me in this writing endeavor. Debbie Ruel from Lawrence Erlbaum Associates provided much help and assistance in the last step of work. Thanks are also due to Cornelia Daub-Metz, whose competent secretarial assistance in preparing the many drafts of these chapters was invaluable. Nicole Aengenheister assisted me in preparing the epidemiological data presented in chapter 3; Katja Waligora checked again the references. Tanja Nieder and Antonia Schwabenland spent long hours preparing the author and subject indices for publication. I wish to express my gratitude to all of them. My thanks also to Linda Lewis and Rachel Bond, who competently assisted me in preparing the translation of the present book.

—Inge Seiffge-Krenke

# 1

# Theoretical Perspectives on Health and Illness

A formal, comprehensive definition of *health* was adopted in 1946 in the original constitution of the World Health Organization (WHO): "Health is a state of complete physical, mental, and social well-being and is not merely the absence of disease or infirmity." This definition represents efforts to conceive health in positive terms rather than as the absence of poor health status and in relation to psychological, physical, and social dimensions. Although such a concept is most closely related to the psychological orientation toward health endorsed in this book, it is embraced by other disciplines concerned with health and health-related activities (e.g., social medicine, epidemiology, and medical sociology). The interdisciplinary nature of this concept is reflected in the various theoretical models of health that are briefly outlined in this chapter. It will become clear that developmental aspects are largely neglected in most theoretical approaches toward studying health. Thus, models that explicitly follow a developmental psychological perspective are highlighted, especially those that attempt to explain the relationships between healthy or normal and ill or pathological processes, as have, for example, been worked out in the field of developmental psychopathology.

## SUBJECTIVE CONCEPTS OF HEALTH AND ILLNESS

A major problem in understanding subjective concepts of health and illness is related to the fact that they are strongly influenced by social or normative factors, that is, society dictates how healthy or ill people should feel and biologically function. Also, subjective concepts of health greatly vary from individual to individual. Furthermore, children's, adolescents', and adults' beliefs and assumptions about these concepts dramatically differ, often in unexpected ways. Unfortunately, subjective concepts of health and illness often are vastly different from the operational definitions used by health care professionals and investigators who are often unaware of how differently individuals construe health and illness, depending on their developmental stage.

### Lay Conceptions of Health and Illness

Subjective concepts of health have not been investigated very often, although they undoubtedly play an important role in how an individual concretely deals with health and illness. One reason may possibly be related to the unconscious attitude most people have about health: Good health is simply taken for granted and only becomes salient when one loses it. Many people think of health as solely being the absence of illness. For example, a Scottish study on persons over 60 years old found that the key dimensions of health mentioned were an absence of illness, a reserve of strength, and a feeling of being generally fit or capable of accomplishing daily tasks (Williams, 1983). Corroborating evidence comes from a study of middle-aged French subjects, who described health in terms of an absence of illness, an equilibrium in daily life, and a capacity to work (Herzlich, 1973; Herzlich & Pierret, 1987). Other researchers found that although both working-class and middle-class people shared the notion that health meant the absence of illness, working-class people tended to emphasize what was essential for their everyday lives: the ability to carry out their daily tasks, especially job and family duties. Middle-class people were more likely to have broader, positive concepts of health that included such factors as energy, positive attitudes, and the ability to cope well and be in control of one's life (Calnan, 1987; Herzlich, 1973). In a study of more than 4,000 people, D'Hontand and Field (1984) found that health concepts varied considerably according to the respondent's socioeconomic status (SES): Skilled workers viewed health in instrumental, negative terms ("absence of illness" or "performance deficit"), whereas individuals with more extensive academic backgrounds viewed health as a personal goal and a state of psychosocial well-being ("happiness").

There are also strong gender differences in people's ordinary concepts of health, especially between mothers and fathers (Versteegen, 1988). Mothers consider their health to be an essential resource; nevertheless, they invest more efforts in protecting and maintaining their children's health than their own. Research has demonstrated, too, that although most individuals have difficulties in articulating their subjective concepts of health, they are quite able to make relatively concrete statements about health-preventive behaviors, such as watching one's diet, getting enough sleep, pursuing athletic activities, relaxing, going for medical checkups, avoiding consumption of health-damaging substances (e.g., cigarettes, alcohol, or drugs), and maintaining social contacts (Freund & McGuire, 1991).

Just as laypeople's notions of health are shaped by their social and cultural background, so too are the ways people understand illness. Individual beliefs about illness are typically drawn from larger cultural belief systems that shape the illness experience, help the individual to interpret what is happening, and offer a number of choices about how to react. Lay conceptions of illness also dictate how an individual responds to disease. For example, a study of middle-class Americans found that people regularly referred to diseased body parts as if they were objects separate from the person (Blaxter, 1983). The concept of disease as a foreign entity reflects a common tendency to understand disease as being caused by some external agent that has invaded the body. Indeed, most people think of disease in terms of what one has, gets, or catches. The causal categories most commonly named in several studies are (a) infection; (b) hereditary or familial tendencies; (c) environmental agents (e.g., toxic wastes or poisons), working conditions, and climate; (d) secondary effects of other diseases; and (e) stress, strain, and worry (Freund & McGuire, 1991). Although causal categories used by lay people may not be correct in medical and biological terms, they are generally rational and are based on the kinds of empirical evidence available to them. In addition, the interpretation of illness is an ongoing process. People reappraise their conditions throughout the various stages of illness.

### Developmental Changes in Conceptions of Illness and Health

A number of investigators studied the development of children's conceptions of health and illness. Most studies have been based on developmental theory as worked out by Piaget. Accordingly, attempts have been made to identify a general congruence between children's conceptions about health and illness and stages of cognitive development, especially with respect to reasoning concerning the physical world. For example, Bibace and Walsh (1981) interpreted the development of health concepts for younger children according to the three broad stages of cognitive development outlined by Piaget (i.e., preoperational, concrete operational, and formal operational). Most younger children (i.e., those between 4 and 7 years old) consider illness to be a magical phenomenon or an act of sorcery; they sometimes view illness as punishment (e.g., the consequence of disobeying their parents). In this developmental period, children begin to acquire an understanding that illness is transmitted from an external source to their own bodies. Nevertheless, they are not always able to understand or explain how illness is spread or they overgeneralize the principle of infection, believing that all illnesses are contagious. In middle childhood (from 7 to 11 years old), children accept the germ theory of illness etiology (i.e., that illnesses are transmitted by germs) but understand that not all illnesses are infectious. They accept a limited number of factors that enhance or reduce the possibility of illness. At about 11 years old, children understand that illness is related to the fact that bodily organs are not functioning properly. At around 14 years of age, they know that an illness may also result from emotional stress. Around the same time, they understand that ordinary definitions of illness also include aspects of a sick person's role (i.e., how someone acts after having been designated as sick). Thus, only when the child has reached the formal operational stage of cognitive development and has acquired more knowledge about internal physiological structures and functions is he or she able to approach understanding illness in terms of complex physiological and

TABLE 1.1
Child and Adolescent Definitions of Illness

| *Topics* | *Adolescents* | *Children* |
|---|---|---|
| Nonlocalized general feelings: "I feel bad." | 39.9 | 60.3 |
| Nonlocalized, specific feelings: "It hurts," "It's sensitive," "I'm dizzy." | 51.9 | 36.6 |
| Localized physical sensations: "I have a headache." | 42.9 | 46.2 |
| Visible signs: "Joints are swollen." | 15.6 | 11.5 |
| Objective but not visible signs: "I have a headache." | 5.2 | 12.6 |
| Illness concept: "Appendicitis." | 10.4 | 9.5 |
| State of feelings: "I'm grumpy, lethargic." | 9.1 | 11.8 |
| Sick role behavior: "I go to bed." | 9.1 | 13.0 |
| Changed conventional role: "I don't go to school." | 28.6 | 10.7 |
| Behavior of others: "The doctor comes." | 2.6 | 8.8 |
| Explicit restrictions: "When I have a cold, I'm not sick." | 0.0 | 2.3 |

*Note:* Table adapted from a table appearing in "Conceptions of Illness in Young Adolescents," by S. G. Millstein, N. E. Adler, and L. E. Irwin, 1981, *Pediatrics*, 68, p. 837. © APA.

psychophysiological processes (C. Eiser, 1985). As Table 1.1 illustrates, the meaning of specific feelings, as well as the inclusion of changed behaviors related to illness or characteristics of a sick person's role, represent some of the most important differences between definitions of illness made by children and early adolescents according to the study of Millstein, Adler, and Irwin (1981).

Observations made about children and adolescents in the hospital setting, documented by A. Freud and Bergmann (1965), shed light on how differently children and adolescents interpret and react to illness and infirmity. Younger children, who are expected to interpret illness as a consequence of disobeying their parents, often felt quite guilty about being ill. For example, they often explained their poor health to be a result of playing outside in the cold without a jacket, although their parents had instructed them to dress warmly. Slightly older children, who would be more likely to accept the germ theory of illness, were extremely careful not to come into physical contact with other ill children. The explanations for illness clearly became more differentiated among the 10- and 11-year-old children, who understand that illness is sometimes caused by bodily organs that do not function properly. Freud and Bergmann described the vigilance with which young patients with heart disease observed the amount, shape, and color of the pills the nurses gave them. Aside from the perceptible changes in heart functioning, these children assessed the gravity of their illness according to the amounts of medication they were required to take. Patients on the orthopedic ward tolerated the long periods of immobilization especially because the physiological reasons for their infirmity were concretely visible and they understood the rationale behind the therapeutic measures involved.

Other empirical studies on the development of health and illness conceptions have shown that both conceptions become differentiated in childhood and adolescence and that this development is associated with personal experiences with illness. For example, Millstein and Irwin (1987) interviewed 11- to 18-year-old adolescents and found that health and illness were different, yet overlapping, constructs. Children's definitions of health and illness became more precise with increasing age, and the focus changed as well. The younger respondents' definitions of health were more strongly bound to personal experiences with illness. In contrast, older adolescents' definitions included more references to physical well-being, the fulfillment of social- and achievement-related norms, and preventive health behaviors. In another study, adolescents typically viewed health as being more than simply the absence of illness: Being healthy meant living up to one's potential, being able to function physically, mentally, and socially, and experiencing positive emotional states (Millstein & Litt, 1990). In fact, "not being sick" accounted for less than 30% of the contents making up adolescents' conceptions of health. Thus, their definitions were more similar to adult conceptions of health and paralleled the formal definition of health laid down by the WHO.

In adolescents, illness and being sick are directly experienced by the manifestation of more or less frequently occurring symptoms of illness. As outlined earlier, their conceptions of health go beyond not being sick and include a variety of aspects of physical, psychological, and social well-being. It should also be pointed out that adolescents often perceive adult encouragement to lead a healthy lifestyle or engage in health-promoting behaviors as attempts of adults to regulate their lifestyles and restrain them from their spontaneous urges to eat, drink, and enjoy the pleasures of life at their will. Indeed, for many adolescents, experiencing health in the sense of well-being includes engaging in various behaviors that are hazardous to their health or are directly opposed to the adult conceptions of illness prevention, in the sense of risk avoidance or reduction. In addition, especially early adolescents sometimes underestimate their potential for becoming ill or injured. This is partly related to the fact that adolescents, due to their lower risk for illness, have generally had little experience with impaired health. Although they share this experience of low risk for illness with children, increased egocentrism—which reaches its greatest levels between 12 and 15 years old and decreases thereafter—contributes to this fallacy of judgment (see chap. 2, this volume). During this age span, adolescents believe they are relatively immune to sickness and injuries. After 16 years old, a more realistic perception of risks develops and adolescents begin to acknowledge and avoid health risks.

Additional changes in the development of conceptions of health and illness in adolescence are related to the sick role and the disruption of control. Although adolescents—compared to children—recognize the sick role as a characteristic of illness, they may not be able to submit to this role easily. Most illnesses disrupt an individual's ability to exercise control, and being disabled or dependent on others can be especially threatening to the adolescent who is making great efforts to achieve independence.

## THEORETICAL MODELS OF HEALTH AND ILLNESS

We are now ready to consider theories generated in the frameworks of various academic disciplines about health and illness. Medical, sociological, and psychological theories are presented and analyzed according to their suitability for a general conception of health in adolescence. It should be emphasized here that the models discussed in this section are oriented toward explaining the general concepts of health and illness; other models that incorporate aspects of health-related behavior, for example, as related to seeking professional care and treatment, are discussed later (see chaps. 8 and 9, this volume).

### Medically Oriented Models

One of the more classic medically oriented theoretical approaches toward understanding health has its origins in the field of virology. The risk-factor model (Abholz, Borgers, Karmans, & Korporal, 1982) is based on the assumption that each illness has a specific cause and is associated with overtly manifest symptoms and physical damage or injury. In its original form, this model proved to have several inherent weaknesses, as Levi (1975) pointed out. For example, it fails to explain why some individuals do not contract an illness, despite exposure to a pathogenic agent.

More recent medical models attempt to compensate for these weaknesses. Compared to earlier models, they are more complex and accommodate for a variety of factors that influence health and health-related behavior. A more comprehensive understanding of health and illness is characteristic of these models. Health and illness are regarded as states determined or influenced by many variables (e.g., the risk of becoming ill and the onset and course of illness being determined by social, psychological, developmental, and physiological factors). More important, illness is regarded as an individual's failure to adapt at various levels instead of primarily being the consequence of bodily damage due to exposure to chronic noxious stimuli, a pathogenic agent, or stress. Thus, health is viewed in relation to an individual's total lifestyle. Additional developments to medically oriented models were drawn from theoretical concepts of psychosomatic medicine, which ascribe much significance to subjective perceptions of illness. Psychosomatic medicine generally has eschewed focusing on monocausal explanations of illness, preferring instead to understand illness in more holistic terms and focusing on the illness in relation to the specific context of the individual.

Antonovsky (1987) followed this approach in developing his salutogenetic model of health. Accordingly, this model attempts not only to describe how illnesses and misdevelopments are generated, but also to explain why some individuals are able to remain healthy or show no signs of illnesses or abnormalities. Antonovsky understands health to represent a dynamic interaction between the various factors that cause or promote stress and those that protect against or relieve the individual from their deleterious effects. This interaction is strongly influenced by the individual's specific life circumstances and personal biography.

Coping processes are strongly emphasized, especially with respect to factors that make an individual less susceptible to the negative effects of stress. Such resistance-promoting factors include an individual's capacities to respond to or prepare for social and biological stressors in a manner promoting self-development. These capacities are reflected in concrete health-promoting or health-preserving behaviors, such as seen in individuals who maintain a healthy diet, take prophylactic measures to avoid certain illnesses, or who consciously avoid stressors, thus reducing the likelihood that they should exert their health-damaging effects.

### Sociologically Oriented Models

Most sociological theories place great emphasis on explaining how social structures, socioecological factors, and socialization affect health and health-related behaviors. For example, according to the socialization theory model, health-relevant behavior is thought to be acquired in a social context throughout the entire life span. This learning process is influenced by social position as well as the access to social and ecological resources (Navarro, 1976). In a more recent overview of "who becomes sick, injured and dies," Freund and McGuire (1991) reported on how mortality and morbidity rates varied depending on race and SES. In particular, not only were individuals living in poverty confronted with additional stressors, but they lacked the resources to deal with health problems.

Whereas earlier sociological theories of health largely neglected the roles of physical constitution and psychological disposition, more recent theories include these aspects. Following the basic approaches characteristic of theories rooted in the fields of medical sociology and personality psychology, theoretical models of stress focused on explaining the relation among stressful life circumstances, behavioral disorders, and the moderating influence of personal and social variables. In his sociologically oriented approach, Pearlin (1987) attempted to integrate various medical and psychological theories of stress. This model of stress acknowledges the importance of life circumstances as defined by a variety of social and economic variables, (e.g., age, gender, SES, occupation, ethnic background, and institutionalized roles associated with the family, workplace, or neighborhood that alone or together may cause stress). In addition, social mediators (especially political, collective, or individually initiated activities that affect the individual's social life circumstances), personal mediators, and self-concept variables determine whether a stressor taxes the individual's adaptive abilities, thus leading to impaired health. Admittedly, definitions of stressors are kept general and the spectrum of stressors is broad (e.g., critical life events, chronic stressors, or difficult life transitions). Consequently, the importance of critical life events become relativized.

A further model was proposed by Badura (1983), who differentiated between acute and chronic stress and acknowledged the moderating influence of social support and coping styles. Social support and coping styles together create a psychosocial immune system insofar as they serve protective functions against psychosocial risks and their effects. Much empirical evidence to support this model was obtained in studies examining the etiologies of various chronic illnesses such as hypertension, cardiovascular disease, bronchial asthma, peptic ulcers, and circulatory disturbances. An individual's lifestyle—in particular, the culturally accepted behavioral strategies used to control and cope with stress—is an important construct in this model. Behaviors manifested as responses to stress that are likely to pose serious risks to health are, for example, excess consumption of alcohol, smoking, or poor eating habits. According to Badura, such potentially health-hazardous behaviors are understood as culturally accepted reactions to complex life circumstances. However, should these strategies become stabilized (i.e., when they no longer represent temporary reactions), then they become "risky lifestyles."

### Psychological Theories

Research in the field of psychology has devoted considerably more attention to developing theoretical models of health that account for the influence of many different variables. In particular, much progress in the study of stress and coping has been made by developmental psychologists. Mounting evidence indicates that the occurrence of psychological disturbances and disorders is more likely when the amount of stress overtaxes an individual's stress-deflecting or buffering capacities. Both a decrease of the protective factors—as, for example, by a change in or loss of social and material support—and the potentiation of stress by the emergence of new or additional stressors thus increases the probability of developing mental illness.

In this context, the concept of vulnerability has been discussed more intensely. It has been observed that some individuals are able to remain emotionally and physically healthy, despite being subjected to great levels of stress. Other vulnerable individuals appear to be particularly predisposed to suffering from stress. Such vulnerability may be very extreme, as seen in individuals who are inordinately sensitive to any kind of negative influence on their lives. These individuals tend to show a relatively unstable personality structure and lowered self-confidence, thus preventing them from making appropriate assessments of reality. Theoretical and empirical research on this phenomenon has attempted to clarify which personality traits, if any, are associated with an increased vulnerability or resistance to stress, and in which manner they may interact with other psychological traits, physical constitution, and social resources (Garmezy & Rutter, 1983).

We consider the increased orientation to developmental psychology, seen in more recent theoretical and empirical research efforts, to be a very decisive advancement. In this regard, the approach adopted by Werner and Smith (1982) warrants particular attention. These investigators put forth a convincing model of health. Based on this model, they conducted well-designed longitudinal studies of health, illness, and development of the entire population of the Hawaiian island of Kauai. A focal point of the study was based on a group of individuals born in 1955, who were observed and interviewed regularly for a period of 20 years. The investigators also relied on information provided by the subjects' parents and teachers, as well as that obtained from pediatric and psychological examinations. In the early phases of the investigation, 72 of the 695 children were selected for further inquiry. These children showed a marked accumulation of serious risk factors, such as family poverty, birth defects, genetically related handicaps, or maternal illness, yet revealed no signs of serious psychological disturbance. It appeared as if—by virtue of certain physical, psychological, and social characteristics—these children developed resiliency forces against unfavorable life circumstances that protected them from developing mental illness. Werner and Smith's study showed that grave risk factors did not, as was expected, necessarily lead to behavioral and emotional problems; in fact, these children enjoyed a rather healthy psychosocial development. As adolescents they proved to be psychically resilient and invulnerable because they were able to cope with highly stressful situations in an active and productive manner and to establish positive, compensatory relationships with others. Accordingly, these authors attempted to describe and differentiate between stressful and protective factors in the child's sozialization process that reinforce or weaken the potential of risk factors to promote mental and behavioral disorders. The following circumstances are some examples of stress-inducing factors:

- Prolonged separation from the primary reference person during the first years of life.
- Birth of siblings during the first 2 years of life.

- Serious or recurrent illnesses in childhood.
- Siblings with handicap or psychic disorder.
- Continuous familial discord.
- Absence of the father.
- Parental unemployment.
- Relocation of the family household.
- Change of school.
- Divorce of parents.
- Stepfather or stepmother joins household.
- Departure or death of older sibling.

Protective factors are represented by the following life circumstances:

- Siblings at least 2 years older or younger.
- Ample attention to child during the first years of life.
- Positive parent–child relationship during the first years of life.
- Other significant reference persons besides mother.
- Adequate care by siblings and grandparents.
- Relatives and neighbors providing emotional support.
- Clear structure and rules in the family household.
- Close friendships with children of the same age.
- Good opportunities for families to obtain advice and counseling from professional day-care providers, teachers, clergy, etc.
- Good access to special organizations and services (e.g., health office, counseling centers, etc.)
- Maternal satisfaction due to continued employment.
- Shared values and life perspectives in the family.

A comparison with a similar study of children living on the Isle of Wight and in inner London (Rutter, 1985b) showed that the most resilient adolescents from Kauai were subjected to fewer cumulative stressors than British adolescents. Nevertheless, some of the risk factors that Rutter found (e.g., marital discord, lower social status, limited space in the family home, parent or parents suffering from emotional illness, or child becoming a ward of the state) were also found to differentiate between resilient Kauain adolescents and those with serious emotional and behavioral problems. This is a surprising finding, because the two populations represent two completely different ethnic groups. In any case, it appears that being exposed to risk factors that endanger normal development does not automatically lead to symptoms of deviancy or other psychosocial abnormality. Indeed, the effects of such exposure are moderated by positive styles of coping and protective social resources.

This theoretical approach places much importance on considering the process of how psychic disturbances and behavioral abnormalities begin and develop. Abnormal behavior is regarded as a symptom or reaction to stress overload such that the individual's capacities to adapt to such stress are overtaxed. Children and adolescents may, for example, be unable to meet the demands that arise in the family or educational contexts. This goodness-of-fit position was also followed in more recent theories on adolescent development (Lerner, 1982), thus reflecting similarities with sociologically oriented theoretical approaches.

In summary, three classic groups of models can be identified according to their scientific orientations to health. Classic medical models are based on the assumption that an illness is a result of specific injury or damage to the organism; health and illness are clearly separate states. According to the classic sociological models that explain social deviancy in relation to political, social, and cultural structures, illness and health are interpreted as reflecting the effects of prevailing social conditions (e.g., as borne from differences related to socioeconomic class or the distribution of power). Classic psychological models take into account genetic and acquired disturbances whose development or promotion may be related to intrapsychical tension and conflicts.

Each of these models, however, focuses on a limited aspect of reality in that they overemphasize one particular aspect of health. These aspects must be integrated if one is to arrive at a truly comprehensive concept of health. As pointed out earlier, newer, more differentiated theoretical approaches are marked by their attempts to integrate theories and paradigms stemming from various disciplines. This has resulted in the fact that the traditional, medically oriented concept of illness, once strictly tied to physiological and genetic risk factors, has expanded to include psychosocial risk factors. In addition to the pathogenetic-curative approach, more emphasis is being placed on the salutogenetic conceptualizations of health, which seek to acknowledge the influence of certain kinds of lifestyles, protective factors, and variables promoting invulnerability to illness. The expansion of sociological models to include factors of social support and social networks and, in others, the inclusion of a positive definition of emotional and physical health are indicative of how conceptions of health and illness, developed independently within the frameworks of various academic disciplines, have begun to parallel each other.

## NEW APPROACHES: DEVELOPMENTAL PEDIATRICS AND DEVELOPMENTAL PSYCHOPATHOLOGY

In this section, two relatively new fields of research are presented that have pursued questions of health and illness from a developmental perspective.

### Developmental Psychopathology

Developmental psychopathology emerged as an organized field around 1970, combining theoretical approaches and empirical methods applied in the disciplines of developmental psychology, traditional academic psychology, clinical psychology, and psychiatry. Whereas in the previous decades medicine and psychology tended to develop more specialized subdisciplines, work in developmental psychopathology represented a hierarchical integration. In 1984, the journal *Child Development* devoted an entire issue to the work being done in this field, and the Rochester Symposium on Developmental Psychopathology in 1987 welcomed the participation of renowned scientists associated with various academic disciplines such as Thomas Achenbach, Norman Garmezy, Marian Radke-Yarrow, Lee Robins, Michael Rutter, and Alan Sroufe, who met to discuss the central aims and themes to guide research and the building of theory, specific research problems, and future developments. In the years thereafter, new journals (e.g., *Developmental Psychopathology* and *Development and Psychopathology*), books, and monographs (e.g., Cicchetti, 1984; Nannis & Cowan, 1988; Rutter, 1986; Sroufe & Rutter, 1984) documented the field's independent status. Because developmental psychopathology and developmental pediatrics have followed an appropriate approach and generated important findings with respect to issues of health and illness in adolescence, a brief description of the historical developments in these disciplines, as well as the current and planned research efforts, is warranted.

The guiding principle for the work done in these fields is "that we can learn more about the normal functioning of an organism by studying its pathology and, likewise, more about its pathology by studying its normal condition" (Cicchetti, 1984, p. 1). The idea of viewing psychopathology as a mirror of normal development was already inherent in S. Freud's and Rapaport's earlier works. This principle acquired recognition in the field of medicine as research work revealed that the study of pathology of embryonic development (Weis, 1961) or of diseased nervous systems reflects more about normal development and psychobiological functioning than the study of normal, healthy organisms. Nevertheless, clinical psychologists and psychiatrists continued to be primarily interested in studying and developing treatments for mental illness and disorders. The research interests and methods of clinical and developmental psychologists thus remained distinct and independent; that is, clinical psychologists showed little interest in addressing developmental issues, and developmental psychologists were generally unconcerned with psychopathology.

Developmental psychopathologists attempted to apply classic psychological methods to understand how mental illness and behavioral disorders develop. Thus, the field of developmental psychopathology was an attempt to rectify theoretical and methodological diversity, thereby hoping to encompass a wider range of approaches for studying mental health. To this end, many developmental psychopathologists began to incorporate concepts and methods common to other disciplines, such as psychiatry, epidemiology, and sociology, into their research efforts. For example, Tom Achenbach was the first to develop an inventory for classifying psychological disorders in adolescence based on a developmental perspective; Norman Garmezy systematically compared resilient children with those at risk for psychic disturbances, in relation to specified developmental criteria. In addition, Alan Sroufe studied the longitudinal development of adaptation and dysfunctioning in relation to mother–child interaction from childhood into adolescence. Prospective studies of high-risk populations, follow-up studies, and studies of the continuity and change in development of normal and pathological conditions are typical designs (Rutter, 1985a). The approach taken by Werner and Smith (1982) can be considered paradigmatic insofar as a large, unselected group of children was studied over many years in order to better observe exactly when and how psychological disorders develop. This study encouraged the idea that knowledge about normal development is critical for understanding disturbances to development. Thus, information about continuities and discontinuities throughout the life span or the presence of risk and protective factors became more relevant than prevalence rates.

Much interest was focused on studying the specific pathologies and the developmental histories of individuals belonging to high-risk populations. In this process, it was found that some individuals were able to successfully adapt to great levels of stress and aversive life conditions, from which the concepts of invulnerability (Werner & Smith, 1982) and risk and resiliency (Garmezy & Rutter, 1983) were developed. In an attempt to understand the mechanisms and processes that are involved in the generation of illness (Rutter, 1988) and to sufficiently recognize the interaction between the individual and the environment, the pathology itself received less attention. This represents an especially appropriate approach for the study of health in adolescence. It is also noteworthy to mention that in addition to the Werner and Smith model presented, various other models were worked out—for example, the compensation model and the challenge model. The compensation model designed by Garmezy, Masten, and Tellegen (1984) proposes a linear relation between adaptation and stress. Accordingly, if adaptation is not held constant, competence negatively covaries with the level of stress.

The challenge model proposes that when stress increases, competence grows in a curvilinear fashion. Garmezy also presented a third model, the compensative challenge and protective factor model, in which the relations among stress, competence, and adaptability are even more complex. Future research will show which of these models is more adequate.

### Developmental Pediatrics

Following the history of developmental psychopathology, the influence of psychological thought in the field of pediatrics gave rise to the formation of the subdisciplines developmental pediatrics, health care pediatric psychology (Wright, 1979), and pediatric behavioral medicine (Melamed & Siegel, 1980). These fields attempted to integrate the relative contributions of theory and knowledge generated by work in developmental psychology and pediatric medicine. Despite the call for standards and aims laid down by the Society of Pediatric Psychology and the improved information network made available by the *Journal of Pediatric Psychology*, Karoly (1982) doubted that pediatricians routinely consult psychologists, teachers, and other health care professionals in dealing with the treatment of chronically ill children and adolescents. This unfortunate situation would certainly benefit from increased interdisciplinary cooperation between professionals and investigators concerned with pediatric health care. For example, many specific problems and tasks related to the health care of children and adolescents (e.g., the counseling of families with ill children who are noncompliant; preparing children and adolescents before planned hospital stays, medical tests, and operations; the continuing education of health care professionals; and teaching health-promoting attitudes to the lay population) are better approached by improved cooperation between psychologists and practicing pediatricians. One reason for this lack of academic and practical cooperation is linked to the prevailing influence of pathology-oriented models of health care in medicine and psychology, which contribute little toward understanding the relation between physical and psychological development and how illness influences and is influenced by processes of physical, social, and cognitive maturation. In this regard, studies of child and adolescent health benefit little from using cross-sectional designs or by comparing different illness groups. In contrast, longitudinal investigations appear better suited for defining and understanding the factors related to child and adolescent health, of which illness is only one, and perhaps not even the most important, factor.

## WHY IS A DEVELOPMENTAL PERSPECTIVE NECESSARY?

It has become clear that the majority of theoretical models of health and illness lack a developmental approach, especially one that incorporates a life-span developmental perspective. If one works with the life-span concept it becomes clear that risk factors in behavior, health-promoting behavior, awareness of health and illness, health care resources, coping with illness and handicaps, and compliance—to mention only a few aspects of health psychology discussed by Weinman (1990)—must be approached differently according to the age of the individual in question. In each developmental phase, there are specific problems that affect an individual's compliance with treatment, cooperation with health care professionals, or ability to cope with illness differently (Seiffge-Krenke, 1990).

The encompassing definition of health, put forth by the World Health Organization (WHO), takes into account developmentally determined differences in attitudes about health and health-related behavior patterns as well as the importance of social relations. Whereas in the preschool years, the attachment processes are centrally important, as can be seen in cases of separation experiences due to necessary medical procedures in the hospital setting (see the summary of Hall & Stacey, 1979), school-aged children are more likely to be confronted with problems related to being unable to cognitively differentiate between healthy and sick, thus making it difficult for them to understand a diagnosis, recognize the agents that cause or promote illness, or impede health-promoting behavior. The consequences are seen in poor abilities to cope with the illness or in low compliance. As a rule, discussion of the concepts health (Natapoff, 1978) and illness (Potter & Roberts, 1984) are oriented to Piaget's stages of cognitive development (see the critical review by C. Eiser, 1990) and neglect alternative approaches that include emotional and social aspects. In adolescence, the specific dynamics of autonomy from the parents and the increased orientation toward peers may have negative consequences for health or in dealing with illness (Seiffge-Krenke, 1990). In contrast, as Baltes and Wahl (1987) documented, the health behavior of individuals in mid- and late adulthood is determined by other factors, above all by the increased likelihood of multimorbidity and the decline of physical and intellectual abilities. Thus, childhood, adolescence, and the various phases of adulthood are each characterized by different kinds of threats, limitations, and losses, each of which entails a changed dependency on others.

The strong dependency of children and adolescents on their parents is often discounted. Practically all medical procedures and health-related behaviors (e.g., eating habits, personal hygiene, athletic activities, visits to the physician, adherence to physician's instructions, or seeking psychotherapeutic care) are monitored or mediated by the parent. Although the adolescent is able to receive medical care without the consent of the parent upon reaching the legal age (normally between 16 and 18 years old), most adolescents remain dependent on their parents for financial support for health-care-related measures until they finish their schooling. This financial dependency is probably less serious than the problems related to emotional and social dependency. From a sociological point of view, the family is understood as having the character of a forced social unit. The living conditions created by the family, the resources made available, the family attitudes toward health and illness, and the actual health behaviors exhibited in the family are defining in that they exert a considerable influence on the adolescent's well-being. Many psychological, psychiatric, and psychosomatic theories stress the negative effects exerted by certain types of family systems on adolescent health, as for example proposed in the concept of the schizogenetic mother (Watzlawick, Weakland, & Fish, 1974) or the psychosomatogenic family (Minuchin, 1974), the anorexic family (Bruch, 1982), or the diabetic family (Minuchin, Rosman, & Baker, 1978). These theories are primarily concerned with the nature of the family's interaction patterns and regard the psychological or somatic symptoms as having a functional significance in stabilizing and maintaining the familial status quo. Studies based on these theories not only show how certain family dynamics promote illness, but also how family members may be hindered by other family members in seeking medical or psychosocial care. This strong dependency of the adolescent's health behavior on the parents has not been satisfactorily included in definitions and conceptualizations of health behavior. In addition, little research has addressed the importance of peer influence on health behavior.

# 2

# Problems in Assessing Health-Related Information

Without doubt, diagnostic information is necessary for the prevention and treatment of illnesses as well as for the determination of factors contributing to health-risk behaviors. Despite this critical importance, not much research in health psychology deals with diagnostic aspects. One exception is the work of Karoly (1985, 1988), whose publications about health-related diagnostics in children highlight the importance of developmental factors. In the following, typical barriers that arise during the assessment of health-relevant information in adolescents are examined and the possible consequences emanating from these changes are discussed. This chapter adopts the perspective that developmental issues must be recognized in interaction between health experts and adolescents. This interactional perspective is already apparent in the very early process of communication between health experts and adolescent patients on diagnostic issues.

## THE SIGNIFICANCE OF DIAGNOSTIC INFORMATION IN HEALTH PSYCHOLOGY

According to Matarazzo (1980), every area of health psychology profits from diagnostic information. However, the interest in diagnostic questions is low, and only a few comprehensive instruments for the diagnostics of health exist. Most instruments assess deviations, troubles, or symptoms; for example, *health* is assessed as a deviation from a disease-related mean. As outlined in chapter 1, the perception of health in instrumental, negative terms (such as *absence of illness*) is also characteristic of many lay conceptions of health. Positive aspects of health, such as physical and emotional well-being, are more difficult to define and assess.

Beyond measuring the extent of illness, how can physical well-being be quantified? Ryff and Keyes (1995) outlined the various conceptual and methodological problems in assessing the indicators for well-being. Health defined in positive terms, rather than by the absence of symptoms, includes reasonable energy levels, enjoyment of life, and the capacity to participate in normal social activities, such as seeing friends and working at one's usual tasks. Such descriptions of physical well-being, or quality of life, are very similar to the definition of emotional well-being, also expressed in terms of satisfying social relationships, self-confidence, energy for living, and sense of mastery and competence (Strupp, 1989). In fact, hardly any instruments exist, at present, that are based on a definition combining psychological health, physical health, and a state of well-being, corresponding, for example, to the definition of health set forth by the WHO. Admittedly, the assessment of such a global health concept is complex and difficult, perhaps an almost unattainable ideal.

Another problem of health diagnostics is that of determining which behaviors, feelings, or coping strategies are healthy or desirable in which persons. A strictly normative approach that does not recognize individual variations or fails to give them sufficient consideration is particularly inadequate for adolescents. In this regard, many theories of development are deficient, especially those based on a normative comparison with adults, thereby overlooking youth-specific needs and developmental processes. Health diagnostics should always be multivariate (not only in adolescents) and rely on physiological methods, systematic observations, tests, interviews, and self-ratings. Although this aspect is sufficiently considered in assessing psychological well-being, the application of psychological methods is still rare in medicine. Family diagnostics play an important role in adolescent health research (McCubbin & McCubbin, 1988), but the assessment of other social support systems is also extremely relevant for all etiological and intervention-oriented questions. In the following, developmental changes in adolescents are linked with aspects of the doctor–patient communication to illustrate the typical problems health experts are faced with when trying to assess diagnostic information in this age group. We start by outlining the distinctive characteristics of doctor–patient communication and interaction, which strongly deviate from everyday experiences.

## DISTINCTIVE CHARACTERISTICS OF DOCTOR–PATIENT COMMUNICATION: A BREACH OF EVERYDAY INTERACTION

The average duration of contact between physician and patient is limited to a few minutes (Freund & McGuire, 1991). In a German survey of 5,711 patients of general practitioners, Moehr and Hahn (1977) found that only 5.4% of the doctor–patient contacts lasted more than 10 minutes. Of course, the length of contact between physician and patient varied depending on the patient's ailments; nevertheless, long-lasting doctor–patient contacts were the rule only in patients with chronic illnesses or in rural regions. This finding indicates that patients' needs for information, explanations, and care may be neglected and that they must describe their health problems under considerable time pressure. In view of the medical consequences that result from an overly short interview, it becomes obvious that the restrictions of time can frustrate and irritate patients. In addition, the physician's role in the physician–patient relationship is such that the physician may need to physically examine the patient. The physician's right to observe and touch the patient's body at will transgresses the normal, socially accepted bounds of everyday physical contact in our culture (Argyle, 1972). In addition, the specific characteristics of communication between physician and patient differ from daily social contacts. Before focusing on this topic more deeply, it is important to understand that the tradition of medical consultation as a problem-solving task for the doctor is valid but narrow. It neglects the interactional perspective.

The patient-centered perspective provides a wider view. In fact, to a greater extent than is often acknowledged, most of the information requested and provided during the consultation is of a psychological rather than biological nature. As Winefield (1992) showed, many symptoms presented to doctors, such as headaches, sleeping difficulties, weight loss, nausea, and pain, signify either organic or emotional dysfunction. Also, a patient's decision to seek medical treatment for minor symptoms (e.g., for common respiratory infections) may be related to underlying emotional distress (such as job dissatisfaction). Some patients present physical symptoms in an attempt to find solutions for interpersonal problems. Moreover, interpersonal stress can aggravate sensitivity to physical dysfunctions, and chronic physical conditions can be exacerbated by anxiety and depression. Often, medical care consists mainly of emotional support, especially when neither effective treatment nor cure is available for the illness or ailment. In addition, most medical care for psychological symptoms is provided by general physicians. Owing to the highly psychological nature of medical care as outlined earlier, it seems important to explore the physician–patient relationship on a broader basis, including aspects from the therapeutic relationship and psychological counseling as well.

Information about the patients, their family backgrounds, their symptoms, the geneses of their diseases, and their current living circumstances are assessed in various ways. In a medical interview, the physician usually makes use of a catalog of structured questions whose order is exactly determined, supplemented by medical data resulting from the physical examination. Psychological or psychiatric first interviews differ in their degree of structuring, depending on the therapeutic approach. Accordingly, a broad variety of instruments are used, ranging from a catalog of issues that are fixed in their order and contents (e.g., anamnestic interviews) to semistructured interviews (e.g., behavior diagnostics or functional analysis of behavior; see Kanfer & Saslow, 1969) to widely unstructured communication in which the patient determines the course of the interview. In this last approach—the psychoanalytic first interview (Balint, 1964)—important conclusions about the genesis of a disorder are deduced from three sources: objective biographical data, their subjective meaning to the patient, and the situational evidence of an unconscious conflict that might manifest itself in the interview situation. As a rule, these psychoanalytic and psychiatric interviews are supplemented by diagnostic tests in order to clarify specific diagnostic questions.

However, it is necessary to consider that all these types of interviews—even those that are rigidly structured—entail elements that represent a breach of everyday communication and interaction. According to observations made by Parrott, Burgoon, Burgoon, and Lepoire (1989), most patients are afraid of their physicians. The patients may fear painful interventions, be apprehensive about the diagnosis and its consequences, or feel helpless and dependent on a powerful physician. The patient's apprehension in the first interview with a psychologist or psychiatrist may even be greater. Insufficient differentiation between physicians and psychologists or psychiatrists contributes to the patients' feeling uncomfortable in the first contact with therapists and counselors. Although the patients are not required to undress and must not be physically examined, they feel exposed psychologically. The questions they are asked (e.g., about their troubles, worries and sorrows, or their sexuality and body image) involve topics that are usually not discussed with a stranger and perhaps only with family members, friends, or relatives. Given these conditions (i.e., a help-seeking, emotionally ambivalent patient and a therapist who is ascribed with an expert status), an unusual communicative situation is created. The communicative situation is asymmetrical from the beginning. The patient is requested to divulge personal information, receiving various amounts of assistance to structure his or her report. The patient must talk about sorrows and problems, while the therapist usually refrains from doing the same. The therapist listens, asks a question now and then, and keeps silent. The patient may be especially irritated by the lack of reciprocity, that is, the fact that communicative acts are not balanced. This basic rule of everyday communication has been termed the *dyadic effect* (Chelune & Waring, 1984).

An asymmetric communicative situation involving one-sided self-disclosure is also typical of the interview with the physician, in which the physician, often under a higher time pressure, remains silent most of the time, listens, or takes notes. At the end of the interview, the physician makes recommendations or gives further orders. The very nature of the physician–patient relationship also affords little opportunity to avoid personal questions or to withhold intimate information if effective diagnosis and treatment are to be achieved. Thus, patients must often share private thoughts and feelings despite their concern about the physician's ability to treat such information with utmost confidentiality (Parrott et al., 1989).

These issues of privacy entail both *informational privacy* (which relates to an individual's right to determine how, when, and to what extent data about the self is released to another person) and *psychological privacy* (i.e., the right to determine with whom and under what circumstances one shares thoughts and feelings or reveals intimate information). Psychological privacy explains why patients withhold information from physicians or are sensitive about the physician's evaluation of their health. One further dimension of privacy—*physical privacy* (the degree to which one is physically accessible to others)—is mostly confined to physician–patient interaction. During the medical interview and examination, patients have limited physical privacy. The physical examination often involves intimate contact; nevertheless, the procedure is usually conducted in a formal, rule-governed fashion, thus explaining the interpretation of the touch. However, according to the study of Parrott and his colleagues (Parrott et al., 1989), violations of physical privacy include having to undress and reveal parts of the body unrelated to the purpose of the medical visit or having to undress while the doctor or nurse is present.

In summary, three basic characteristics of the communication and interaction between health experts and patients deviate from everyday experience: asymmetric power relations, the fact that private information is not shared in a reciprocal way, and the possibility that the health expert may also violate physical privacy. This departure from the everyday communicative norms and boundaries is characteristic of all interviews with health experts and has only a few variations, depending on the amount of structure of the interview and the health expert's role.

## DEVELOPMENTAL BARRIERS IN ASSESSING DIAGNOSTIC INFORMATION

### Adolescents' Reservations in Communicating Private Information

As detailed earlier, these unusual forms of communication and interaction make adult patients rather uncomfortable. As far as adolescent patients are concerned, the specific dynamics of their developmental changes might make the assessment of diagnostic information even more difficult. Due to a shift in preference of self-disclosure partners from parents to peers, adolescents have great difficulty in talking frankly with an adult person. As early as 12 years old, adolescents begin to differentiate between private and public information and are no longer willing to talk with everybody about private, intimate topics (Laufer & Wolfe, 1974). As Broughton (1981) described in his concept of the "divided self in adolescence," adolescents learn to distinguish between an inner "true self" and an external facade. In front of adults, they adopt styles of self-representation that prevent them from becoming hurt because, as Winnicott (1969) outlined, "the adolescent does not wish to be understood" (p. 209). At around 15 years old, the change in preferred partners of self-disclosure becomes more and more visible. Until then, the child prefers to talk with parents, especially the mother, about his or her sorrows, problems, and intimate experiences, whereas from this age onward, adolescents choose (more and more often) peers of the same gender or, later on, heterosexual partners for intimate self-disclosure. Readiness to accept the parents as disclosure partners clearly wanes, and peers increasingly assume this function.

My fellow researchers and I were able to confirm this finding in a study of 241 adolescents aged 12 to 17 years old. The disposition to disclose personal information was assessed by using the Letter test by Koch (1977). The adolescents were asked to share various topics of self-disclosure (such as intimate personal information or public information like career plans and future perspective) with several addressees via letters. Figure 2.1 shows the preferences for various self-disclosure partners, over the years, based on the total scores for self-disclosure.

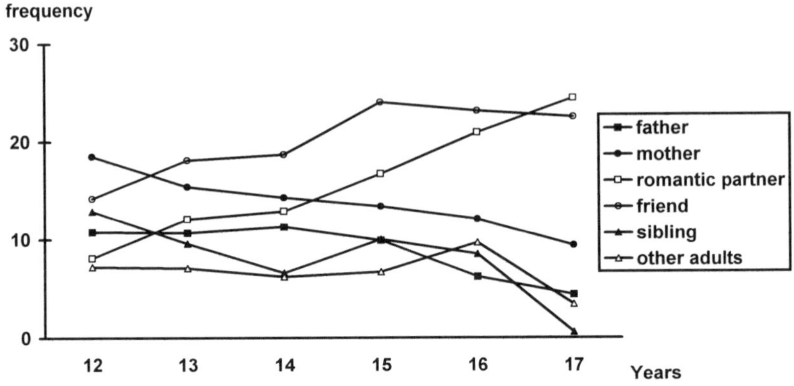


FIG. 2.1. Changes in disclosure partners during adolescence ($N$ = 241).

Inspection of the data reveals that adolescents talked more frankly with their mothers than with their fathers. As they grew older, the preference for both parents clearly dwindled but increased for male and female peers. In general, adults were not chosen very frequently as disclosure partners. The readiness to share information more often with the mother than with the father was also dependent on the self-disclosure topic—self-disclosure to the father was generally lower. Furthermore, only certain topics, such as professional plans and goals, were discussed with fathers. Very personal thoughts and feelings became increasingly reserved for peers. These findings are substantiated by the study of Papini, Farmer, Clark, and Snell (1988). Their results reveal that adolescents engage in more sexual disclosure with their friends than with their parents. In addition, significantly greater disclosure about sexually related topics took place between adolescents and their friends of like gender than between those of the opposite gender.

Several studies showed that adolescents feel better understood by their friends (Millen & Roll, 1977) and that mutual disclosure becomes an essential characteristic of close friendships (Buhrmester & Furman, 1987). This change of preferred disclosure partner and the process of selecting which information is considered suitable for which target person is generally regarded as an indicator of social maturity (Chelune & Waring, 1984). However, it inevitably gives rise to diagnostic difficulties when trying to assess the health status of adolescents. Moreover, it can be considered a barrier in cases of seeking and accepting help. For example, in one study of highly stressed adolescents, we observed that they were caught in a dilemma between the desire to get help and the inhibition to talk about themselves (Seiffge-Krenke, 1989). On the one hand, the general readiness for self-disclosure increases with the pressure of problems, as Cozby (1973) showed. On the other hand, the need to protect one's own privacy also increases. These apparently contradictory tendencies are related to the fact that in our society, low self-disclosure is judged to be socially appropriate. In studies on adolescents, we demonstrated that this dilemma between the desire to get help and the inhibition to talk about private issues becomes particularly salient because adolescents are quite guarded in their styles of self-representation with adults. In the study of highly stressed adolescents, desire and inhibition to talk were exactly balanced, thus hindering therapeutic help and counseling (see chap. 6, this volume).

### Dealing With Nudity

Strong reservations about discussing physical symptoms are also common. As mentioned in the preceding section, adult patients are very sensitive to violations of psychological privacy in physician–patient relationships. In addition, patients may feel insulted by violations of physical privacy. In a study conducted by Parrott and his colleagues (Parrott et al., 1989) on privacy between physicians and patients, age and gender differences emerged in the boundaries of psychological and physical privacy. Younger patients (16–29 years old) were more likely than older patients (30–60 years old) to regard the practice of having to undress before seeing the physician or having to reveal parts of the body unrelated to the purpose of the medical visit as violations of physical privacy. Females were more likely to regard this practice as invasive; younger females objected most. Females were also more uncomfortable about having to undress when a nurse was present. Patients may become socialized to the fact that they must undress when they visit the doctor, but this does not mean that they are comfortable in the situation. Greater sensitivity to this issue seems warranted, especially with respect to adolescent patients.

In a study conducted by Schulz (1991), it became obvious how important it is for adolescents to protect their physical privacy. Similar to acts of verbal self-disclosure, the adolescents often took the initiative to control physical contact and nakedness. In interviews with 15-year-old girls, marked changes in physical contact with the family members emerged. Adolescents reported that as they grew older, physical contact with their parents not only decreased, but also became less desirable. A strong association was found between a drastic reduction in physical contact and physical maturity. Around the onset of menarche, the previous forms of close physical contact (e.g., sitting on the lap, embracing, and kissing) with the father were drastically reduced and replaced by ritualized physical contact such as hugging at departure. Half of the girls refused to engage in any physical contact with their fathers; contact with the mother was tolerated, but also reduced. Additionally surprising was the avoidance of any physical contact in the bathroom. Two thirds of the girls avoided any visual or physical contact with their parents while undressed. This shows that changes resulting from maturational processes make girls more sensitive about this aspect of physical interaction than physical contact per se, which is at least maintained in a ritualized form (see chap. 4, this volume). The reduction in physical contact with the father is much more marked than with the mother, and it is mostly initiated by the young girl and only to a small extent by the father himself.

Similar trends were identified in a study of father–son body contact. Salt (1991) asked fathers and their 7- to 12-year-old sons to rate the acceptability of affectionate touch between father and son. In addition, the joint play of fathers and sons in various physical games was videotaped. Results show that as the sons grew older and approached adolescence, both father and son reported and showed a decrease in the amount and acceptance of touch between them.

In summary, the results reported thus far demonstrate that physical contact with both parents is reduced during adolescence and replaced by ritualized forms of physical contact. In addition, the manner in which nudity is dealt with changes dramatically such that any encounter with the parents while naked is avoided. This finding suggests that general practitioners, pediatricians, and above all gynecologists are confronted with strong inhibitions about physical exposure. Physical examinations including diagnostic first interviews on physical symptoms and psychological problems are extremely difficult to carry out in the adolescent. Based on the studies previously cited, it seems that female adolescents are more sensitive about any violation of physical privacy than males. They are, however, more ready to disclose personal or private issues; that is, their need for psychological privacy is less (Parrott et al., 1989). Norell (1984) also noted that adolescent females divulge more personal information, a finding that is probably related to their higher rates of seeking and accepting offers of professional help (when needed) compared to male adolescents (see chap. 8, this volume).

### Changes in Referential Norms: Egocentrism and Risk-Taking Behavior

Additional problems for diagnosis might arise in connection with other developmental dynamics particular to adolescence. Daydreaming and fantasizing increase in early adolescence. According to a study by Giambra (1974), intense daydreaming is characteristic through adolescence; a reduction in the frequency of daydreaming becomes evident around 20 years old. In addition, increased egocentrism during the period of early to mid-adolescence may prevent adolescents from perceiving symptoms as dangerous or behaviors as risky. In particular, intense daydreaming and fantasizing are closely related to egocentric behavior in early adolescence. The adolescent becomes able to perceive aspects of his or her own psychological self from the other's point of view (Broughton, 1981), a development that is frequently linked with a period of extreme sensitivity and self-centeredness. Around 13 years old, when this egocentricity is at its peak, adolescents are intensively concerned about the integrity of their body image and extremely sensitive to the prospect of physical disruption or distortion. At the same age, this preoccupation with the self easily gives rise to misjudgments about real dangers.

Elkind (1967) and Elkind and Bowen (1977) described two main manifestations of egocentrism: the *imaginary audience* (e.g., the feeling of always being observed and judged by others) and the *personal fable* (the perceived uniqueness). The personal fable phenomenon ("such things cannot happen to me"; see Elkind, 1967) is held partly responsible for increased risk-taking among adolescents. In the previously mentioned study on 241 adolescents 12 to 17 years old, egocentrism was investigated by means of the Personal Fable Questionnaire designed by Sanok (1975), which assesses the estimates of certain risks. The results are presented in Fig. 2.2.

A systematic tendency was found among healthy adolescents, especially the younger age groups, to underestimate the likelihood that they themselves might become ill. The possibility of being involved in an accident also continued to be misjudged, even among the older age groups. Other authors assume that the phenomenon of the personal fable in early and mid- adolescence is responsible for the high incidence of accidents (Amir, 1987) and pregnancies (Urberg & Rosen, 1987) in this age group. It must be mentioned, however, that this is only a temporary phenomenon: From 16 years old onward, the unrealistic perception of risk factors gives way to a more objective and appropriate view. Nevertheless, it must be kept in mind that adolescents' health-related and illness-preventive behaviors deviate from those seen in general population. Although the knowledge about risk factors influencing morbidity and mortality has led to a positive change of lifestyle in most adults during the past decades, the percentage of adolescents who consume alcohol, drugs, and nicotine or are involved in dangerous

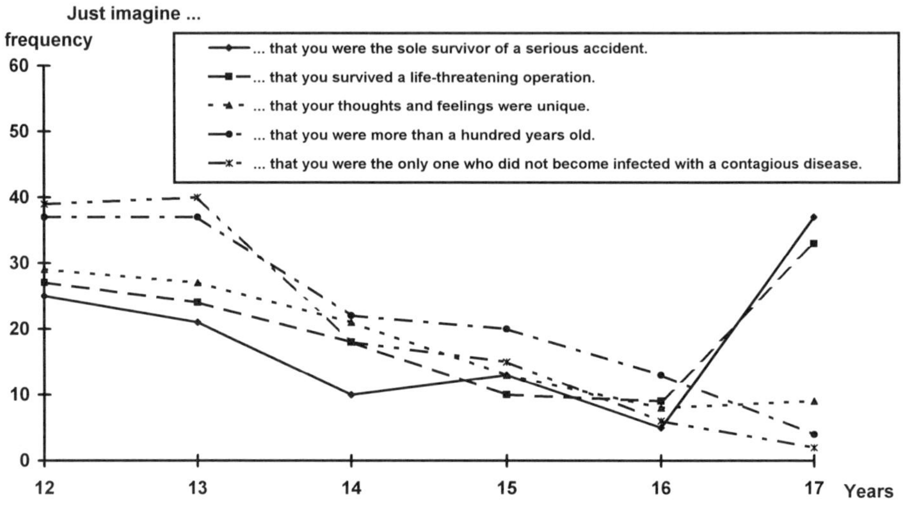


FIG. 2.2. Changes in egocentrism (personal fable) during adolescence ($N = 241$).

driving has increased (Jessor, 1986). This can be traced to age-related differences in the manner in which such risk-taking behavior is perceived and evaluated. Even when young people are able to adequately perceive a behavior's potential risk, risk-taking is an integral part of the adolescent lifestyle. Taking on excessive risk is seen as a demonstration of adult status. Longitudinal studies conducted by Kandel (1986) and Jessor (1986) show that much of this risky behavior fades out as adolescence comes to a close.

## SOME CONSEQUENCES OF DEVELOPMENTAL CHANGES FOR THE DIAGNOSTIC PROCESS

### Misjudgment of Symptoms and Communication Problems

In the previous section, the following developmental changes emerging in early and mid-adolescence were found to impede the assessment of diagnostic information about the health status: change in self-disclosure partners, changes in physical privacy, temporary egocentrism, and risk-taking behavior. These developmental changes are limited to a certain period of time and vanish in late adolescence. From a developmental perspective, the onset of these changes is considered to be positive; however, such changes lead to difficulties in assessing symptoms and making proper diagnoses.

Each aspect of health service is adversely influenced by problems in communication and interaction between health care experts and adolescents. Medical diagnosis, for example, is influenced by the physician's skills in eliciting symptoms and by the manner in which such symptoms are reported and conceptualized by the patient. Despite this importance, little empirical work has investigated the patient's role in conceptualizing, labeling, and reporting symptoms. The adolescent's increasing reluctance to speak frankly and the vague statements about physical problems and psychological symptoms create many problems for general practitioners, psychologists, psychiatrists, and other health care experts.

Two studies to date have dealt with this issue on adolescent samples. Silber (1982), as well as Dirks, Schraa, and Robinson (1982), reported that adolescents often present themselves in the doctor's office with a variety of complaints that are vague, recurrent, and ranging from mild and transitory to fairly severe, leaving it to the physician to describe and interpret them more precisely. In both studies, the adolescent's strong inhibitions about revealing personally important information lead to erroneous reports of symptoms as well as communication and interaction problems between the physicians and their adolescent patients. Dirks et al. reported a high incidence of mislabeling of symptoms due to imprecise reporting by adolescent patients. In particular, the patients' mislabeling of symptoms had a negative effect on medical outcome. Silber reported that the vague symptoms presented by the adolescent patients often received equally vague attention and responses from the physician who might have dismissed them as psychogenic or fake. In both studies, countertransference reactions were present in the attending physicians. Silber noted a large number of evasive answers made by physicians. In addition, the physicians often trivialized their adolescent patients' problems. The doctors reported that they preferred to examine patients with more concrete symptoms.

Similarly, Dirks et al. found that, owing to the sheer number of problems reported, the vague descriptions of symptoms, and the painstaking efforts involved in eliciting diagnostically relevant information from their adolescent patients, physicians were often prompted to devote their attention to other patients who were "really ill." This tendency has unfortunate consequences for the adolescent's health. The experienced general practitioner must learn to recognize and correctly assess symptoms that are neglected by the adolescent. For example, the adolescent patient may exhibit self-destructive behavior (e.g., scratching or substantial weight loss) that indicates severe psychopathology. In such cases, consultation with a psychologist or psychiatrist is recommended.

### Discrepancies in the Evaluation of Symptoms by Adolescents, Parents, and Health Care Experts

Further consequences of the developmental dynamics of adolescence for the assessment of health-relevant information become evident in the different evaluations of symptoms made by adolescents, parents, and health care experts. These discrepancies are especially salient in the domain of psychological disorders but are also obvious in the assessment of physical symptoms. In the study by Dirks et al. (1982), one fourth of the 587 asthma patients regarded such general troubles as tiredness or changes in body temperature as "asthmatic." Even larger distortions can be expected in adolescents' accounts concerning the psychodynamics and psychogenesis of their disorders. Snyder, Handelsman, and Endelman (1978) came to the pessimistic conclusion that adolescent patients are able only to a limited extent to provide the kind of information about themselves that physicians need to appraise the illness.

This points to the necessity of using several sources when assessing health-relevant information. Parents are often called on to provide information that may be relevant to the diagnosis (Offord et al., 1987). It is uncertain, however, whether parents are the most reliable sources of information that contribute to an appropriate assessment of symptoms in the adolescent. As we outlined earlier, the developing adolescent becomes less inclined to share private information or discuss personal problems with his or her parents and prefers to entrust such knowledge to close friends and peers. In addition, adolescents become more and more reserved in dealing with physical symptoms and with nudity. Several studies have demonstrated considerable discrepancies among adolescent patients, their parents, and health care experts with respect to their respective judgments of the type and severity of psychological disorders. In the study by Pierce and Klein (1982), parents and adolescents agreed on only 7 out of 52 items on a Behavior Rating Scale. Only with respect to clearly observable behavior disorders (e.g., social isolation, eating disorders, theft, or enuresis) did adolescents describe themselves in the same way as did their parents. All in all, the adolescents perceived themselves to be more anxious, more depressive, and more ill than their parents considered them to be. In contrast, in the study by Adelman, Taylor, Fuller, and Nelson (1979), adolescents described their problems as being less grave than did their parents and teachers. These results suggest that parents and adolescents perceive the latter's behavior differently and adolescents do not disclose many of their problems to adults. Especially as they grow older, adolescents increasingly keep such feelings as sadness and anxiety to themselves. This has resulted in the opinion that adolescents overreport symptoms and exaggerate the severity of their problems (Garber, 1984).

Achenbach, McConaughy, and Howell (1987) conducted a meta-analysis of cross-informant agreement based on 119 studies carried out from 1967 to 1984, employing a self-report (YSR), a parent report (CBCL), and a teacher report (TRF) on adolescent symptomatology (Achenbach, 1991b, 1991c, 1991d). Their analysis resulted in correlations in the .20 to .30 range among different informants. Specifically, the correlation between parent and teacher reports of problem behavior was .27, between teacher and adolescent the correlation was .20, and between parents and adolescent it was .25. These results confirm that each informant's perspective of the adolescent's health is valid in its own right, but multiple sources of information are necessary in order to obtain a comprehensive picture of an adolescent's health problems. The question remains, however, "What variables contribute to low cross-informant agreement?" Low self-disclosure rates in adolescents may contribute to these results. Another factor is related to the type of problem being evaluated. Most studies show higher cross-informant agreement for externalizing behaviors as compared to internalizing behaviors. In particular, agreement about depressive symptoms is low (Achenbach et al., 1987). This emphasizes that especially for those health problems that are hidden from adult views, the adolescent's perspective is indispensable.

Some studies also have shown that parental perceptions of adolescent health problems may be more a function of parents' own psychological adjustment than of the child's level of symptoms. Studies comparing fathers' and mothers' ratings consistently showed that mothers report higher rates of problem behavior in their children than do fathers. Whereas fathers' ratings are not much influenced by their own problems, maternal depression, maternal anxiety, as well as marital discord were found to influence mothers' perceptions of their children's health status (Reid & Crisafulli, 1990; Renouf & Kovacs, 1994; Seiffge-Krenke & Kollmar, 1997). Webster-Stratton (1988) found that fathers' perceptions of their children's health status and problem behaviors were relatively unaffected by personal adjustment measures such as marital dissatisfaction, depression, and life stress. Although mothers are usually used as informants, their evaluation might be influenced by their own problems. Assuming that mothers and fathers have different relationships with their children, that mothers usually spend more time with their children, and that adolescents are more likely to discuss intimate problems with their mothers than with their fathers, we would expect that mothers are better able to recognize their children's health problems. Maternal concern with their own problems, however, suggests that fathers can provide a different, and not necessarily inaccurate, picture of the adolescent's health status and problem behavior.

Additionally, the adolescent's physician judges the specific symptoms, any underlying conflicts, and the seriousness of the illness differently than the patient or parents. The specific nature of interaction between adolescents and their doctors, however, leads to countertransference reactions that might bias the diagnosis and selection of kind of treatment. Due to these problems, it has become more common to employ cross-informant data, for example, in assessing psychological symptoms. With respect to the assessment of psychological symptoms, health care professionals surely benefit from using information provided by others related to or involved daily with the adolescent patient.

### Deficiencies in the Diagnostic Process and the Diagnostic Classification

Interestingly, health care experts have paid little attention to the adolescent's disinclination to self-disclosure and to the discrepancies in the assessments of psychological disorders and physical symptoms made by different sources. When asked to explain the low concordance between the diagnoses made by their colleagues, most health care professionals ascribed discrepancies to the diagnostic system; only a small minority thought that the discrepancies were related to the patients' or their families' reports (Seiffge-Krenke, 1986). Some authors have suggested that clinicians have difficulty in agreeing about their diagnostic impressions, that diagnoses tend to be inconsistent over time, and that diagnostic labeling is not particularly helpful in predicting various parameters of psychological disturbances (e.g., Zubin, 1967). In 1970, Weiner reviewed findings on the classification of psychological disturbances in adolescence and found that one third of the diagnostic disagreements observed in empirical studies were attributable to varying abilities of diagnosticians, for example, to elicit concealed information from the patient and identify the predominant pathology in mixed pictures. According to his review, many empirically demonstrated deficiencies of the diagnostic process could be eliminated by improved training of diagnosticians and relatively minor alterations in the medical nomenclature.

Also, the procedures by which classification systems were established in the past showed considerable deficits, with respect to the intuitive collection, assessment, and subjective weighting of symptoms, the confounding of description and interpretation at an early stage of classification, as well as the use of potentially nontypical samples, that might bias the classification. In particular, the medical classification model, according to which persons are differentially assigned to syndromes, can easily lead to incorrect diagnoses because there are only a few empirically confirmed syndromes in childhood and adolescence that can be dissociated from each other.

The currently leading general systems of psychiatric classification—the *International Classification of Diseases, Injuries, and Causes of Death* (*ICD–10;* Chapter F; WHO, 1992) and the *Diagnostic and Statistical Manual of Mental Disorders* (*DSM–IV;* American Psychiatric Association, 1994)—have tried to make up for these deficits by including thorough literature reviews, re-analyses of data on psychiatric disorders, and field trials in their recent, revised editions. Based on former editions of these classification systems, research on diagnostic and nosological implications of most types of disorders has increased substantially during the past 10 years. The results of these comprehensive research activities were analyzed during the revision processes of *ICD* and *DSM* and combined with field trials. For this reason, in the *ICD–10* and *DSM–IV*, empirically confirmed syndromes and disorders prevail, whereas new diagnoses with a yet insufficient base of empirical data were excluded from consideration. Both systems were developed in parallel and interdependently at the beginning of the 1990s, in order to establish a unified—or at least two compatible—referential system(s) useful for research, diagnostic, and therapeutic settings.

Both systems adopted a multiaxial classification procedure in order to accommodate for the complexity of clinical situations and the heterogeneity of individuals presenting the same symptoms. In 1993, WHO published the additional multiaxial presentation of the *ICD–10* in which psychiatric disorders and somatic illnesses are coded on axes Ia and Ib. Axis II includes registers of social handicaps; axis III assesses factors of the social environment and individual coping with general life circumstances.

The *DSM–IV* system, on the other hand, requires the simultaneous classification of individual functioning on five axes. Most mental disorders listed in the manual are coded on axis I (clinical disorders), while only personality disorders and mental retardation are coded on axis II, ensuring that these domains of psychic dysfunction are not overlooked in the presence of other more florid disorders represented on axis I. Axis III is reserved for the individual's general medical conditions; axis IV considers all relevant psychosocial and environmental problems during the last year before the diagnosis, and axis V represents a 100-step global rating scale (GAF) of the individual's psychological, social, and occupational functioning at the time of the diagnosis. Besides these common general psychiatric classification systems, numerous special classification schemes were developed for different purposes. For example, a multiaxial diagnostic system (MAS) was developed in parallel for the assessment of psychological disturbances in childhood and adolescence. The classification developed by Rutter and his colleagues featured developmental deficits as a descriptional category (Rutter, Tuma, & Lann, 1988; van Goor-Lambo, Orley, Poustka, & Rutter, 1994). Rutter and coworkers presented their approach as basically descriptive and not theory bound. Achenbach (1991b, 1991c, 1991d) proceeded similarly in developing self-ratings for children and adolescents, as well as ratings destined for other informants, assessing externalizing and internalizing syndromes. In the instruments designed by him and his research group, disorders and competencies are assessed simultaneously. The advantage of such methods of assessment is that it is possible to make a differentiated diagnosis of a disorder based on information about the patient's general background.

Since the advent of former versions of the *DSM–III* and *DSM–III–R*, clinicians and researchers have shown increasing interest in the significance of comorbid disorders in children and adolescents. Evidence accumulated that comorbidity (i.e., the co-occurrence of several disorders) is pervasive in adolescence. Many concerns have been advanced that the nosological system's inherent weaknesses account for the high rates of comorbidity (Achenbach, 1990; Caron & Rutter, 1991). With respect to adolescence, these concerns intersect with developmental and methodological issues. From a developmental perspective, comorbidity may reflect amorphous, nonspecific expressions of psychopathology in younger age groups, in contrast to more clearly articulated clinical presentations by older adolescents and adults. Clinical features for drawing clear boundaries between distinct disorders are lacking. A closely related issue concerns the point at which boundaries are drawn between the normal and pathological range of functioning (Nottelmann & Jensen, 1995).

### Low Reliability, Validity, and Stability of the Diagnosis

Other authors have strongly objected to efforts to apply traditional nosological concepts in diagnosing adolescents. For the most part, these objections stem from the notion that adolescence is a turbulent, unpredictable time of life in which apparent psychopathological behavior may occur as transient developmental phenomena. Laufer and Laufer (1984), for example, argued that accurate, differential diagnoses of adolescent disorders require careful assessment of the interplay between basic pathology and adolescent dynamics. Concerns about the appropriateness and utility of diagnostic classification in adolescents are by no means limited to psychoanalytic authors. Weiner (1970) argued that there are few reliable constants of a physical or psychological nature that would allow one to construct a model for matching the individual against such constants or scores. The increased availability of such data during recent years, however, does not alter the fact that diagnostic labeling of adolescents is deprecated in some way as an inexact and inappropriate procedure.

Even if an appropriate classification system existed and sufficient information from different sources was available, diagnoses would have to be made carefully: Adolescence is a transitional period in the human life cycle in which rapid and momentous changes occur simultaneously in different important areas of development. Furthermore, developmental progression does not necessarily follow a linear course in adolescence. Even regressive processes engender subsequent progression (Blos, 1973). Anna Freud (1960) outlined that although developmental changes account for some disorders, they also lead to the solution of former conflicts and health problems. The spontaneous remission rate during adolescence is quite high, amounting to 39% (McMahon & Peters, 1990). In addition, it is also necessary to consider the low stability of diagnoses in adolescence. For example, diagnoses remained stable in only one third to one half of the cases examined by Nottelmann and Jensen (1995).

Another striking aspect of the epidemiology of adolescent psychopathology is the emergence of transient, unclearly defined disorders. According to Weiner (1970), it is the most common diagnosis for adolescent patients in psychiatric hospitals in the United States. In an extensive study of 1,334 patients 12 to 18 years old, Weiner and Del Gaudio (1976) documented that uncertain, transitory disorders accounted for 27% of the cases. Rosen, Bahn, Shellow, and Bower (1965) reported similar results based on the data of 41,496 adolescent patients. Uncertain, transitory personality disorder was the most common diagnosis, seen in 37% of the female adolescents and 36% of the male adolescents. In contrast, in adult patient samples, this diagnosis was made for only 2% of the sample. A more recent overview (Nottelmann & Jensen, 1995) showed that the situation has not changed much over the years. Similarly, in a study on German adolescents, 20% of the clients seeking help from counselors and psychotherapists were assigned with the diagnostic label "uncertain transitory disorder." Again, no gender differences in the distribution of the diagnoses were found (Seiffge-Krenke, 1989). Health care providers also tend to believe that adolescent problems are more attributable to their developmental stage than to other causes and that adolescents outgrow their psychiatric disturbances (Lavigne, 1977).

All in all, these studies reflect how difficult it is for health care providers to correctly assess the variety of symptoms presented by adolescent patients or discern between normal and pathological functioning. Adolescents' low willingness to disclose information about themselves further contributes to this difficulty. The problems of comorbidity, as well as unclear diagnostic categorization, have not yet received much attention in the medical literature. The fact that *somatization* (i.e., physical complaints for which medical evaluation reveals no explanatory physical pathology) is frequently polysymptomatic suggests that similar processes are at work in medical diagnoses (Campo & Fritsch, 1994).

### Change of Symptoms and Comorbidity

In most studies, strong age and gender differences emerged in adolescents' symptomatology. Male adolescents tend more often to show externalizing, socially disruptive behaviors (e.g., increased aggressivity, hyperactivity, and socially deviant behavior); in females, higher rates of internalizing disorders (e.g., depression and anxiety) have been found (Achenbach, 1991d; Rutter, Shaffer, & Sturge, 1976; Rutter, Tizard, Yule, Graham, & Whitmore, 1977). In the preceding section, it was shown that unreliability of psychological and psychiatric diagnoses was generally thought to be a result of deficiencies in diagnostic procedures, whereas the contribution of the vague and imprecise communication characteristic of adolescents was mostly overlooked. Recently, health care professionals are becoming increasingly aware that there are changes in symptoms of some disorders, which makes it increasingly difficult to put forward an appropriate diagnosis in spite of improved diagnostic instruments. In the following text, these changes are illustrated by referring to two types of disorders, anorexia nervosa and depression, both of which show increased prevalence in female adolescent patients. First, however, a brief discussion of the issue of comorbidity in adolescent patients is warranted.

### Comorbidity of Disorders

The tendency for several emotional and behavioral problems to cluster or co-occur in the same individual is now widely recognized as a diagnostic problem (Maser & Cloninger, 1990). *Comorbidity* refers to this co-occurrence of two or more diagnostic categories. Many children and adolescents with diagnosed conditions have more than one disorder. Comorbidity has been documented not only in referred samples, but also in several population samples (Nottelmann & Jensen, 1995). In particular, adolescent psychopathology is marked by the coexistence of disorders. For example, several studies have reported high correlations between depression and anxiety disorders in adolescence (for a review, see Kovacs, 1990). Also, the correlation between depressive and conduct disorder symptom scores reported by adolescents in a nonclinical community sample was high ($r = .73$; see Verhulst & van der Ende, 1993). In a review of community epidemiological studies of adolescent depression, Fleming and Offord (1990) reported that estimates of comorbidity of depression with any other disorder ranged from 33% to 100%. With respect to depression specifically, it is safe to say that comorbidity is the rule rather than the exception.

Although comorbidity rates for depression are particularly high in adolescence, other disorders also show considerable overlap. Multivariate studies of adolescents' behavioral and emotional problems have repeatedly identified two major groupings of problems, designated as *externalizing* and *internalizing* behaviors (Achenbach, 1991a). The *externalizing* syndromes include aggressive and delinquent behavior, as well as attention problems and hyperactivity. The *internalizing* syndromes include anxiety, depression, somatic complaints, and withdrawal. These groupings have different implications for intervention and therapeutic programs. For example, whereas children and adolescents with externalizing syndromes are more frequently referred for therapy, there is a tendency to underreport internalizing symptoms, especially by teachers.

Although the terms *externalizing* and *internalizing* describe different types of problems, these two patterns of behavior often co-occur in many children and adolescents. For example, Achenbach (1991a) reported correlations ranging from .45 to .63 between parents' ratings on the externalizing and internalizing scales for nonreferred and clinically referred samples of children and adolescents between of 4 and 18 years old.

Recent studies have analyzed the comorbidity between internalizing and externalizing syndromes measured according to the CBCL, TRF, and YSR for matched general populations and clinical samples of American children and adolescents 4 to 18 years old. The general population sample of 2,705 children and adolescents investigated by Achenbach and coworkers was representative of 48 contiguous states with respect to ethnicity, SES, geographic region, and area of residence. On the CBCL, comorbidity ranged from 40% to 44% for the aggressive behavior scale with the anxious-depressed scale and from 25% to 31% for the delinquent behavior scale with the anxious-depressed scale. Thus, there was a moderate to high overlap between the two externalizing syndromes and the internalizing syndrome based on parents' reports. Compared to the CBCL, comorbidity rates were somewhat lower on the TRF, which assesses teachers' ratings of child and adolescent symptomatology. Using the same general population sample, McConaughy and Skiba (1993) also computed comorbidity rates for deviance on the higher order externalizing and internalizing syndromes. For these analyses, clinical deviance was defined by scores at or above 82% ($T > 60$). Results showed that for children and adolescents who were deviant on the CBCL externalizing syndrome, 51% were also deviant on the internalizing syndrome. Conversely, 52% of those deviant on the CBCL internalizing syndrome were also deviant on the externalizing syndrome. In addition, comorbidity rates were higher for adolescents than for children.

The moderate to high comorbidity of externalizing and internalizing problems not only has important implications for designing intervention strategies and determining outcome, but it also challenges the specificity of the stress–symptomatology relation. As is discussed in chapter 5, stressful events are related to symptomatology. However, the specificity of this relation and the mechanisms underlying this association remain poorly understood. It is noteworthy to add that one of the theoretical models for explaining comorbidity designed by Caron and Rutter (1991) explains comorbidity in terms of shared and overlapping risk factors. Different types of stressors, the general stress level, and cumulative changes all affect the adolescent and lead to a generalized and varied picture of coexistent disorders.

### Historical Changes in the Symptoms of Some Illnesses

From an epidemiological perspective, there has been a shift in the relative incidence of acute physical illnesses toward chronic conditions (see chap. 3). Similarly, a change in the incidences of certain kinds of psychological disorders has occurred; at least, there seems to be an increase in the comorbidity of certain disorders. This shift in disorder types has been recognized for several years. Kohut (1977), for example, claimed a gradual decrease of classical neuroses (such as hysteria or phobia) and a simultaneous increase of disorders of the self, such as narcissistic disorders. Classical neuroses caused by conflicts seemed to decrease. In contrast, severe personality disorders, in which deficits of the patients' identity and structure become salient enough to negatively influence their ability for social relations and work, occur more frequently. The symbolization of a psychological conflict has also declined and has been replaced by vague psychosomatic and vegetative symptoms that cannot be linked to a nuclear conflict but rather represent diffuse equivalents of anxiety or tension. Today, the disorders are also judged to be considerably more severe than they were 30 or 40 years ago. In particular, the increase in comorbidity is regarded as reflecting more severe psychopathology (Nottelmann & Jensen, 1995; Verhulst & van der Ende, 1993). The Dunedin Health and Development study (Frost, Moffitt, & McGee, 1989) indeed shows that 13-year-olds with multiple diagnoses (25%) were significantly more impaired than peers with a single diagnosis. Bird, Gould, and Staghezza (1993) reported, for the Puerto Rico Child Psychiatric Epidemiological study, that 23% of the children and adolescents with one diagnosis were under treatment compared to 77% with two or more diagnoses. Thus, comorbidity seems to be related to the increased rates of professional mental health care.

In the following subsections, the aspects of comorbidity and symptomatology are illustrated by referring to two types of disorders—eating disorders and depression. From a historical perspective, it is obvious that the co-occurrence of disorders is not a recent development.

***Eating Disorders.*** From a historical point of view, anorexia nervosa is not a new disorder. Already in the 17th century, Morton presented a first description of the disorder by means of a case study. Nearly 200 years later, Gull (1873), in England, and Lasègue (1873), in France, speculated about the psychological cause of anorexia. Their descriptions of the symptoms remain valid and correspond to the criteria postulated by Feighner et al. (1972). In contrast, bulimia nervosa was described much later, around 1932. In an analysis of 32 publications between 1873 and 1960, Caspar (1983) noted that the symptoms of self-induced vomiting, binge-eating, and weight phobia were classified only since the 1940s. He concluded that bulimia came into existence as a subtype of anorexia. The symptoms of anorexia nervosa are inherent in the syndrome of bulimia: attacks of binge-eating, induced vomiting, and the abuse of laxatives occur both in the bulimic patient at normal weight and in more than half of all anorexics. Bulimia was described in single cases until Russell's report (1979) of the syndrome and the later inclusion of bulimia nervosa in the *DSM–III* in 1980. From this point on, the literature on bulimic disorders dramatically increased. Bulimia is currently considered to be an eating disorder that shows high increase rates comparable to those for anorexia nervosa (see *DSM–IV* and *ICD–10*).

In this context, it is important to recognize that abstention from and complete refusal of nutrition has been practiced by young women for centuries and has generally received high levels of social approval. In his book *Holy Anorexia*, Bell (1985) analyzed the biographics of female saints, dating back to the 12th century, and found that 39% of these women showed striking parallels to present anorexics; 26% fasted obsessively. Incidentally, Bell noted that many of these women showed symptoms of classical hysteria, such as paralysis, pain, dizziness, nausea, and convulsions. Almost all of these women had these symptoms during puberty (e.g., in a phase where the development toward the sexually and socially mature woman is at stake). Thus, the particular proneness of adolescents to a certain defense mechanism, asceticism (that is, rigorous self-denial and extreme abstinence; A. Freud, 1936), was historically confirmed.

Since the beginning of the 1980s, bulimia has become a fashionable topic of scientific and popular literature. It is, therefore, difficult to ascertain its true incidence; that is, the increased rate of bulimic female patients may be related to the fact that bulimia is popularized in the mass media. Furthermore, it is not clear whether bulimia is a variant form of other disorders (especially anorexia and adipositas; i.e., extreme overweight) or a genuine "new" illness. In anorexia nervosa, a historically older and more comprehensive disease, covariations with other psychological disorders were apparent quite early on. Since the first cases of anorexia nervosa, covariations with hysteria ("anorexie hystérique," according to Lasègue, 1873) and borderline conditions were found.

Halmi (1974) discovered hysterical complications in about 25% of his female patients; the simultaneous occurrence of depression and anorexia nervosa was discussed more recently. After a guiding study on eating disorders by Morgan and Russell (1975), who found depressive moods in 34% of their anorexic patients, more and more reports of the co-occurrence of anorexia nervosa and depression were published. In several studies, from 35% to 67% of the anorexic patients also showed dysphoric moods (Cantwell, Sturzenberger, Buroughs, Salkin, & Green, 1977; Hendren, 1983; Hudson, Pope, & Jonas, 1984). Additionally, in relatives of anorexic patients, there were twice as many people with affective disorders than in healthy control groups (Winokur, March, & Mendels, 1980). Comorbidity between eating and affective disorders not only presents diagnostic problems, but also has consequences for treatment and prognosis. Depressive symptoms, for example, might continue after the decline of anorexic symptoms, thus making a favorable prognosis unlikely.

***Depression.*** Depression is another illness for which changes in its presentation and comorbidity with other disorders can be verified. A further aspect becomes salient, which makes the diagnostic classification of depression even more difficult—namely, its overlap with normal developmental course. Although the classification of depression in childhood and adolescence has only been a diagnostically independent category for 30 years, some descriptions of the disease date back to the 19th century (Berkhan, 1863; Emminghaus, 1887). During the last 20 years, numerous articles on the phenomenology, diagnostic assessment, and risk factors of depressive disorders in childhood and adolescence were published. Petersen (1993) reported that 2,000 articles on this subject were published between 1987 and 1991.

Due to the acknowledged bias in clinical samples, studies on nonclinical samples have been carried out as well. The number of reports of depression and depressive mood in early adolescence are increasing, especially in female adolescents. The prevalence of depressive disorders in early adolescence currently matches prevalence rates for mid- and late adolescence (Fleming & Offord, 1990; Rutter, 1991). The typical clinical symptoms of depression for adults, that is, negative self-evaluation, anhedonia, loss of interest in daily activities, as well as loss of appetite, insomnia, and decreased energy, are rarely seen during adolescence and hardly ever seen before 17 years of age (Kovacs, 1989). However, there are other kinds of symptoms that are often erroneously ascribed to physical changes. Such symptoms were termed "depressive equivalents" (Toolan, 1969) or referred to as signs of "masked" or "larvate" depression (Glaser, 1967; Kielholz & Adams, 1988). This diagnostic uncertainty is reflected in the variety of published prevalence rates, ranging from 10% to 40%.

In the following, the phenomena of changes of disorders and comorbidity with other disorders is discussed for depressive syndromes or depressive disorders that were ascribed with a definite clinical significance. If, as previously mentioned, comorbidity is the rule for depression in adolescence, it becomes very difficult to offer adequate and comprehensive treatment. Comorbidity with phobias and anxiety disorders was found in 30% to 75% of patients with clinical depression (Kovacs, 1990); comorbidity with behavior disorders and obsessive disorders varied between 14% and 33% (Fleming & Offord, 1990; Mitchell, McCanley, Buke, & Moss, 1990). As already mentioned, comorbidity exists between depression and eating disorders (Hoffmeyer, 1988; Morgan & Russell, 1975). More recent findings show an increasing comorbidity with externalizing behavior, which was previously considered to be independent of depression or other internalizing behaviors. The comorbidity with alcohol and drug abuse is 23% to 25% (Fleming & Offord, 1990) and with delinquency 12% (Rohde, Lewinsohn, & Seeley, 1991). These findings may reflect a shift toward more externalizing symptoms in depressive disorders.

From a diagnostic standpoint, it is important to recognize that clinically relevant externalizing syndromes found in depressive adolescents may "mask" the depression. Externalizing behavior disorders are often the reason for consulting psychologists or psychiatrists, whereas the depression itself remains unrecognized and untreated. Furthermore, some externalizing behaviors are transitory in nature and can vanish during adolescence. Should depression during adolescence be untreated, there is a high risk for the onset of depressive disorders in adulthood (Compas, Ey, & Grant, 1992). This illustrates again that adolescent patients with mixed disorders can have a worse outcome, partly because it is difficult to treat the divergent symptoms adequately.

# 3

# Epidemiological Findings on Health Problems, Diseases, and Health-Risk Behavior

In this chapter, data on causes and rates of mortality in adolescents are presented first, followed by prevalence rates of acute and chronic physical diseases, symptoms, and subjective health status. Then, typical health hazards of adolescence, such as eating disorders, suicidal and risky sexual behavior, as well as patterns of substance abuse are analyzed.

The majority of the epidemiological statistics presented here were obtained from the U.S. Center for Disease Control and Prevention (CDC) and the National Center for Health Statistics (NCHS), based on findings from nationwide surveys on health and drug abuse and from cross-sectional and longitudinal health studies on community-based samples of children, adolescents, and young adults. Some international comparisons with similar data for European countries (in particular, Germany) are also provided. It should be pointed out that the statistics obtained in the framework of large surveys represent rough estimates of adolescent health status. This is not only related to the inherent weakness of some methods used to assess health status per se (e.g., self-reports versus health agency documentation), but also is a result of, as outlined in chapter 2, the fact that adolescents may be reluctant to disclose information about their health.

## CAUSES OF DEATH AND RATES OF MORTALITY IN ADOLESCENCE

In adulthood, the principal causes of death are disease-related. In contrast, the most frequent cause of death in adolescence is related to injuries resulting from violence. Accident-related injuries were the leading causes of death in young people aged 15 to 24 years old in the United States (42.0 per 100,000 in 1991), followed by homicide (22.4 per 100,000 in 1991) and suicide (13.1 per 100,000 in 1991) (National Center for Health Statistics, 1993a). Sells and Blum (1996) pointed out that violent injuries, accidents, homicides, and suicides account for 77% of adolescent deaths in the United States.

Similar trends were documented for European countries, where most adolescent deaths are caused by accidents, especially motor vehicle accidents. Homicide is the second leading cause of death in adolescents in the United States, and in Germany and most other European countries, suicide is the second leading cause of death in adolescents (Statistisches Bundesamt, 1992). In many countries, the rates of death caused by accident and acts of violence are higher for male adolescents, for example, in Germany (Bundesminister für Gesundheit, 1991) and the United States (NCHS, 1993a). SES and race are frequently found to be associated with increased mortality rates. For example, a close relation between low SES and increased injury risk was documented by Newacheck (1994). In North American samples, the mortality ratio of Black to White males is approximately 2 to 1 (Singh & Stella, 1996).

In the United States, 78% of all adolescent deaths resulting from accidental injuries are caused by motor vehicle accidents, with males accounting for three fourths of these deaths (National Safety Council, 1993). A disproportionate percentage of fatal motor vehicle injuries occur at night and in rural areas. The number of adolescents in the United States, aged 15 to 24 years old, who died from injuries sustained in motor vehicle accidents decreased by 38% from 1979 to 1992 (NCHS, 1993a). Nevertheless, 78% of all deaths caused by motor vehicle accidents were suffered by adolescents under 19 years old (National Safety Council, 1993). A number of factors have contributed to this improved outcome, including passive restraints, safer automobiles, reduced speed limits, and the nationwide increase in drinking age to 21 years old (Sells & Blum, 1996). Although the alcohol-related traffic fatality ratio decreased by more than one third between 1987 and 1992 for 15- to 24-year-olds (from 21.5 to 14.1 per 100,000; Centers for Disease Control and Prevention, 1994a), the consumption of alcohol still represents one of the leading causes of fatal traffic accidents involving adolescent drivers.

As previously mentioned, homicide is one of the leading causes of death in American youths. In 1991, more than 8,000 adolescents, aged 15 to 24 years old, were victims of homicide, reflecting a 54.5% increase in the homicide rates for this age group since 1979. Most homicide-related deaths occur in 15- to 19-year-old males; between 1985 and 1991, the annual homicide rate for this group increased by 154% (from 13.0 to 33.0 per 100,000). Correspondingly, age-specific arrest rates for murder and nonnegligent manslaughter increased by 127% for males 15 to 19 years old, and 43% for males 20 to 24 years old during the same period. In 1991, 15- to 19-year-old males were more likely to be arrested for murder than males in any other age group (CDC, 1994a). Firearm-related homicides accounted for 88% of all homicides documented for this age group in 1991. This overall increase in homicide, especially by the use of firearms, represents a dramatic change from the pattern observed during 1963 to 1984.

Although homicide and violent death are currently not a major cause of adolescent deaths in other countries, over the past 15 years, increased violence gained recognition as an important public health and social problem (see chap. 5, this volume). Although the immediate and specific causes of the dramatic increase in violent deaths in the United States are unclear, it is speculated that it may be the result of the relative ease with which many young people obtain firearms in their own homes (American Academy of Pediatrics and Center to Protect Handgun Violence, 1994). In addition, more young people are lured into drug-dealing rings, where the use of guns is common (Blumstein, 1994). Factors underlying the immediate precursors include poverty, social and family instability, and frequent exposure to violence as an acceptable or preferred method of resolving disagreements (Reiss & Roth, 1993). The homicide rate for males is more than 400% higher than for females, and Black youths are disproportionately represented in national homicide rates (National Safety Council, 1993). Homicide is the leading cause of death for Black males (158.9 per 100,000) and females (21.6 per 100,000) 15 to 24 years old (NCHS, 1993a).

The leading causes of death in adults, such as cardiovascular disease or cancer, also rank among the leading causes of death in adolescents, although the prevalence rates are comparatively lower. In Germany, 1 in 100,000 adolescents dies from cancer or heart disease. In 1991, cancer and heart disease were the fourth and fifth leading causes of death among American adolescents. Acquired immunodeficiency syndrome (AIDS) ranked as the sixth leading cause of death in young people, accounting for 1.6% of all deaths in 1989 through 1991. The mortality rates for adolescents with AIDS have increased worldwide; in the United States, the rate increased by 38% between 1987 and 1993. Congenital anomalies, pneumonia and influenza, stroke, and chronic obstructive pulmonary diseases were the seventh through tenth leading causes of death between 1989 and 1991, respectively (Singh & Stella, 1996). Whereas at the beginning of this century, acute infections, congenital abnormalities, and serious physical illnesses accounted for the highest mortality rates, these causes of death are now relatively seldom. One exception, of course, is the emergence of new infectious diseases, such as AIDS, which shows dramatic increases in incidence in adolescents and young adults.

In interpreting national mortality statistics (e.g., those published by the CDC or NCHS), it is important to recognize that younger adolescents are usually assessed together with children (age group 5–14 years old). The death rate for this age group of older children and young adolescents historically was the lowest of all age-specific death rates in the United States and has consistently declined since 1950 at an average rate of 2% per year (NCHS, 1995). It tends to be 40% to 60% higher for boys than for girls. Between 1989 and 1991, 24.5 per 100,000 older children and young adolescents in the United States died. Black children and young adolescents have the highest mortality rates (35.1 per 100,000), followed by Native Americans, Whites, and Hispanics. Compared with the mortality rates in early and late adulthood, the likelihood that an adolescent in this age group will die is quite low.

## MORBIDITY IN ADOLESCENCE

### Hospitalization and Doctor Visits

Although adolescents are comparably healthy and bear a fairly low risk of mortality in relation to adults, they nevertheless have experience with diseases and hospitalization. However, they are less frequently affected by serious or chronic illnesses than are other age groups. German adolescents between 12 and 16 years old are hospitalized to receive outpatient hospital care on the average of 1.6 times. Thirty to thirty-five percent of all inpatient hospital care is related to accidents. Due to increased and improved medical prevention, the rate for hospitalization in this age group has decreased (Mrazek, 1987a). Similar trends exist in the United States: between 1983 and 1987, the rate of children's and young adolescents' hospital stays fell from 7,076 to 5,130 per 100,000. Respiratory conditions, injuries, and digestive conditions accounted for more than 50% of these hospitalizations (Hodge, Dougherty, & Pless, 1995). The hospitalization rate for asthma in the United States, for example, remained relatively constant for persons 5 to 24 years old between 1980 and 1993 (approximately 18–22 per 10,000 5- to 14-year-olds and 8–10 per 10,000 15- to 24-year-olds annually). In the younger age group, boys were 1.3 times more likely than girls to be hospitalized for asthma, whereas among older adolescents and young adults, females were 2.1 times more likely to be hospitalized than males (CDC, 1996).

Nonfatal injuries are a frequent cause of hospitalization, especially among adolescent males. The most common causes of injuries were due to motor vehicle accidents, accidents with motorized bicycles, athletic and recreation injuries, falls, lacerations, burns, animal or insect bites, and accidental poisoning. The estimated national annual incidence rate for such injuries in 10- to 13-year-olds was 17.8 per 100 adolescents and 22.5 per 100 older adolescents 14–17 years old. About 60% of these injuries occurred in males, and about one third of all injuries reported was considered to be severe, whereas two thirds were classified as minor injuries (Scheidt et al., 1995).

Older children and adolescents (6–18 years old) also have the lowest annual rates of physician visits in the United States and Canada (mean is 3.33 visits per year in Canada and 2.73 per year in the United States; the total population means were 4.82 and 4.05, respectively; Katz, Hofer, & Manning, 1996). According to the National Health Interview Survey (NHIS) in 1988, White adolescents reported a mean number of 2.6 visits to a physician in the previous year, whereas Black and Hispanic adolescents were in a physician's practice only 1.8 and 1.7 times, respectively (Adams & Hardy, 1989). White adolescents spent an average of 4.6 days in bed and missed an average of 5.2 days of school per year due to poor health, whereas Blacks only stayed 3.1 in bed days per year and missed school 3.8 days per year. Hispanics reported being in bed for 3.9 days and absent from school on 6.6 days per year. Although White adolescents made use of medical services more often, 83% of them judged their health status to be excellent or very good, compared to 61% of the Black and 74% of the Hispanic adolescents.

Seventy-seven percent of all adolescents stated that they had made use of ambulatory health care services for routine care during the past 2 years (Igra & Millstein, 1993). Eighty-one percent of the White adolescents visited a physician's office, private clinic, or health maintenance organization, whereas only 59% of Blacks and 58% of Hispanics made use of these services. They either went to a neighborhood or hospital clinic (21% and 15%, respectively), or reported having no access to services providing routine care (11% of Whites, 13% of Blacks, and 22% of Hispanics; Lieu, Newacheck, & McManus, 1993). In this regard, it is important to mention that these rates of visits to providers or facilities for routine health care corresponded to the adolescents' insurance coverage. According to the NHIS conducted in 1988, 11% of White, 16% of Black, and 22% of Hispanic adolescents residing in the United States had no health insurance coverage. Thus, these rates reflect the impact of financial barriers on Black and Hispanic adolescents seeking health care.

### Infectious Diseases

Due to progress in medical research and improved hygienic conditions, diseases caused by bacterial or viral infections rarely occur today. Nevertheless, new or previously unrecognized strains of viruses, such as the Hanta virus or Ebola virus, the latter of which has been linked to the recent outbreak of hemorrhagic fever in Zaire, still pose direct or potential threats to individuals living in both industrialized and nonindustrialized nations. Furthermore, less dramatic but recurrent epidemics or pandemics of influenza continue to pose a serious health risk, especially among high-risk groups (Pinner et al., 1996).

Methodologically, morbidity and mortality rates for infectious diseases are difficult to assess. Epidemiological information is usually documented for each infectious disease separately, thus obscuring their aggregate impact. Furthermore, in contrast to other disease categories, such as cancer or heart disease, infectious disease trends are susceptible to rapid shifts. Finally, they are often classified as organ-system diseases despite their infectious etiologies, obscuring the assessment of their prevalence even more.

Pinner et al. (1996) reviewed the mortality rates for the general U.S. population between 1980 and 1992 and found that the mortality rate due to infectious diseases increased by 58%, from 41 to 65 deaths per 100,000 inhabitants. The increase varied among different age groups. Among individuals 65 years old and over, the mortality rate increased by 25% (from 271 to 338 deaths per 100,000). A 63% increase (from 6 to 38 deaths per 100,000) was documented for 25- to 44-year-olds; most of the deaths in this age group were AIDS-related. The lowest infectious mortality rate was found for children, adolescents, and young adults 5 to 24 years old (approximately 3–4 per 100,000). This rate remained constant between 1980 and 1992.

Despite the increased risk of contracting AIDS in adolescence, infectious diseases are rarely seen in adolescence. According to statistics published in 1992 by the Society for Adolescent Medicine (SAM; 1992), most childhood infections continue to occur at low endemic rates in adolescence. For example, only 0.10 cases of rubella per 100,000 were reported in 1988, and the CDC registered 4 cases nationwide among 10- to 14-year-olds in 1994 and 11 cases in the age group 15 to 19 years old in 1994 (CDC, 1995b). An incidence of 0.6 per 100,000 adolescents was documented in 1983 for measles (rubeola). However, there was a notable increase at the end of the 1980s, with a peak in April 1989, occurring in highly vaccinated populations of adolescents (SAM, 1992). In 1994, the CDC register documented 128 cases of rubeola in 10- to 14-year-olds and 255 cases in 15- to 19-year-olds (CDC, 1995b).

Poliomyelitis, tetanus, and diphtheria have more or less vanished in the United States, but still continue to threaten millions of children and adolescents in underdeveloped countries. The incidence of tuberculosis has also decreased dramatically over the past 100 years as a result of several factors that include pasteurization of milk, improved living conditions, as well as the development of effective pharmacotherapy. In 1986, only 1.4 cases per 100,000 were reported for children and adolescents 5 to 14 years old and 4.4 cases per 100,000 for adolescents and young adults between 15 and 24 years old. In 1994, 272 cases of tuberculosis were registered for adolescents between 10 and 14 years old and 544 cases in adolescents from 15 to 19 years old (CDC, 1995b). Hepatitis B was registered in 165 10- to 14-year-olds and in 807 15- to 19-year-old American adolescents in 1994.

### Chronic Illnesses

Chronic illnesses are distinguished from acute diseases and handicaps by their duration or recurrence as well as the extent to which they influence individual functioning. In adults, the incidence of acute illnesses tended to decrease over the past few decades; in contrast, chronic illnesses, such as coronary disease or cancer, have become more common. This trend is less distinct in adolescents because they are generally less affected by these diseases. Also, many chronic diseases develop latently over a long period of time, only becoming manifest during middle or late adulthood. Nevertheless, an increase in chronic conditions impairing the general health status of children and adolescents was observed during the past and present decades.

Most health surveys on the epidemiology of chronic illnesses fail to provide separate data for adolescents. Adolescents are either lumped together with children (including newborns, infants, toddlers, etc.) or divided into groups including young children and young adults (e.g., age groups of 5–14 years old and 15–24 years old; Westbrook & Stein, 1994). Moreover, the chronic conditions under scrutiny vary considerably, depending on the focus of the study and the definition of chronic conditions or diseases. In the NHIS, the term *condition* was chosen to include physical diseases and illnesses as well as injuries and impairments, and conditions were considered to be *chronic* if the onset was more than 3 months before the interview or if known to be chronic by nature (Adams & Hardy, 1989).

In the NHIS of 1988 (Adams & Hardy, 1989), 31% of all children and adolescents in the United States, or almost 20 million nationwide, were reported to be affected by one or more chronic health conditions. Twenty-one percent of these children and adolescents reported two and 9% reported three or more chronic mental or physical conditions. This rate is somewhat higher than in other industrialized countries. The rate of chronic conditions for most European countries ranges between 10% and 16% (Eiser, 1990). However, the sequence of rankings for most illnesses basically parallels North American figures.

As shown in Table 3.1, the most commonly reported chronic conditions in the United States included respiratory allergies (including hay fever), asthma, frequent or severe headaches, eczema and skin allergies, and repeated ear infections. Respiratory allergies affected 130.3 out of 1,000 adolescents, and each of the other relatively common conditions had a prevalence ranging between 30 and 50 per 1,000 adolescents. Chronic diseases of low prevalence included diabetes, sickle cell disease, and cerebral palsy, each of which affected fewer than 2 of every 1,000 adolescents in the United States. Chronic conditions were more prevalent in boys and male adolescents than in females and also occurred more frequently in Whites than in Blacks. Although most of these chronic conditions require continuous or frequent medication, frequent hospitalization is generally limited to adolescents afflicted with diabetes (36% hospitalized in the previous year), epilepsy and seizures (19%), cerebral palsy (12%), heart disease (8%), or asthma (7%) (Newacheck & Taylor, 1992). Beside these classic physical chronic illnesses, disabilities are also regarded as chronic conditions. In 1992, 30% of all U.S. children and adolescents were diagnosed with a learning disability, and 13% were diagnosed with a speech disability (CDC, 1995a). Mental retardation was diagnosed in 7% and emotional disorders were diagnosed in 6% of the U.S. adolescents. Other chronic disabilities include blindness or vision problems, deafness or serious hearing defects, paralysis of any kind, deformed or missing limbs, autism, head or spinal cord injury, heart trouble, or cancer (all of the latter occurring in 0.5% to 3% of all children and adolescents in the United States).

Measures of SES, including income, education, and occupation, are strongly related to mortality and morbidity rates for chronic diseases (Lowry, Kann, Collins, & Kolbe, 1996). Newacheck (1994) compared children and adolescents from families with different economic backgrounds and found that individuals from poor families exhibited a higher risk of severe chronic conditions. Simultaneously, poor families

TABLE 3.1
Prevalence of Childhood and Adolescence Chronic Conditions in Cases per 1,000 by Age, Gender, and Race

| *Condition* | *Age* | | *Gender* | | *Race* | |
|---|---|---|---|---|---|---|
| | *Under 10 Years* | *10 to 17 Years* | *Boys* | *Girls* | *White* | *Black* |
| All children with chronic conditions | 302.2 | 315.0 | 326.2 | 288.2 | 324.4 | 246.5 |
| *Impairments* | | | | | | |
| Musculoskeletal impairments | 10.9 | 20.9 | 16.7 | 13.6 | 15.9 | 10.5 |
| Deafness and hearing loss | 14.1 | 17.0 | 18.3 | 12.3 | 17.7 | 6.0 |
| Blindness and vision impairment | 10.3 | 16.0 | 11.4 | 14.2 | 13.9 | 8.4 |
| Speech defects | 31.6 | 18.9 | 35.3 | 16.7 | 25.9 | 33.5 |
| Cerebral palsy | 2.2 | 1.2 | 2.0 | 1.5 | 1.9 | 0.5 |
| *Diseases* | | | | | | |
| Diabetes | 0.6 | 1.5 | 1.5 | 0.5 | 1.2 | 0.1 |
| Sickle-cell disease | 1.3 | 0.9 | 0.9 | 1.4 | 0.1 | 6.9 |
| Anemia | 11.0 | 5.8 | 8.4 | 9.1 | 8.6 | 10.0 |
| Asthma | 39.3 | 46.8 | 50.7 | 33.9 | 41.0 | 51.4 |
| Respiratory allergies | 71.8 | 130.3 | 106.5 | 86.7 | 106.1 | 53.2 |
| Eczema and skin allergies | 31.1 | 35.2 | 30.1 | 35.8 | 34.3 | 22.8 |
| Epilepsy and seizures | 1.7 | 3.3 | 1.7 | 3.1 | 2.5 | 2.3 |
| Arthritis | 1.5 | 8.7 | 4.2 | 4.9 | 4.5 | 5.3 |
| Heart disease | 13.6 | 17.4 | 16.4 | 13.9 | 17.3 | 7.5 |
| Frequent or repeated ear infections | 120.6 | 33.6 | 88.5 | 78.1 | 91.6 | 53.2 |
| Frequent diarrhea/ bowel trouble | 22.6 | 9.6 | 18.1 | 15.9 | 17.8 | 13.6 |
| Digestive allergies | 23.2 | 21.1 | 25.6 | 18.9 | 24.5 | 9.7 |
| Frequent or severe headaches | 9.9 | 45.8 | 22.8 | 27.9 | 26.5 | 21.9 |
| Other | 12.1 | 30.0 | 19.3 | 20.3 | 21.9 | 9.9 |

*Note.* Data from National Center for Health Statistics (1988), *Vital statistics, morality data, multiple cause of death detail* (pp. 26, 48), Hyattsville, MD: U.S. Department of Health and Human Services.

were confronted with substantial barriers to obtaining appropriate care, most were uninsured and also lacked access to health care services (see chap. 8, this volume). Although poor families seldom used ambulatory health care services, they received more inpatient hospital care than more well-off families.

## PSYCHOLOGICAL PROBLEMS AND DISORDERS

### Prevalence of Psychological Symptoms and Disorders

Most adolescents pass through their teenage years without salient psychological problems or behavioral disorders. Large epidemiological studies (see, e.g., Offord, Boyle, & Racine, 1990b; Rutter, Graham, Chadwick, & Yule, 1976) demonstrated that the prevalence rates for psychological disturbances during adolescence only slightly differ from the rates for childhood and adulthood; however, the manifestation rates and peaks of particular syndromes vary with age. Disorders frequently seen in childhood, such as enuresis, hyperactivity, or conduct disorders, decrease in adolescence (Kashani, Carlson, & Beck, 1987). Simultaneously, adolescence is characterized by first manifestations of depressive syndromes, schizophrenia, obsessive–compulsive disorders, anxiety disorders, eating disorders, drug abuse, or suicidal behavior. Sixty percent of these disorders develop during puberty; they are rarely seen, for example, in 10-year-old children (Rutter et al., 1977).

These diagnoses are also made in psychiatric examinations of unselected samples. Kashani et al. (1987) assessed a community sample of 150 adolescents 14 to 16 years old. Using structured psychiatric interviews, they established that about 9% of the adolescents had anxiety disorders, 9% had depressive disorders, 6% had oppositional disorders, and 5% to 6% were alcohol and drug abusers. Many of the individuals had multiple diagnoses (see chap. 2, this volume). In a cross-cultural comparison of psychiatric epidemiological studies (Florenzano, 1991), about 2% to 3% of adolescents were diagnosed with schizophrenia and personality disorders.

Beside these clearly defined disorders, the prevalence rates for vague or transitory disorders are high, accounting for about one fourth of all diagnoses of psychiatric symptomatology in adolescence (Weiner & Del Gaudio, 1976; see also chap. 2, this volume). Moreover, adjustment disorders were diagnosed in 4% to 10% of adolescents in general population samples as well as in 15% to 42% of adolescents from clinically referred samples (Cohen et al., 1993).

Whereas before 15 years old, more male children are brought to the attention of psychologists and psychiatrists, in adolescence, a higher proportion of females seeking professional help becomes apparent. In addition, gender-specific patterns of adolescent symptomatology begin to emerge. Male adolescents more frequently show externalizing behavior syndromes (e.g., aggression, dissocial behavior, hyperactivity, or delinquency); female adolescents show higher prevalence rates for internalizing disorders (e.g., depression and anxiety) as well as somatization disorders (Graham & Rutter, 1985; Kashani et al., 1987; Offord, Boyle, & Racine, 1990a, 1990b; Rozario, Kapur, Rao, & Dalal, 1994). Cohen et al. (1993) reported prevalence rates in a general population sample for anxiety disorders to be 14% in young adolescent girls and 5% in boys 14 to 16 years old. The rates for older adolescents (17–20 years old) were 14% in females and 5% in males. The prevalence rates for attention deficit disorder (ADD) and conduct disorder were about one third higher in younger male adolescents (11% and 16%) than females (6% and 9%), but these differences were more or less leveled out in later adolescence. Oppositional disorder occurred in 2% of all adolescents, and the rate remained constant with age. In most studies, it was found that psychiatric symptomatology in adolescence peaks in its early phase. For example, Rozario, Kapur, and Kaliaperumal (1990) found the highest rates of psychological disturbances were shown by younger adolescents around 13 years old (11%). The percentage of adolescents with psychological problems or symptoms declined by about 2% to 4% annually. In the following text, affective disorders including depression and suicidal behaviors are discussed in more detail. Because bipolar affective disorders rarely occur in adolescence (Lewinsohn, Klein, & Seeley, 1995), we focus our attention on unipolar depression.

***Depression.*** As detailed in chapter 2, the problem of comorbidity makes the diagnosis of depressive symptoms difficult. The large variety of depressive symptoms is grouped into depressive moods, depressive syndromes, and severe depressive disorders (see Compas et al., 1992). These symptoms are identical to those exhibited by adults suffering from affective disorders, namely cognitive features such as rumination, negative self-evaluation, anhedonia, loss of interest in daily activities, and vegetative features such as loss of appetite, insomnia, and decreased energy. However, adolescents usually show fewer classic vegetative signs. Whereas depressed adults often suffer from hyposomnia, hypersomnia can be a major sleep disturbance in adolescent depressives. Adolescents also report unspecific depressive complaints and feelings of emptiness, irritability, or boredom (Carlson & Kashani, 1988; Kutcher, 1986).

Depressive moods and depressive symptoms are common in adolescents, but prevalence figures largely vary, ranging from 20% to more than 50% (Kutcher & Marton, 1989; Stavrakaki & Ellis, 1989). Different diagnostic criteria, different methods of assessment (structured interviews vs. self-report measures), and different sources of information are responsible for this variability in epidemiological findings. A large-scale North American epidemiologic survey of high school students (Kandel & Davies, 1982) revealed a prevalence of depressed mood to be about 25% among 14- to 18-year-olds. Similarly, Pearce (1978) found depressive symptomatology in 25% of postpubertal individuals receiving care at Maudsley Hospital. In the Ontario Child Health Study (Offord et al., 1987), symptoms of depression were reported by 37% of boys and 56% of girls between 12 and 16 years old. Thus, one fifth to one half of the adolescent population experience some symptoms of depression at any given point in time.

The same study that surveyed a sample of over 3,000 Ontario children and adolescents (4 to 16 years old) reported a prevalence rate of only 3% for depressive disorders in adolescent boys and 7% in adolescent girls. Kashani et al. (1987) examined a community sample of 14- to 16-year-olds in a Missouri high school and found that 3% of male and 13% of female adolescents were diagnosed with a major depression or dysthymic disorder, the gender difference being significant. In 14 studies reviewed by Fleming and Offord (1990), lifetime prevalence rates of about 8% and prevalence rates of current depression ranging from 0.4% to 6% were found.

Nearly all studies converge in the overall trend that depressive symptoms, as well as depressive disorders, increase from the preadolescent to adolescent years and that the increase is most marked in girls (Kutcher & Marton, 1989). The prevalence of depressive symptomatology seems to peak among persons of both genders between 18 and 24 years old, with the absolute rate being higher in females (Moreau, 1990). Research examining some earlier theories of adolescent development led to major revisions of our understanding of both normal development and psychopathology during adolescence. In particular, many analyses of the processes and determinants of adolescent depression were carried out during the past 10 years (for a summary, see Kutcher & Marton, 1989; Petersen, 1993). Other investigations made significant contributions toward understanding the relations among stress appraisal, certain coping styles, and the emergence of depression (see chaps. 2 and 6, this volume).

***Suicide and Suicidal Behaviors.*** Special focus on adolescent suicide was prompted by increases in the adolescent suicide rates for highly industrialized areas of North America and Northern Europe. In comparing 19 countries, Diekstra (1989), for example, found that the adolescent suicide rate in Finland has tripled, and the suicide rate in the United States has quadrupled over the last 40 years. This rise in adolescent suicide in the United States is a singular phenomenon; the rates for other age groups over these years either declined or remained constant (Ryland & Kruesi, 1992). Suicide is now the third greatest cause of death in older adolescents in the United States (Berman & Jobes, 1995), following accidents and homicide (Hodgman, 1990), whereas it is ranking second place among European adolescent mortality rates. In 1950, 2.7 per 100,000 persons between 15 and 19 years old committed suicide in the United States; in 1980, 8.5 per 100,000 committed suicide, and in 1988, 11.3 per 100,000 committed suicide (CDC, 1986; NCHS, 1988). Suicide does not occur equally across ages; it is extremely rare in prepubertal children. The rate of male suicide sharply increases during adolescence, peaks around 23 years old, then levels off until 65 years old, when the rate rises again. For women, the rise is less dramatic during the adolescent years, nevertheless, the rate continues to slowly rise during her late 20s and 30s, peaks between 45 and 55 years old, and decreases thereafter (NCHS, 1988).

Internationally, adolescent males commit suicide more often than females, although females attempt suicide more often than males. In most countries, the ratio between male and female suicides ranges from 2 to 1 to 7 to 1 (Diekstra, 1989). For example, suicide rates in the United States are over four times greater for males than females (18.0 per 100,000 vs. 4.4 per 100,000), and Whites commit suicide twice as often as non-Whites (12.3 per 100,000 vs. 6.0 per 100,000; NCHS, 1988). White males show the highest risk for suicide. In 1990, 73% of all suicides among 15- to 24-year-olds were committed by White males (Berman & Jobes, 1995). According to the NCHS (1988), White male adolescents have the highest suicide rates (19.6 per 100,000) and non-White females have the lowest suicide rates (2.5 per 100,000). As mentioned, the increased suicide rates are largely a male phenomenon.

Australia, New Zealand, and Northern European countries show similar rates and experienced similar increases in adolescent suicide (Diekstra, 1990). Suicidal ideation is also very frequent. In a recent epidemiological study of 15- to 19-year-old high school students (CDC, 1991), 27% of the students seriously thought about attempting suicide in the previous year, and 8% actually attempted suicide. Suicidal thoughts were identified in 76% of the subjects in a community sample of depressed adolescents, and 27% reported having attempted suicide in the previous month (Hoberman, 1989).

Gaining insight into adolescent suicide requires understanding the associated risk factors that include psychiatric disorders such as depression, anxiety, conduct disorder, and alcohol or substance abuse (Marttunen, Aro, Henriksson, & Lonnqvist, 1991; Shafii, Carrigan, Whittinghill, & Derrick, 1985). Although the existence of depressive disorders is frequent among suicide victims, the coexistence of affective disorders with antisocial behavior, conduct disorder, or alcohol abuse is even more common (Marttunen et al., 1991). Family environment is also thought to influence the suicide risk among adolescents. The families of adolescent suicide victims were shown to be marked by intrafamilial turmoil and a history of parental psychiatric disorders. Discordant family relations (Rich, Sherman, & Fowler, 1990), a history of suicide in the family (Roy, Segal, Centerwall, & Robinette, 1991), and exposure to suicidal behavior in the personal environment (Pfeffer, 1990) were also frequently found. For example, among studies of adolescent suicide victims, prevalence of family discord ranged from 11% to 80%. In addition, Runeson (1989) noted that 71% of the families of suicide victims consulted a physician or psychotherapist for a mental disorder, and 52% of the families had at least one other member suffering from substance abuse. Problems of sexual identity, or more specifically homosexuality, were increasingly recognized as a risk factor for suicidal behavior (Ryland & Kruesi, 1992). Psychological and psychophysiological disorders also play a role; for example, low concentrations of monoamine metabolites in the cerebrospinal fluid were related to suicide in adolescent populations (Kruesi et al., 1992). Each of these factors contribute to suicidal behavior, however, specific suicidogenic factors have yet to be discovered (Khan, 1987).

In the United States, most male and female adolescent suicides involve the use of firearms. The next most frequently employed method is hanging (for males) and jumping from a height (for females; Shaffer, Garland, Gould, Fisher, & Trautman, 1988). In Oregon, where legislation mandates that all suicide attempts by persons under 18 years old be documented, Andrus et al. (1991) found that most unsuccessful attempts to commit suicide were related to drug overdose (76%), followed by laceration or stabbing (10%); those adolescents who were successful chose "more reliable" methods like shooting (72%) or hanging (17%). Males were far more likely to choose more fatal methods than females, and choice of method was the strongest predictor of outcome in this study ($p < 0.0001$). The rise in suicide rates of adolescents is not easy to explain. Whereas some authors pointed out that cohort effects play some role in suicide, others (e.g., Diekstra, 1989) suggested that cohort effects are altering the suicide rates. Wetzel, Reich, Murphy, Province, and Miller (1987) argued that social factors are most likely responsible for increased suicide rates because biological and genetic changes would not proceed rapidly enough to explain the change in suicide rate patterns.

Support for the view that social changes exert a significant influence on suicide rates, however, comes from studies of native populations undergoing cultural alterations. For example, Micronesia experienced a 10-fold increase in the male youth suicide-behavior rate from 1960 to 1970, during which time the islands underwent rapid industrialization. Similar patterns of increasing adolescent male suicide during periods of rapid social change were observed among Greenland Innuits, aborigines in South Australia, and native North Americans (Ryland & Kruesi, 1992). The enormous influence of macrosocial changes and stressors on the life of adolescents is dealt with more specifically in chapter 5.

## HEALTH RISK BEHAVIOR

### Weight Problems and Eating Disorders

Eating disorders such as obesity, anorexia nervosa, and bulimia nervosa are steadily increasing in industrial nations. Whereas *obesity* is characterized by extreme overweight, *anorexia nervosa* is distinguished by an all-consuming pursuit of thinness, by means of excessive dieting, abuse of laxatives or diuretics and physical activity, overriding the patient's physical and psychological well-being, and eventually becoming the only focal point of attention in the patient's life (Garfinkel, 1990). Anorexia is frequently associated with serious electrolyte imbalances and sometimes with amenorrhea (Siegel, 1992). *Bulimia nervosa*, on the other hand, is characterized by episodic patterns of binge eating, alternating with extreme efforts to lose weight (e.g., fasting or vomiting).

Whereas obesity is a health problem affecting the overall population of the United States, bulimia and anorexia nervosa are conditions seen primarily in adolescence and young adulthood, almost exclusively affecting females (90% to 95%; Siegel, 1992). Even if they do not meet the strict DSM-IV criteria for eating disorders, up to 20% of randomly selected adolescent girls score in the abnormal range on standardized tests of eating attitudes and behaviors; up to 50% to 60% of adolescent girls consider themselves overweight and attempt to diet (Fisher et al., 1995). Many of those females who have eating problems on a subclinical level might still suffer from a similar level of psychological distress seen in clinical cases (see chap. 4, this volume). The study conducted by French, Story, Downes, Resnick, and Blum (1995) investigated the correlates between frequent dieting, vomiting, and purging with negative psychosocial and health behavior outcomes. About 12% of females and 2% of males dieted 10 or more times during the previous year, and 15% of females and 7% of males reported vomiting or purging behavior of some type. Both dieting frequency and vomiting or purging status were independently associated with increased psychosocial and health behavior-risk factors. The dieting frequency was associated with a history of binge eating, poor body image, lower connectedness to others, as well as greater alcohol and tobacco use.

Incidence rates for anorexia nervosa increased steadily from 1955 to 1990 among adolescent girls 10 to 19 years old, but not among adults. The current prevalence rate of 0.5% among 15- to 19-year-old females probably underestimates the real occurrence among youth (Fisher et al., 1995). According to their literature review, approximately 1% to 5% of adolescent girls were reported in studies conducted during the 1980s to meet strict DSM-III-R criteria for bulimia nervosa, whereas as many as 10% to 50% reported occasional self-induced vomiting or binge-eating. Garfinkel (1990) found a prevalence rate of 2% to 3% for bulimia nervosa in young women, with mild variants occurring in 5%; the prevalence rate for anorexia nervosa in female adolescents was 1%.

Being overweight, on the other hand, is associated with serious health risks such as coronary heart disease, hypertension, diabetes mellitus, gallbladder disease, joint disease, and an increased mortality in adulthood. Because being overweight in adolescence is a significant predictor for being overweight in adulthood, the prevalence rates among U.S. youth have to be observed carefully. During the time period of 1988–1991, 21% of all adolescents between 12 and 19 years old were clinically overweight. Gender-specific prevalence of overweight adolescents was 20% for males and 22% for females (CDC, 1994b). Mexican American boys (27%) and Black girls (30%) 12 to 17 years old had the highest prevalence rates for being overweight in the National Health and Nutrition Examination Survey (NHANES) of 1991 (Troiano, Flegal, Kuczmarski, Campbell, & Johnson, 1995). Both the overall prevalence rate, as well as particular subgroup rates of obesity, steadily increased in children and adolescents since the first national surveys in the 1960s, with an overall increase of one third to one half. Black adolescents show both the highest increase rate and the highest ratio of obese adolescents in the course of the NHANES surveys. Other data from these studies from the past 30 years suggest that this tendency is not only caused by a dramatic increase in caloric intake, but also by a simultaneous decrease of physical activity.

### AIDS, Sexually Transmitted Diseases, and Risky Sexual Behavior

Since the 1980s, the risk of contracting sexually transmitted diseases (STDs)—for example, venereal diseases and especially AIDS (Acquired Immune Deficiency Syndrome)—has become a serious problem, particularly for adolescents and young adults. Nevertheless, studies of sexual risk behaviors among teenagers related to the transmission of the AIDS virus (Human Immunodeficiency Virus, HIV), other STDs, and unintended pregnancy indicate that young people continue to practice high-risk behaviors, despite widespread knowledge about HIV infection (CDC, 1992b; Stiffman, Earls, Dore, & Cunningham, 1992). In 1991, HIV infection was the sixth leading cause of death among 15- to 24-year-old males and females in the United States (NCHS, 1993a). By the end of 1993, 1,554 cases of AIDS in the age group of 13- to 19-year-old, and 13,890 in the age group of 20- to 24-year-olds, were reported to the CDC (CDC, 1994d). In comparison, in 1992, it was estimated that between 550,000 to 700,000 men and 120,000 to 160,000 women were infected with HIV (Karon et al., 1996), which corresponds to prevalence rates of 5% to 7% in men and 1% in women. At the end of 1994, there were 1,965 registered cases of AIDS among young people 13 to 19 years old, and 66% of these cases were males. Eighty-three percent of these male cases were infected through blood transfusion for the treatment of coagulation disorders, homosexual contact, and intravenous drug use. Most females became infected through heterosexual contact (U.S. Department of Health and Human Services, 1994a).

Because of the long period between infection with HIV and the onset of AIDS, many people diagnosed with AIDS in their late 20s were probably infected during their teenage years. Back calculation models of age-specific AIDS incidence suggest that age at onset of HIV infection has declined during the last 15 years, with 25% of new infections from 1987 to 1991 occurring in persons younger than 22 years (Rosenberg, Biggar, & Goeddert, 1993). As many as 25% of all AIDS patients who were infected through heterosexual contact are estimated to have been infected when they were 13 to 19 years old (Byers, Lindegren, Hanson, Sweeney, & Onorato, 1992).

Sweeney, Lindegren, Buehler, Onorato, and Janssen (1995) analyzed health surveys from 130 clinics, juvenile correctional facilities, and homeless and runaway youth centers in 24 cities across the United States. Among 79,802 serum specimens from teenagers 15 to 19 years old, 591 of them were positive for HIV-1 antibody. The median clinic-specific prevalences were 0.2% (range was 0% to 1%) in 22 adolescent medicine clinics, 0.3% (range was 0% to 7%) in 33 correctional facilities, 0.5% (range was 0% to 4%) in 70 STD clinics, and 1.1% (range was 0% to 4%) in five homeless youth centers. Rates were highest among young men who reported having sexual contact with men, with clinic rates ranging from 16% to 17% in two homeless youth centers and 13% to 17% in two STD clinics. Surveys in homeless youth centers generally resulted in higher infection rates (median was 4% in males and 0.9% in females). In addition to male homosexual activity, the sharing of needles among intravenous (IV) drug users represents another risk factor for the adolescents as do risky sexual behaviors such as prostitution. This tendency among adolescents to engage in multiple-risk behaviors may account for the higher prevalence rates for HIV-infection in homeless and runaway youth centers or correctional facilities. Infection rates for male and female adolescents with heterosexual contact as the only risk factor were generally low.

It should be pointed out that these official figures are probably not accurate estimates; the real percentages of infected persons may be much greater (Glasner & Kaslow, 1990). There is a long latency period of about 2 to 8 years between infection with HIV and first manifestation of AIDS symptoms. Moreover, adolescents are especially reluctant to take the HIV test, in part because of their low awareness of the increased risk for this age group (see chap. 2, this volume).

On the other hand, the highest increase in HIV-prevalence rates took place during the 1980s; incidence rates have shown less dramatic increases since the beginning of the 1990s (Karon et al., 1996). Simultaneously, the awareness of the risk for HIV infection has mounted, which has spurred an increased use of condoms. The percentage of adolescents who reported using a condom during the most recent act of sexual intercourse significantly increased from 46% in 1991 to 53% in 1993. However, subgroup analyses indicated a significant increase in condom use only among females (from 38% to 46%) and Blacks (from 48% to 57%) (CDC, 1995c). These findings suggest that HIV infection and AIDS have not become epidemic in the general population, as previously feared. Nevertheless, AIDS still represents a serious threat for certain risk groups like IV drug users or individuals engaging in risky sexual practices.

Besides the threat of becoming infected with HIV, risky sexual behavior is associated with a higher risk of contracting other STDs (e.g., gonorrhea, chlamydia trachomatis, syphilis, or trichomonas vaginalis). Gonorrhea is the most frequent communicable disease reported to the

CDCs. Because the actual number of cases is probably twice the reported rate, an annual incidence of 500,000 cases is estimated to occur among adolescents (SAM, 1992). Risk factors for its acquisition include low SES, urban residence, and early onset of sexual activity. Chlamydial genital infection is the most common STD with an estimated 3 to 5 million cases occurring annually. Because such cases must not be reported to the CDC, accurate national statistics regarding prevalence rates are not available, but prevalence rates among adolescents are estimated to range from 14% to 26%, dependent on demographic background, number of sex partners, and contraceptive use. The incidence of syphilis in adolescents is unknown, too. It has been estimated that it occurs in about 0.1% of adolescents and young adults (SAM, 1992), the risk for an infection being highest among homosexual males and Blacks residing in large, poor urban areas. Thus, STDs are common causes of morbidity in adolescents and therefore should become a major public health concern. Adequate screening procedures already exist but are not administered regularly to risk groups. Consequently, appropriate treatment for many STDs often comes too late.

Another issue related to adolescents' risky sexual behavior is the frequent occurrence of adolescent pregnancies and abortions, especially in the United States (Petersen, 1993). In 1989, 1,043,600 women residing in the United States under 20 years old became pregnant. Of these, 27,810 were 15 years old or younger. Nearly half of these females gave birth, 37% had legal abortions, and an estimated 14% miscarried (Henshaw, 1994). Pregnancy rates for all women between 15 and 19 years old increased by more than 5% between 1985 and 1989 to a level of 114.9 per 1,000, their highest level in nearly 20 years (Sells & Blum, 1996). Pregnancy and birth rates differ markedly for different ethnic groups. The pregnancy rate for non-White adolescents from 15 to 19 years old was 184.3 per 1,000 in 1992 and almost twice as high as for White adolescents (93.4 per 1,000). For teens under 15 years old, the pregnancy rate was 4.9 per 1,000, 90% of them being non-White (NCHS, 1993b). The rates for teenage abortion have steadily decreased over the past decades; nevertheless, 24% of all abortions in 1989 were performed on women under 20 years old (CDC, 1992a).

Although adolescent pregnancy and abortion rates in other developed countries (e.g., in Europe) do not match U.S. rates (Petersen, 1993), they are considered to reflect health problems. With respect to the decreasing numbers of live births and abortions in adolescents, in relation to the total prevalence rates in Germany, adolescents do not represent a major risk group. Only 2% of all abortions in Germany are performed on 15- to 18-year-olds (Statistisches Bundesamt, 1991); only 3% to 9% of all mothers between 15 and 50 years old are 15 to 19 years old. An increased risk for pregnancy and birth-related complications exists for the younger mothers, because they often conceal their pregnancy or do not seek or receive adequate prenatal care.

### Consumption and Abuse of Alcohol, Tobacco, Illicit Drugs, and Medically Prescribed Substances

Adolescents are considered to be a risk population for the consumption and abuse of legal and illegal drugs. However, methodological problems render the analysis of data on adolescent substance abuse difficult. It is not easy to obtain validation of self-reports, with respect to the information provided in the comparison of cross-sectional and longitudinal data and the prevalence rates among different cohorts are subject to pitfalls. Furthermore, the consumption of individual substances must be seen in the context of general use patterns for different subgroups of adolescent drug users.

***Consumption of Alcohol.*** Alcohol is the most common substance abused by adolescents. The average age of first drinking alcohol outside of family-sanctioned use or religious occasions has decreased to 12 years of age. Almost 50% of sixth graders in a national survey conducted in the United States reported feeling peer pressure to experiment with alcohol, and 40% had already tried beer or wine, yet only 15% perceived any risk of harm from using alcohol daily (National Survey on Drugs and Drinking, 1987). In 1993, 67% of eighth graders, 81% of tenth graders, and 87% of high school seniors had already experimented with alcohol (O'Malley, Johnston, & Bachman, 1995). More than one fourth of eighth graders (26%) had used alcohol in the previous month, as had 42% of tenth graders and 51% of high school seniors. Ten percent of all sixth graders, one third of all eighth graders, and 75% of all twelfth graders had been intoxicated at least once. These rates are about 10% lower for Blacks and Hispanics than for Whites (Oetting & Beauvais, 1990). Although only 1% of adolescents consider themselves to have a drinking problem, 23% often had driven a motor vehicle after excessive drinking, 17% report problems in peer relationships because of drinking, and 10% had been criticized by a close friend for drinking (Werner & Adger, 1995).

Although nearly all U.S. high school seniors report experience with alcohol, heavy alcohol use among adolescents dramatically decreased during the 1980s. The percentage of seniors who engaged in daily drinking especially declined, from a peak of 7% in 1978 to less than 3% in 1994 (Johnston, O'Malley, & Bachman, 1995). A similar trend was documented for German youths whose alcohol consumption steadily decreased between 1970 and 1990 (Institut für Jugendforschung, IJF, 1990). Cross-national studies showed that daily consumption of alcohol and drinking to intoxication are more common among males than females. Whereas alcohol use appears to be similar in metropolitan and rural or suburban areas, regional differences are found in American samples, with the highest use occurring in the Northeast and the lowest use occurring in the West (Johnston, O'Malley, & Bachman, 1994). According to the Bogalusa Heart study (Johnston et al., 1995), adolescent drinking was more prevalent among males than females ($p < .001$) and more prevalent among Whites than Blacks ($p < .01$). In all surveys, White male adolescents of all ages showed the highest rates (31%–35% across ages and surveys) and Black females showed the lowest rates (approximately 10%) for the once weekly consumption of alcohol. Between 81% and 87% of the males reported drinking once or twice a week, whereas 10% to 17% drank three to four times a week. The percentages of males consuming alcohol weekly increased dramatically through adolescence and young adulthood, peaking at 18 to 20 years old. In females, alcohol consumption increased marginally with age and showed a significant decrease after 20 years old.

Alcohol abuse is a major factor contributing to the deterioration of the health status of adolescents and young adults (Rogers & Adger, 1993). Approximately one half of all fatal motor vehicle accidents and homicides, as well as a substantial proportion of suicides, are associated with the use of alcohol and other drugs (CDC, 1990; Garrison, McKeown, Valois, & Vincent, 1993). In addition, alcohol has been implicated in a majority of drownings, fire-related deaths, and fatal falls (U.S. Department of Health and Human Services, 1990). Moreover, adolescent alcohol users often engage in other risk-taking behaviors, especially risky sexual behavior (Mott & Haurin, 1988).

***Tobacco Smoking.*** Today, tobacco smoking represents the largest avoidable health risk. Long-term smoking has been implicated as a causal factor for several types of cancer, cardiovascular disease, hypertension, and other diseases. In 1988, 435,000 deaths in the United States were due to smoking (Fiore, 1992). Since the 1960s, the smoking prevalence rates in the overall population of the United States have steadily declined (Orleans & Slade, 1993), whereas the percentage of adolescents experimenting with cigarettes and beginning to smoke on a regular basis has remained, more or less, constant (CDC, 1992c). Eighty-nine percent of all smokers report having tried their first cigarette by the age of 18 (U.S. Department of Health and Human Services, 1994b). The median age of initiation to smoking has dropped to 16 or 17 (CDC, 1994; Lee, Gilpin, & Pierce, 1993).

Results of several national surveys on health behavior and drug use, summarized by Oetting and Beauvais (1990), reveal that one half of all adolescents were already smoking cigarettes in the eighth grade (49%–55%). The lifetime prevalence rate of adolescent smoking only increases slightly to about 65% during high school senior years, which corresponds to the findings previously mentioned. About 62% of tenth-grade students report that they already smoked at least one cigarette, and 50% report that they had smoked their first cigarette by the seventh or eighth grade (Orleans & Slade, 1993). About 50% of both men and women report that they started to smoke regularly by 18 years of age; about 90% report that they started by age 21. In 1994, adolescent-lifetime prevalence of cigarette smoking was 62%, and 31% of all adolescents reported having smoked during the last 30 days before the survey (Johnston et al., 1994). Cigarettes continue to be the most common substance used daily by adolescents. Although daily cigarette smoking declined for adults, the rates for high school seniors have remained constant for more than 10 years (between 18% and 19%). Since 1992, cigarette smoking among adolescents has consistently increased, with males still being slightly more likely to smoke than females (Sells & Blum, 1996).

Considering the strict antismoking campaigns that were launched in the United States in recent decades, this finding is somewhat perplexing. In other countries, cigarette smoking in the general population has declined slightly; however, the proportion of adolescents who smoke has remained relatively large. The number of German adolescents who smoke ranks about average when compared to other countries, whereby the ratio of adolescent smokers to nonsmokers in Germany is clearly greater than that of American adolescents (Lopez & Fuchs, 1990). At the beginning of 1990, nearly 40% of German 14- to 25-year-olds smoked regularly and nearly 50% smoked occasionally (IJF, 1990). Most adolescents start smoking between 15 and 17 years old. One other trend that deserves particular mention is the finding that in Germany and in most other European countries, the number of female adolescent smokers is increasing.

Racial differences in the number of adolescent smokers were reported in the United States. In 1991, fewer Black than White adolescents smoked. However, these findings must be interpreted with caution: Bauman and Ennett (1994) found that Black adolescents significantly underreported their smoking habits compared to White adolescents.

Unfortunately, systematic surveys of smoking behavior for the total population of adolescents in the United States have not been conducted on a regular basis over the last 25 years. One exception is the study conducted by Nelson et al. (1995), who analyzed the changes in patterns of adolescent smoking between 1974 and 1991, based on national health data for this period. They found a slight decrease in the respective numbers of both male and female adolescents between 1974 and 1985, whereas the rates remained relatively constant during the past 10 years (see also CDC, 1995d).

Adolescents often underestimate the danger of becoming addicted to cigarette smoking. Nearly a third of high school seniors who smoke one pack or more of cigarettes a day think they probably or definitely will not be smoking in 5 years, and the less adolescents smoke, the more they feel certain about not smoking a couple of years later (CDC, 1994c; Pierce & Gilpin, 1996). Yet, in fact, most adolescents who experiment with cigarettes for more than a short period of time will remain smokers during their adult years, as prevalence of smoking is highest between 20 and 35 years old and only declines gradually in middle and late adulthood (Pierce & Gilpin, 1996).

***Illicit Drugs.*** Nationwide, illicit drug use poses a significant health problem for adolescents. According to one study (Chen & Kandel, 1995), both incidence and prevalence rates for illegal substance use peak during adolescence and early adulthood, whereby adolescents 14 to 19 years old are the most likely to use illicit substances. Most of them only experiment with harder illegal substances and abstain from regular use in adulthood, but a small percentage of adolescents become addicted to illicit drugs, thus threatening their health and psychosocial functioning.

Reported annual and 30-day prevalence rates for illicit drug use have fallen since peaking in 1979. For example, the reported 30-day prevalence rates for illicit drug use among high school seniors declined significantly, from 39% in 1979 to 22% in 1994 (Johnston et al., 1995). However, the reported use of illicit drugs has started to show a slight increase again. The annual prevalence rates for illicit drug use among high school seniors are highest for White adolescents (31%) and Hispanic adolescents (29%), whereas the lowest rates were reported by Black teenagers (17%).

Marijuana is still the most commonly used illicit drug. In the United States, the lifetime prevalence rate for marijuana use is 15% for eighth-grade adolescents and between 30% to 35% for tenth-grade high school students. Forty-seven percent of all adolescents in the twelfth grade report having used marijuana at least once (Oetting & Beauvais, 1990).

The prevalence rates for regular marijuana use show a peak in late adolescence and early adulthood, steadily declining after the age of 25 (Chen & Kandel, 1995).

The lifetime prevalence rates for harder drug use vary between 1.7% and 5% among adolescents attending eighth grade, increases to between 2% and 9% for tenth graders, and peak in twelfth grade. Eleven percent to 12% of high school seniors report having used cocaine, and between 9% and 12% have experimented with hallucinogens. The lifetime prevalence rate for crack use amounts to 5% in twelfth grade. According to the American Drug and Alcohol Survey conducted in the late 1980s, the lifetime prevalence rates for heroin use were the highest for adolescents in the seventh to ninth grades (3%–4%), whereas only 2% of the seniors stated that they tried heroin at least once in their lives.

The most frequently used substances are essentially the same for minorities as for White American youth. There are some differences, but the most notable point is probably that the use of most of these drugs is lower in Black American and Asian adolescents and slightly lower for Mexican American youth, corresponding with the findings on alcohol and tobacco use mentioned earlier. In a comparison study by Chavez and Swaim (1992), Mexican American eighth graders reported significantly higher lifetime prevalence rates for using marijuana, cocaine or crack, heroin, and steroids than White eighth graders, who reported higher rates for alcohol and tobacco use. In contrast, White twelfth graders reported significantly higher lifetime prevalence rates for the use of a wide range of substances. This suggests that Hispanic adolescents begin to experiment with drugs at an earlier age. However, the overall incidence and frequency during adolescence is higher in Whites. On the other hand, the prevalence rates for drug use among many Native American adolescents surpass those of other ethnic groups, especially for those living on reservations (Oetting & Beauvais, 1990).

***Abuse of Inhalants and Medically Prescribed Substances.*** When the topic of substance abuse among adolescents is discussed, drugs such as opiates, LSD, crack, and amphetamines tend to become focal points. One group of substances that receives only marginal attention is known as *inhalants* (i.e., volatile substances capable of being inhaled in order to achieve an intoxicated state). In the adolescent population, abuse of inhalants steadily increased during the past decades.

In the United States, the abuse of inhalants is approximately as popular and as widespread as the consumption of the drugs just mentioned (Johnston, O'Malley, & Bachman, 1987; Oetting & Beauvais, 1990), although this fact is generally ignored by the public. This trend is evident in Germany, too, although the prevalence rates are somewhat lower with lifetime prevalence rates of 2% to 4%. About 25% of drug-use-experienced adolescents, between 14 and 25 years old, report having used inhalants once or more (Bundesminister für Gesundheit, 1991).

Lifetime prevalence data from the High School Senior Survey (Johnston et al., 1987) indicate that inhalant use among high school seniors increased between 1976 (10%) and 1986 (16%); based on the researchers' corrections for suspected underreporting, the figures came close to 20% in 1986. The 1988 National Household Survey on Drug Abuse reported that 9% of the 12- to 17-year-olds stated that they abused inhalants at least once in their life. For those in the 18- to 25-year-old age group, the lifetime use rate was 13% in 1988. According to the cross-sectional data obtained in the 1988–1989 American Drug and Alcohol Survey (Oetting & Beauvais, 1990), 17% of students in Grades 7 to 12 ($N = 103{,}073$) abused inhalants; the highest percentage of lifetime prevalence was found among eighth graders (19%) and the lowest rates among students in grades 7 and 12 (15%). This suggests that initiation to inhalant abuse is occurring at younger ages than before and that inhalant abuse is still on the rise.

There are about 700 different substances capable of being inhaled in order to achieve an intoxicating effect (Whitaker, 1987). They can be classified into three broad categories: solvents (e.g., common household items like glue, shoe polish, paint, and paint thinner), aerosols (e.g., hair spray, adhesives), and nitrates (e.g., preservation substances). According to the 1988 National Household Survey, the inhalant of choice among 12- to 17-year-olds is gasoline (used by 42% of those reporting lifetime use), with glue coming second (32%); the 18- to 25-year-olds prefer substances categorized as amylnitrates and commonly used by medical professionals to dilate blood vessels (about 41%; Gorny, 1994).

The use of legally prescribed medication also has a high lifetime prevalence rate among adolescents. In several national health and drug use surveys, 5% to 6% of all eighth graders, 12% to 13% of tenth graders and 18% to 20% of adolescents in twelfth grade reported using stimulants, a rate which is comparable to the use of inhalants for intoxicating purposes. Tranquilizers are used about half as often by adolescents. Ethnic distributions of prevalence rates correspond to those found for other substances (Oetting & Beauvais, 1990).

### Developmental Patterns of Drug Involvement

Epidemiological research has identified developmental stages in involvement with drugs. The use of noncontrolled substances, such as tobacco and alcohol, tends to precede and increase the use of illicit drugs. Adolescents are very unlikely to experiment with marijuana if they did not previously experiment with alcoholic beverages or cigarettes; very few try illicit drugs without first experimenting with marijuana (Donovan & Jessor, 1983; Kandel & Faust, 1975).

Crack, which suddenly appeared in urban centers in the 1980s, was considered to represent a completely new pathway of entry into drug use, but this hypothesis remains to be confirmed (Fagan & Chin, 1991). Kandel and Yamaguchi (1993) postulated a model of subsequent stages of drug initiation. In their sample, marijuana was first tried at an average age of 14.6 years old (*SD* = 2.0), 2.5 years later than cigarettes (mean age was 12.9 years old, *SD* = 2.4) or alcoholic beverages (mean age was 12.5 years old, *SD* = 2.6). Cocaine (mean age was 15.9 years old, *SD* = 1.6) and crack (mean age was 15.8 years old, *SD* = 2.0) were used for the first time slightly more than 1 year later than first-time marijuana use. Adolescents who used both alcohol and cigarettes were most likely to try marijuana, but only a small proportion of adolescents who used all three substances before were likely to experiment with cocaine and crack. The age for first-time drug use was an important factor for the progression of later drug use: On the average, adolescents who progressed to using cocaine, and especially crack, began smoking cigarettes, drinking alcohol, or smoking marijuana 2 years before those who did not go on to use cocaine.

In Bailey's study (1992), adolescents who increased their levels of alcohol or cigarette consumption after some period of light or infrequent use were more likely to begin using other substances than those participants who began using alcohol or cigarettes very frequently or heavily. This indicates that a gradual increase in substance abuse bears a higher risk of progression in regular and heavy multiple drug use than an intense consumption of alcohol or cigarettes at the time of initiation.

In spite of these findings, however, we must keep in mind that the use of alcohol, cigarettes, or even marijuana, does not necessarily predict the use of harder drugs, as the differences in prevalence rates already show. It is now widely accepted that multiple risk factor models are required in order to understand adolescent drug use (Vega, Zimmerman, Warheit, Apospori, & Gil, 1993). Bry, McKeon, and Pandima (1982) stated that drug use is best understood as a general coping mechanism. Furthermore, multiple risk factors play a role in promoting adolescent drug use. Vega et al. (1993) suggested that a cumulation of risk factors, such as peer approval and friends' use of drugs, low family cohesion, delinquency, and willingness to engage in nonnormative behavior, as well as substance abuse by other family members, are associated with an increased likelihood to use alcohol and illicit drugs during adolescence.

In summary, adolescents' illness has changed dramatically in most Western industrialized nations during this century. In the United States and Europe, in particular Germany, acute and chronic disorders are no longer leading causes of death in this age group. Infectious diseases, which claimed the lives of thousands of adolescents during the early 20th century, have been largely eliminated through improvements in infectious disease control, sanitation, housing, and medical care. Mortality rates fell from 870 per 100,000 children, 1 to 14 years old, in 1900 to 33 per 100,000 in 1987 (Adams & Hardy, 1989).

Nevertheless, although adolescent health has progressively improved, closer inspection of data on the leading causes of death in adolescence in North America and Europe is disquieting. In contrast to adult mortality, adolescent mortality is primarily associated with preventable social, environmental, and behavioral factors. Behavioral factors rank high among causes of morbidity in adolescence, with accidents, substance use, and sexual risk-taking behaviors being leading causes. It is important to note, however, that some aspects of adolescent mortality and morbidity seen in the United States are not typical of other developed countries (Petersen, 1993). The rates of adolescent homicides and pregnancies in the United States far exceed the rates for Europe. Nevertheless, increasing violence has a strong impact on the mortality rates for adolescents in Europe.

As Sells and Blum (1996) noted, the only individuals in the United States that have not experienced improvement in their health status over the last 30 years are adolescents. In particular, they pointed out that violence has emerged as the primary cause of death among young persons, with accidents, homicides, and suicides accounting for two thirds of adolescents' deaths in the United States. Of the three possible causes of death, suicide is perhaps the most disturbing because it involves some voluntary elements. It raises the question of why young people, who are just beginning to experience life, choose to end it. The answer to this question may emerge in the next chapter, in which I discuss the challenges and frequently experienced stressors with which adolescents are confronted and often unable to cope.

# 4

# Dealing With the Body

Adolescents are intensely preoccupied with the processes of physical maturation and with physical attractiveness. From the perspective of health psychology, changes in body self-image and the timing of physical maturation are highly relevant because they are accompanied by various somatic complaints or behaviors that are potentially hazardous to one's health.

This chapter addresses aspects of timing in physical maturation and body concept and their bearing on the adolescent's psychosexual development. Research findings are presented on how changes in body image, occurring in adolescence, affect relationships with others, especially with respect to physical contact and nudity. The relation between physical maturation and sexual development, as manifested, for example, in first experiences with coitus, is also examined, and adolescents' contraceptive practices are analyzed.

## PHYSICAL CHANGES IN ADOLESCENCE: PUBERTAL STATUS AND TIMING

Physical maturation heralds the beginnings of sexual maturation and the transition to the reproductive life phase. Puberty is indeed unique in that it involves biological and social changes. Some cultures attribute much importance to puberty and openly celebrate it with traditional rites and ceremonies. In Western societies the transition remains a private experience. Nevertheless, even in Western societies, the consequences of this transition become inevitably apparent: Puberty introduces a new definition of roles, and bodily changes affect the adolescent's social relations and life planning.

Many psychoanalytically oriented authors stressed the importance of the body for the development of cognitive abilities, in particular for perception and reality testing (Blos, 1973; A. Freud, 1958). Similarly, psychologists generally uphold the view that physical changes stimulate developments in cognitive, emotional, and social areas; conversely, these developments in turn influence physical development (Stattin & Magnusson, 1990). From a health psychology perspective, the topics of pubertal status and the normal timing of development are particularly important, because they are associated with certain risk behaviors.

### Pubertal Status and Timing

*Pubertal status* usually refers to the level of physical development attained during adolescence. The kinds of physical changes that were studied vary considerably. Because pubertal maturation was found to be highly related to ossification, x-rays of the wrist have sometimes been employed to determine an adolescent's level of maturation. Maturational level is also assessed according to changes in secondary sex characteristics (e.g., pubic hair growth, breast development, or change in pitch of voice). As a rule, the criteria set forth by Tanner (1972) are used to assess pubertal status. Whereas most investigators have reported the mean age for menarche to be 12.5 years (for summaries, see Brooks-Gunn, 1988; Paikoff & Brooks-Gunn, 1991), the mean age for semenarche (the first ejaculation) has yet to be firmly established. To date, only a few researchers have dealt with this topic, and most of these studies were based on small samples (e.g., Gaddis & Brooks-Gunn, 1985; Stein & Reiser, 1994). In general, semenarche appears to occur later (mean age 12.9 years), however, variability is the rule rather than the exception for all pubertal processes. In girls, the time lapse between the first signs of puberty and complete maturity varies from 1.6 years to 6 years. Corresponding variations in rate and order of changes have been observed in boys (Nottelmann et al., 1987).

Pubertal timing may be conceived as a measure of individual development in relation to expected pubertal maturation at a given age or to some reference group. Pubertal timing is usually calculated according to age- or school-related criteria. Because social comparison is so common in adolescence, pubertal timing is generally regarded as a more crucial aspect of pubertal development than pubertal status (Simmons, Blyth, & McKinney, 1983). According to the concept of the *social clock*, defined by Neugarten (1979), adolescents may be "in time" or "off time." More recently, this concept was revived by Galambos and Tilton-Weaver (1996), who studied how adolescents perceive their own and others' developmental timing. The adolescent's perception of timeliness in pubertal development is typically influenced by others' reactions, especially by other adolescents in the peer and social reference group and by the prevailing sociocultural norms about pubertal status. Thus, whereas one female adolescent may perceive herself as being off time, with a menarche after 14 years, another, who is a ballet dancer, may perceive herself as being in time because a considerable number of ballet dancers have a delayed menarche (Brooks-Gunn & Warren, 1985).

Marked gender-specific differences in the perception of pubertal timing have been documented. Early maturing boys have an advantage relative to late maturers in many aspects of social-emotional functioning. Early maturation does not seem to be socially advantageous for girls (Paikoff & Brooks-Gunn, 1991). A considerable amount of the research conducted by Anglo-American investigators has been concerned with issues of early maturation, especially in girls (Brooks-Gunn & Warren, 1985; Petersen & Crockett, 1985). Based on the findings obtained in these studies, it is possible to conclude that early maturing girls (menarche before 11.6 years old) perceive menstruation more negatively than those menstruating for the first time between 11.6 and 14 years old or late maturers (menarche after 14 years old). For early maturing females, the feeling of being off time is associated with a negative perception of one's own development and attempts to conceal breast growth. In contrast, boys who mature early experience greater social acceptance and are behaviorally more stable (Brooks-Gunn, 1987). Petersen and Crockett (1986) have reported that early maturing female adolescents exhibit more deviant behavior, have more conflicts with family members, and have more problems in school. In a study of German adolescents, Schulz (1991) examined how female adolescents perceived the timing of their physical development. The mean age of menarche was 12.6 years in the sample, which suggests that most girls were in time. However, subjective evaluations of this event differed. Thirty percent of the adolescents reported that they felt that menarche had occurred too early, and 30% thought it had occurred normally. Forty percent of the girls thought it had occurred too late, which reflects the great normative pressure on girls to achieve physical maturity.

Different psychosocial models and hypotheses have been developed to explain physical development in relation to social and cultural contexts. In this regard, it was established that subjectively perceived timing is more important than the norms established for certain age groups (Rierdan & Koff, 1985). In addition, it was reported that the perceptions of physical changes in adolescents influence adults' reactions, and these reactions are possibly more important than the actual changes themselves (Petersen & Taylor, 1980). Furthermore, because role definitions in adolescence are often quite undefined, others' expectations of adolescents vary greatly. In addition, there may be differences related to context and culture. For example, based on his interviews with young girls in 23 different countries, Logan (1980) found striking cultural differences in female adolescents' reactions to menarche.

Three important hypotheses were worked out by developmental psychologists studying the timing of physical maturation in adolescence. The *stage-termination hypothesis* proposes that each development requires sufficient time to unfold and that premature physical development impairs or curtails developments in other areas. Differences between early and late maturers are a function of the amount of time available for psychosocial development prior to the onset of puberty. This perspective posits that early maturation interrupts the acquisition and consolidation of adaptive skills. According to this hypothesis, girls and early maturers, in general, are at greater risk for adjustment problems. Unfortunately, little empirical work has been done to test this hypothesis (for details, see Petersen & Crockett, 1985). The *deviance hypothesis* assumes that early versus late maturers differ in adjustment because of their status relative to the rest of the peer group. Early or late maturation places the adolescent in a socially deviant category. Research has provided a mixed pattern of support for the deviance hypothesis. Finally, the *goodness-of-fit* hypothesis proposes that an optimal adjustment between the adolescent and his or her sociocultural environment must be achieved. A girl who matures normally may nevertheless experience difficulties if the sociocultural context places great emphasis on childlike bodies, as was shown in a study of young female ballet dancers (Brooks-Gunn & Warren, 1985).

### Pubertal Timing and Psychological Maladjustment

There is a general consensus that physical maturation and timing affect the adolescent's general adjustment and that such effects are different for boys and girls. Recent Anglo-American studies have been oriented to identifying problem behaviors or psychopathology related to aspects of physical maturation. As pointed earlier, these studies show that the effects of early physical maturation are negative in girls and positive in boys. Early maturing boys are more relaxed, more self-assured, better adjusted, and less dependent than early maturing girls (Petersen & Taylor, 1980). Early maturing girls may engage in adult behaviors (e.g., smoking, drinking, and sexual intercourse) at a younger age than late maturing girls (Brooks-Gunn, 1988). Interestingly, early maturing boys and late maturing girls correspond in essential behavior patterns and in the positive effects on overall development.

Another focal point of research is to establish how physical maturation, especially with respect to its timing, may potentiate psychological problems that typically occur in adolescence. A great body of literature exists pertaining to the association between early physical maturation and the incidence of depression (Rierdan, Koff, & Stubbs, 1987; Rutter, 1986), negative self-concept and emotional problems in female adolescents (Susman et al., 1985), and externalizing behavior patterns (e.g., aggression and delinquency) in male adolescents (Olweus, Mattson, Schalling, & Low, 1988). Also, higher values for depression, a greater number of psychosomatic symptoms, and a more intense preoccupation with dieting in early maturing girls have been reported (for a summary, see Stein & Reichert, 1990). Other studies analyzing the effects of physical maturation on nonconforming behaviors have found that such effects have a greater bearing on the incidence of delinquent behavior (e.g., theft, alcohol, and drug abuse) in girls than in boys. However, in their longitudinal study, Magnusson, Stattin, and Allen (1986) noted that the effect of early maturation in girls on increased abuse of alcohol or drugs was temporary. In addition, it should be noted that the results of the Early Adolescence study (Petersen & Crockett, 1985) suggest that the belief in pubertal development as a primary influence on adjustment must be modified. Whereas effects of pubertal timing emerged for three aspects of adjustment (i.e., school achievement, impulse control, and psychopathology), effects of grade level were found for most aspects of adjustment (e.g., school achievement, psychopathology, peer relations, family relations, and body image) except impulse control. That is, grade in school influences more aspects of adjustment than does pubertal timing.

In summary, interactions between pubertal changes, their timing, and gender have been demonstrated repeatedly. In particular, the negative effects of early maturation in girls are striking. One must remember, however, that many aspects shown to be centrally important in female adolescents (e.g., body weight, physical attractiveness, timing, etc.) have not been studied as extensively in male adolescents. In addition, the male experience of the first ejaculation has received little attention (Stein & Reiser, 1994). Thus, it is inappropriate to draw conclusions for male adolescents, who were generally studied less frequently and in smaller numbers. Furthermore, most studies on physical maturation were conducted on young girls growing up in Anglo-American cultures. Methodological problems must also be considered, because the variables age, pubertal development, and timing of development are closely interrelated and make interpretation of results difficult.

## DEVELOPMENT OF BODY IMAGE

### The Concept of Body Image

*Body image* refers to a person's subjective concept of his or her body, including its physical appearance, internal organs, functions, and capabilities (Schonfield, 1969). The mental representation, which may be realistic or unrealistic, is constructed from self-observation, the reactions of others, and a complex interaction of attitudes, emotions, memories, fantasies, and experiences—both conscious and unconscious. Body image is understood as being a part of a hierarchically organized concept of self, because the body is a fundamental element of identity. Although gender differences in the level of esteem for one's own body exist from childhood on (Vaugham, Stabler, & Clance, 1981), these become more marked during early adolescence. The importance that bodily changes during puberty have for the overall perception of the self was already demonstrated in the early Schonfield study. However, little systematic, empirical work has been done on this topic since then. This is surprising, considering that physical changes occurring in this developmental period are related to fundamental changes in social roles; that is, social roles covary with body image.

Mrazek (1987b) conducted one of the few studies on the structure and development of body image in adolescence. He investigated 1,026 German adolescents between 12 and 16 years old, using a scale for assessing one's own body. Factor analysis revealed the following eight dimensions:

1. Fitness and sports (e.g., "I exercise my body regularly").
2. Maintaining personal appearance and hygiene (e.g., "I use a deodorant regularly").
3. Weight and figure problems (e.g., "I count calories").
4. Narcissism (e.g., "I think I have a nice body").
5. Alienation from the body and health problems (e.g., "My body sometimes does what it wants").
6. Cigarette smoking and consumption of alcoholic beverages (e.g., "I often smoke a cigarette").
7. Avoidance of body contact (e.g., "I don't like it when my parents or relatives embrace me").
8. Snacking (e.g., "I like to eat sweets").

It should be pointed out that the dimensions 5 and 7 were not been found in similar studies conducted on adults (Brähler, 1988). An important finding in the Mrazek study was that the structure of body image did not change much, despite the increasing preoccupation with personal appearance between 12 and 16 years old. In contrast, many clear gender-specific changes were found, above all, in the domains of appearance, figure, and fitness. Compared to boys, girls between the 12 and 16 years old paid more attention to their physical appearance. However, they had more problems with their figures, did less for their physical fitness, and considered themselves to be physically weaker. Girls felt more alienated in their bodies and assessed their bodies less positively. An analysis of sociodemographic variables showed that adolescents from higher social classes had fewer problems with their weight and physique, felt less alienated in their bodies, and paid less attention to their physical appearance.

Similarly, in the study carried out by Koff, Rierdan, and Stubbs (1990) on 169 American high school students in the ninth grade, males were more positive about their bodies than were females. Moreover, females had more differentiated body images than males. In an earlier study analyzing the representation of the female body by early and late adolescent girls, Rierdan and Koff (1980) found that girls in the sixth grade included more explicit illustrations of breasts in their drawings of body image than girls in the eighth grade. This result suggests that early adolescent females are more preoccupied with those parts of the body whose changes signal the beginning of puberty, whereas late adolescent females have more integrated body images. With respect to females' representations of their inner genital space, the study conducted by Amann-Gainotti, Di Prospero, and Nenci (1989) demonstrated a very slow integration of inner genital space in the body image. The authors analyzed the drawings made by 275 females aged 11 to 18 years, who were requested to illustrate how they viewed their bodies and sexual organs. Only the 17- and 18-year-olds consistently integrated their internal sexual organs into their drawings.

### Satisfaction With the Body and Physical Attractiveness

Most studies on physical attractiveness have been conducted in the United States (see the summary by Lerner & Karabenick, 1974). As previously documented, females are taught early in life to comply with society's standards of beauty. In their review of the literature, Feldman, Feldman, and Goodman (1988) noted that by the age of 6, girls seem to have internalized cultural perceptions of attractiveness and understand its relation to popularity. Research findings obtained in these studies indicate that physical attractiveness is significantly related to self-concept of females, but not males (Lerner & Karabenick, 1974). In an extensive interview study of 1,917 adolescents between 12 and 16 years old, Simmons and Rosenberg (1975) found that, compared with boys, girls were more dissatisfied with their sexual roles and the changes in their physical appearance and placed greater value on recognition by peers of the same and opposite gender. Compared with girls, boys were more concerned with formulating their future plans with respect to education and profession; also, they were more optimistic about their futures. In contrast, girls placed greater emphasis on improving the qualities of their interpersonal relationships, acquiring social skills, and maintaining or improving their physical appearance. In addition, girls often appeared extremely concerned with the impressions of others (i.e., they evaluated themselves and their bodies through the eyes of others). This suggests that perceived attractiveness has a greater bearing on female self-concept than other factors, such as academic or job success. Moreover, there are different, gender-specific expectations with respect to physical attractiveness. Beauty and physical attractiveness are not only more important for women than for men, but women have fewer possibilities of compensating for a lack of beauty (Freedman, 1989; Rosenbaum, 1979). Thus, it is not surprising that twice as many girls as boys in high school change their appearance (Musa & Roach, 1973) and that fewer girls are satisfied with their appearance than boys (45% compared to 75%; see Dacey, 1982). Girls think they are less attractive than their female peers, whereas boys think they are more attractive than their male peers (Freedman, 1989). Females also tend to overestimate their body width and underestimate body length. In a longitudinal study, Rauste-Von Wright (1988) investigated satisfaction with one's own body in male and female adolescents who were 11, 13, 15, and 18 years old. Satisfaction with one's own body varied not only with gender—male adolescents were more satisfied with their own bodies at all ages—but also according to age and maturational status. The 18-year-old boys and girls were the most satisfied with their bodies, whereby the late maturers were less satisfied than the early maturers. It may be reasonable to assume that a weight gain associated with physical maturation in adolescence contributed to the different levels of satisfaction with the body in males and females.

As the findings from the studies cited suggest, physical maturation and body image are closely linked. Tobin-Richards, Boxer, and Petersen (1983) and Petersen and Crockett (1985) reported, for example, that early maturing boys have a more positive body image and a more strongly pronounced feeling of attractiveness than late maturing boys. According to these authors, not only the state of having matured early, but also the advantages that are associated with becoming adult make early maturation so positive for boys. Furthermore, these authors observed that facial hair growth in puberty showed the most positive effect on the subjective concept of self in males. Not only is facial hair an overt characteristic of physical maturation, but it is also a symbol of adult status. For female adolescents, the highest values for satisfaction with the body were observed in the middle stages of puberty, especially among the girls who perceived their pubertal development to be in time (Tobin-Richards et al., 1983).

Gender-specific differences in expectations of physical attractiveness were documented for decades. Male adolescents still place great value on pleasant appearance and good figure in their choice of female partners, whereas girls deem intelligence to be the most important quality of their male partners (Freedman, 1989). In the literature, there is a pervasive, uniform view that the female body is used to impress and attract others, whereas the male body is a high-performance instrument capable of influencing the environment (Koff et al., 1990). There is some support for the power of the cultural ideal of thinness in adolescent girls (Blyth, Simmons, & Zakin, 1985). The intense desire in younger girls to be attractive, coupled with their insecurity about their own attractiveness, can create a situation in which their self-esteem becomes largely dependent on their subjective perceptions of physical attractiveness. This may have a pathological outcome, so that in their attempts to achieve culturally defined ideals of physical attractiveness, girls become obsessively preoccupied with the physical appearance of their bodies. An example of this phenomenon is particularly evident in many Western industrialized cultures, in which great emphasis is placed on female thinness. Adolescent females in these societies show an increased rate of eating disorders (e.g., anorexia nervosa and bulimia, see chaps. 2 and 3, this volume).

### Negative Body Image, Physical Maturity, and Dieting Behaviors

Research in the past decades has pointed to a high prevalence of dissatisfaction with the body and dieting behaviors in adolescent females. These findings are a cause of concern because they also are associated with eating disorders in female adolescents. In reviewing the literature, however, it becomes clear that not all studies find similar proportions of subjects reporting body dissatisfaction. Eisele,

Hertsgaard, and Light (1986) found that 78% of 12- to 14-year-old girls wished they weighed less. A similar level (83%) of dissatisfaction with body weight was found by Storz and Greene (1983) in 14- to 18-year-old girls, whereas Desmond, Price, Gray, and O'Connell (1986) reported that 43% of females and 9% of males with normal weights described themselves as heavy. Thus, for the most part, negative body image is seen in young girls, which, as mentioned earlier, is partly related to the timing of their physical maturation. Early maturers have a poorer body image than on-time or late maturers (Brooks-Gunn, 1988). However, negative attitudes about the body and a depressive self-concept have been found to exist in the majority of young girls independently of the timing of physical maturation.

With this connection, reference should be made to the observations documented by several authors of reduced self-esteem (Rierdan et al., 1987) and depressive symptomatology (Noles, Cash, & Winstead, 1985) in adolescent females who placed great emphasis on external physical characteristics and the opinions of others. The correlations between depression and negative body image were found to be evident in early puberty and remained stable throughout adolescence. Depressed girls were not only more dissatisfied with their own bodies and saw themselves as less attractive, but also thought their bodies were deficient in many respects. They described their bodies as less attractive, less competent, and less a familiar part of the self than did nondepressed girls (Noles et al., 1985). Girls not only have a more negative body image than boys, but they are also more dissatisfied with their body weight (Paxton et al., 1991; Richards, Boxer, Petersen, & Albrecht, 1990). Adolescent girls studied by Cohn et al. (1987) wanted to be thinner—even thinner than what they thought men would find attractive. Davies and Furman (1986b) found that 46% of the 12-year-old girls in their study wished to lose weight; about 11% of the girls said that they were currently dieting. By the end of high school, 60% of the girls studied by Freedman (1984) had already been on a "serious" diet, and about 30% were sporadically dieting. Stein and Reichert (1990) confirmed that extreme dieting in females typically begins in the fifth and sixth grades.

Thus, body dissatisfaction increases in girls after puberty. In particular, dissatisfaction with weight in adolescent girls increases with age and is greater postmenarchally than premenarchally. Such dissatisfaction is certainly related to the disproportional weight gain with respect to body height in girls during puberty, as typically manifested by increased body fat around the waist and thighs (Davies & Furman, 1986b). Interestingly, the desire to reduce weight in girls is pervasive and unrelated to actual body weight (Davies & Furman, 1986a). Furthermore, a strong positive relation between girls' subjective perceptions of being underweight and satisfaction with their own bodies has been demonstrated in several studies. In addition, the relation between body weight and overall satisfaction in adolescents differs according to gender. In their study of adolescents, for example, Paxton et al. (1991) reported that two thirds of girls thought that being thinner would make them happier. Whereas girls associated weight loss with positive changes in their lives, boys considered weight loss in solely negative terms. In addition, girls considered thinness and fitness to be related to physical conditions, whereas boys believed they could exist independently of one another. Additional evidence showing that adolescent girls are intensely preoccupied with their bodies and physical attractiveness was obtained in an analysis of diaries kept by 15-year-old girls (Seiffge-Krenke, 1993b). Twenty-eight percent of the diary entries focused on such topics as fashion, body weight, and physical appearance. The close relationship between interest in clothes, body satisfaction, and eating behavior was also confirmed in a study of adolescent females conducted by Littrell, Damhorst, and Littrell (1990).

Body image also varies according to health status. In a longitudinal study of chronically ill and healthy adolescents (see chap. 7, this volume), it was found that a negative body image was uniformly present in both male and female adolescents suffering from chronic illness. These adolescents described their bodies as being less interesting, less developed, and more rigid in comparison to their healthy peers. Indications of a negative body image is also present in the individual assessments of the level of physical maturation. For example, the assessments of menarche and semenarche, made by chronically ill adolescents were much more negative than those of healthy adolescents (Seiffge-Krenke, Schmidt, Kollmar, Floss, & Roth, 1996). Whereas 23% of healthy girls thought positively of their own menarche, only 13% of chronically ill female adolescents had positive attitudes. The differences in attitudes about physical maturation were also striking among boys: 62% of healthy boys viewed their semenarche positively compared to 41% of chronically ill boys. This finding is further evidence that chronically ill adolescents generally view their bodies more negatively, whereby compared to males, females evaluate their physical maturity much more negatively.

In another study of healthy 15-year-old girls, similar negative perceptions of physical maturation processes were found (Schulz, 1991). From a medical standpoint, the age of 15 years is considered to be the time when physical development is more or less completed in girls, with

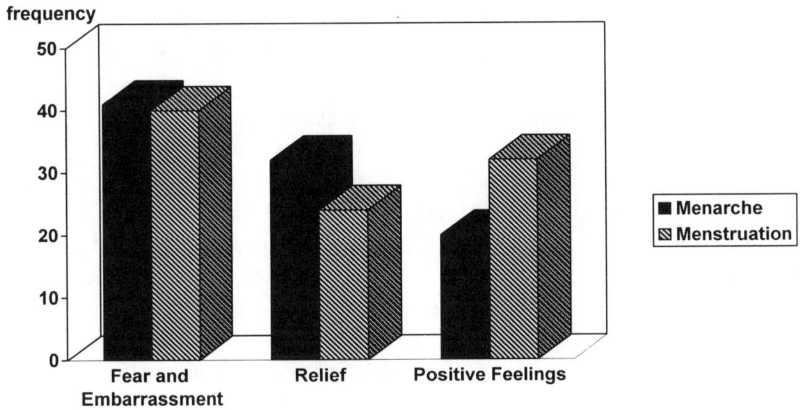


FIG. 4.1. Female adolescents' evaluations of menarche and menstruation ($N$ = 150).

the exception of breast growth, which may continue up until 18 years old. In this German study, over 40% of the girls interviewed were indifferent about or displeased with their breast growth. Even higher percentages have been documented for Anglo-American samples (see Brooks-Gunn & Ruble, 1983). In the Schulz study (1991), only 29% of the interviewed girls, most of whom were late maturers, felt relieved about their breast growth. Also, the correlation between the reaction to menarche and breast development was found to be highly significant ($r$ = .43). Both studies showed that reactions to menarche were ambivalent or negative. Sixty-five percent of female adolescents interviewed in the Brooks-Gunn and Ruble (1983) study made ambivalent or negative statements about menarche. Only 17% of the girls made clearly positive statements, and only 18% made clearly negative statements. In the Schulz interview study (1991), one third of the girls expressed their relief that their first period had taken place (i.e., they were glad to know they were healthy and normal); in contrast, 47% were afraid or embarrassed. Figure 4.1 demonstrates that girls are not only ambivalent towards menarche, but also toward menstruation in general.

These overall negative or ambivalent attitudes might be related to the possibility that the girls are not adequately informed about menstruation. However, 80% of the girls in the Schulz study (1991) claimed that they knew about menstruation before it occurred. Nevertheless, their initial reactions to menarche reflected just how surprised and irritated they actually were. Similarly, Brooks-Gunn (1988) reported that approximately 10% to 15% of White girls in the United States were not prepared for menarche.

## PUBERTAL DEVELOPMENT AND CHANGES IN PHYSICAL CONTACT WITH OTHERS

As discussed in chapter 2, adolescents may find both conversations with health care providers and physical examinations highly disruptive insofar as their individual privacy is violated. It is therefore surprising that so few empirical studies have been conducted on this particularly sensitive matter (Bulcroft, 1991). The basic changes in the relationships with parents and friends—that is, the increasing autonomy from the parents and the orientation toward peers as trusted conversational partners for discussing intimate, personal topics—occur in parallel with and are closely dependent on physical changes. Thus, the reservations adolescents have about being examined by or talking about their bodies with health care providers or other adult individuals may be seen as being related to the normal developmental process of adolescent separation and distancing from parents or authority figures, a process initiated by the adolescents themselves.

### Physical Maturation and Relationships With Parents

As pointed out in the previous section, studies on physical maturation in adolescence in the United States and Germany produced similar findings. The findings of negative assessments of maturational processes in young girls and the different, gender-specific effects of early maturation certainly are important ones for health psychologists. Additional effects of physical maturation in adolescence, which also may be relevant for health psychology, are the changes in the relationships to parents, as seen, for example, in decreasing openness and reduction of physical contact.

Does menarche effect the adolescent girl's relationships with her parents? In the Schulz study (1991), 63% of female adolescents reported that their relationships with their parents did not change after the onset of menarche, 3% reported that their relationships with their mothers deteriorated, and 30% noted an improvement in their relationships with their mothers. None of the girls thought that their relationships with their fathers improved; however, 27% reported that their relationships with their fathers deteriorated. In this regard, it is interesting to note that parents are not necessarily the sources from which girls learn about menstruation. In the Schulz study, most of the adolescents (43%) learned about menstruation in school, 27% from their parents, and 30% from other adults (e.g., physicians, other relatives). In addition, girls invariably approached their mothers first to disclose the news of their first menarche and seek advice. In a review of studies of American adolescents, Brooks-Gunn (1988) reported that although mothers are most likely to be a girl's primary source of information about puberty and menarche, they are less likely to discuss these topics with their early-maturing daughters. Early maturers seldom report that their fathers know about their menarche and are less likely to directly tell their fathers about it. In one of the rare studies of semenarche, Stein and Reiser (1994) found that boys' most common responses to semenarche included surprise, curiosity, pleasure and confusion; some boys were also scared. Most boys did not tell anyone about the event, and some initially confused ejaculation with urination. When a boy did tell someone, it was usually a friend.

Most parents appear to have difficulties in dealing with physical maturation, and they may be unable to talk about it openly with their children. Adolescents may also be quite unwilling to talk about their bodies and the physical changes taking place in them. Indeed, their increased sensitivity about their bodies also manifests itself in other aspects of interpersonal interaction (e.g., activities involving physical closeness and contact with other family members). This aspect is explored in the following section.

### Changes in Physical Contact With Family Members

The nature of physical contact between parents and children changes dramatically during adolescence. In the Schulz interview study (1991), adolescents reported that as they grew older, physical contact with their parents not only decreased, but also became less desirable. This reduction in physical closeness can be interpreted as a sign that the adolescent is in the process of separation from the parental household. Nearly 47% of the girls interviewed in this study generally refused to engage in any physical contact with their fathers; 37% tolerated physical contact only with their mothers. On the average, a decline in physical contact between father and daughter began between 11 and 12 years old, indicating that female adolescents already began to reduce such contact before menarche. Female adolescents did not want to be cuddled anymore and withdrew from physical contact with both parents. Only 11% of the girls reported that their fathers withdrew from physical contact after becoming aware of their physical maturation. As adolescents became older, a new form of physical contact became apparent. Thus, spontaneous cuddling and hugging was replaced by more ritualized contact (e.g., embracing before and after longer periods of separation, on birthdays, and similar occasions). As demonstrated in

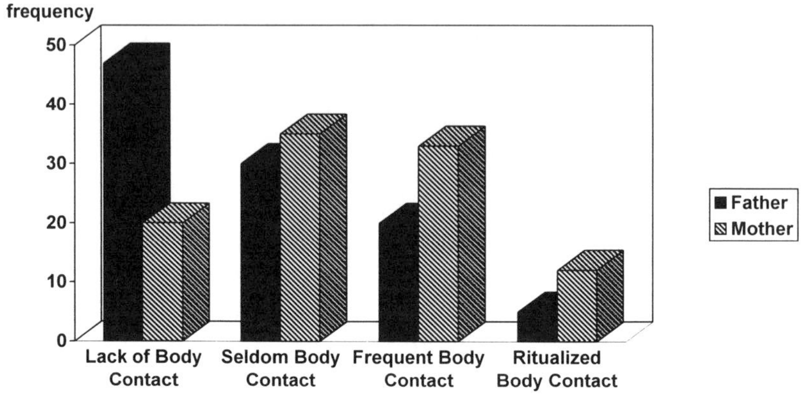


FIG. 4.2. Female adolescents differences in body contact with mothers and fathers ($N = 150$).

Fig. 4.2, this change is more obvious in body contact with fathers than with mothers.

With respect to nudity, 47% of the female adolescents avoided revealing their naked bodies to their parents or seeing their parents naked; 27% tolerated seeing their parents undressed or being viewed by the family members when naked, but were extremely embarrassed when confronted with nudity. Thus, adolescents are even more sensitive about nudity than about physical contact. According to Schulz (1991), the consequences of this changed attitude about nudity were especially obvious in the use of the family bathroom. Forty percent of the adolescents reported that they always locked the bathroom door, and 43% indirectly avoided being observed while naked by showering or bathing only when the parents were not at home. Only 17% of the adolescents were not bothered when their parents happened to enter the bathroom when they were in it.

As detailed in chapter 2, similar changes are observed in males. Salt (1991) reported a decrease (initiated by sons) in the amount and acceptance of affectionate touch between father and son. A change in nudity practice was also reported in the study carried out by Stein and Reiser (1994) of adolescent males who were interviewed about their first ejaculation.

In summary, adolescents are very protective about maintaining their privacy, either by direct or indirect methods, and parents pay more attention to maintaining personal spheres of intimacy, although to a lesser extent than do their children. This changed manner in dealing with one's own body and nudity certainly has consequences in situations involving physical examinations by health care providers, especially gynecologists. Studies of chronically ill adolescents (chap. 7, this volume) revealed that these adolescents were very sensitive about nudity and undressing in front of others. The adolescents were very ashamed by the bruises and scars caused by insulin injections. Thirty-five percent of the adolescents (especially girls) considered their deformed bodies to be a major problem and consciously avoided exposing their naked bodies in the presence of others.

### Pubertal Development and Peer Relations

Only a few studies examined the relation between physical maturation processes and friendships, although social comparison is very common in adolescence. Schulz (1991) found that girls typically refrained from informing their friends about their menarche until some time after its occurrence. Thereafter, they were eager to exchange their experiences with others. In addition, 67% of participating female adolescents reported that they were greatly interested in the status and developments of their female friends' physical maturation. They were also very concerned with physical appearance. Most girls engaged in conversations with their female friends about dieting, weight problems, and athletic activities, especially in connection with weight reduction. Thus, according to this study, the central topics of interest among girls and their female friends concerned weight loss and physical appearance. Moreover, social comparison among these girls involved an inordinate amount of competitiveness and envy.

Seventy percent of the interviewed girls followed a retaliatory dress code, that is, they placed great importance on dressing themselves in a manner most opposed to how their parents preferred. These girls were highly conscious of what their female peers wore and very critical of girls who looked as if "their mothers still dressed them."

Other examples of the importance of friends for the process of physical maturation are found in studies of adolescent diaries (Seiffge-Krenke, 1995). Diary entries made by female adolescents were frequently related to aspects of female identity, the shaping of which is closely tied to experiences and attitudes about the diarist's and her female friends' bodies. Diary entries describing the activities pursued together with other female friends involved experiences related to modeling and experimenting with the body and appearance (e.g., making up each other's faces, sharing clothes, or sharing bathroom facilities). Other entries were related to the first approaches to boys and men. The diarists' best female friends were often present in these situations to provide security. According to an analysis of the diarists' entries, clothing fashions, physical appearance, and changes in the figure and weight were public topics (i.e., they were discussed with other girls). Other topics remained secret, such as those related to eating behaviors, especially when they became pathological—for example, showing signs of anorexia nervosa or bulimia. Nearly 12% of the entries containing reports of pathological or deviant behavior were associated with unusual eating behaviors (e.g., "wolfing down a meal," "puking," "hoarding food," or "stuffing myself"). In another study of adolescent diaries (Soff, 1989), one 15-year-old girl's entries revealed how much she detested her body and how determined she was to control it. Her entries contained regular reports of induced vomiting and regular consumption of appetite suppressants, and she noted her bulimic episodes with the acronym SV ("stuffing and vomiting").

Research on boys' pubertal development has been quite inconclusive. Although we know from the Stein and Reiser (1994) study that the first sign of physical maturity, semenarche, is most frequently shared with friends (if shared at all), information about the meaning and significance of pubertal changes for friendships between males is lacking. One limited generalization that can be made from past research, however, is that early maturation in boys brings about positive changes in peer relations and status (Bulcroft, 1991). Furthermore, it was demonstrated that during puberty, there is a shift in parent–adolescent power relations. A male adolescent's position in the family power structure is enhanced by his development, and he assumes greater independence from his parents. It is hypothesized that the positive effects of pubertal development on boys' peer relationships are largely responsible for the transformation of family power relations (Susman et al., 1985).

In summary, research findings suggest that girls are much more preoccupied with aspects of physical maturation and attractiveness than are boys. Moreover, girls view the process of physical maturation much more negatively and possess a more negative body image. They have ambivalent or negative feelings about menarche and do not necessarily feel that menstruation is evidence of having achieved womanhood, whereas boys express positive feelings such as pleasure and curiosity. Girls are greatly interested in knowing how their peers have physically developed. Social comparison with other girls and a more negative evaluation of their own attractiveness are common. Findings in the adolescents' sources of information about physical maturation are mixed. Some adolescents seem to learn about reproductive processes from sources outside of the family, including peers, health care providers, or teachers. Girls are generally more open with their mothers, but physical contact with both parents drastically decreases in adolescence. Boys also show changes in physical contact with others. In addition, they became increasingly more reluctant to reveal their naked bodies to adults. A distanced, ritualized form of physical contact with family members replaces the spontaneous, close physical contact seen in childhood.

## DEVELOPMENT OF SEXUAL BEHAVIORS

The onset of sexual activity is a normal and important aspect of development, marking in part, the transition to adulthood. Although the average age of the onset of puberty declined in the 20th century (Weddle, McKenry, & Leigh, 1988), the general cultural expectation is that young yet sexually mature adolescents delay sexual activity. However, adolescents are becoming sexually active at earlier ages, and by the end of their adolescent years, more than 80% of all males and more than 70% of all females are sexually active (Scott-Jones & White, 1990). Although research on adolescent sexuality increased in recent years, most investigators focused their efforts on studying individual sexuality. Aspects of sexual relationships (e.g., the dynamics of dyadic interaction and attachment) have hardly been examined. Theoretical concepts tended to uphold the assumption of gender-specific differences in sexuality, and empirical studies consistently demonstrated such differences, which, from a historical perspective, have not changed greatly.

### Theoretical Concepts of Sexual Development in Adolescence

Psychology, psychoanalysis, and sociology ascribe different levels of importance to the study of adolescent sexuality. In addition, the aspects of adolescent sexuality, studied empirically in these domains, differ. Psychoanalytic approaches consider final sexual organization to be the most decisive developmental task, after which, further development in other areas can progress normally or result in "developmental breakdown" (Laufer & Laufer, 1984, p. 5). This task involves the incorporation of the physically mature genitals into the body image. Furthermore, the psychoanalytic theory proposes that the body, which was passive before puberty, becomes active in living out sexual and aggressive fantasies. Although sexual desires exist before puberty, in adolescence they become irreversibly integrated into the individual's sexual identity. When sexual organization in adolescence is complete, this identity cannot be modified. All sexual identifications become part of the "central masturbation fantasy" (Laufer & Laufer, 1984, p. 6). The physically mature genitals become important components of this fantasy. According to Laufer and Laufer, although the fantasy does not change in adolescents, the need to experience it in concrete relationships increases. Thus, physical maturation and sexuality are central aspects in this conceptualization of sexual development. Accordingly, deviant or psychopathological behaviors in adolescence are understood to result from inadequate sexual development. This viewpoint has its roots in earlier theoretical approaches that proposed the existence of a "deadline" (Bernfeld, 1923) or a "second chance" (Eissler, 1958) for resolving oedipal identifications. In his work "Three Contributions to the Sexual Theory," S. Freud (1905, 1952a) described *puberty* as a series of changes through which the infantile sexual life becomes transformed into its final form. The tasks in adolescence include the "subordination of partial drive under the genital primacy" (p. 105), the "creation of this primacy for the purpose of reproduction" (p. 105), the "unification of affectionate and sensual desires of sexual life in a non-incestuous object, the separation from the family, and the differentiation into man and woman" (p. 124). Freud's approach recognizes the complexity of sexual development and its contingency on physical maturity, body image, role expectations, and relationships with others.

According to Freud (1905/1952a), female and male sexual drives differ. Whereas male adolescents in puberty show "a great thrust in libido," girls experience "a wave of repression" (p. 124). Freud never developed a genuine model of female sexuality, preferring to interpret it in terms of a deficient male sexuality. In his later works on female development, he made many references to the deficiencies of female genitals, of the resulting penis envy, and of women's difficulties in suppressing their desires to experience maleness, considering them to represent sources of life-long conflicts (S. Freud, 1933/1952c). Thwarted in their attempts to fulfill these desires, women develop an increased "physical vanity" (p. 562) and a special kind of narcissism (S. Freud, 1914/1952b). The exhibition of a pretty female face and womanly body is interpreted as a displacement for penis envy. Around the end of the 1970s, the French school of psychoanalytic theory challenged the claims of phallic monism (Chasseguet-Smirgel, 1979), and the ethnopsychoanalytic discussion in the 1980s placed the idea of a second chance in a broader cultural and social framework (Erdheim, 1988). Nevertheless, the central position of sexuality in theoretical conceptualizations of adolescent development has not changed over the years. Sexuality is, according to the more recent treatments of the subject (Laufer & Laufer, 1984), the most important determining factor for healthy development.

Although psychological theories are less oriented to concepts of genital primacy, they are generally less complex and frequently exclude considerations of sexuality. Thus, as pointed out in the previous section, most theories of physical maturation and the studies attempting to support them are generally concerned with such variables as weight, height, and growth norms. Other facets include the body self-image and physical attractiveness. Another, partly sociologically oriented facet is the process of fulfilling social role expectations (e.g., sex-typing). However, studies on sex-typing, as well as physical maturation, make little reference to sexuality (see the summary by Udry & Billy, 1987) or physical attractiveness (see the summary by Blyth et al., 1985). Many studies conducted in the United States attempted to establish correlations between problem behaviors and sexual activity in early adolescence. Thus, although psychological studies dealt with important aspects of sexual development, there remains a paucity of interest in examining sexuality. Similarly, when sexuality is incorporated into the research focus, aspects of interpersonal relationships are invariably neglected.

### Adolescent Sexuality

The first comprehensive, representative study on young adults' sexuality was conducted by Kinsey in the late 1940s and early 1950s. Similar investigations conducted on adolescents in Germany (e.g., Sigusch & Schmidt, 1973) were strongly oriented to this approach. In these studies, masturbation, coitus, and the use of contraceptive devices was examined. Since then, a great deal of research was conducted by Anglo-American investigators on reproductive control in adolescence, in part to establish profiles of pregnancy risks. This one-sided focus on adolescents' risky sexual behavior becomes understandable when one considers that the highest percentages for teenage pregnancies and abortions of all Western industrialized societies were documented in the United States (Lief, Fullard, & Devlin, 1990; Weddle et al., 1988). In general, such studies treated sexual behavior in adolescence as a nonnormative event and focused on documenting the dangers of premarital sexual activity (e.g., unwanted pregnancy or AIDS).

***Masturbation.*** According to Sigusch and Schmidt (1973), much of adolescent sexual behavior is made up of substitute activities, including erotic fantasizing, nocturnal emission, and masturbation. Surprisingly, very little research was devoted toward understanding any of these sexual behaviors, perhaps because they were and still are regarded as very private and somewhat shameful activities. A more tolerant approach in dealing with this topic only recently found acceptance in literature. According to Katchadourian (1990), masturbation is the most common cause of orgasm in male and female adolescents. In two out of three cases, a boy's first ejaculation is elicited by masturbation. For most adolescents, masturbation is the first kind of conscious and direct sexual activity they experience. Studies on adolescent masturbation conducted in the 1980s documented that 75% of all male adolescents and one third of all female adolescents between 14 and 17 years old masturbated. According to Moore and Rosenthal (1993), who published an overview of findings on the subject, the frequency of masturbation increases with age. Whereas male and female adolescents continue to show different rates of masturbation, such differences narrowed over the decades. Nevertheless, it seems that young girls begin to masturbate at an earlier age (on average, at 12 years old) than boys (on average, at 14 years old). Both male and female adolescents state that they feel guilty or ashamed about their masturbation behavior, and girls especially are reluctant to report or disclose details about their masturbation experiences. Whether girls' lower rates of reporting masturbation behavior reflect a real difference or simply a difference in willingness to admit to a stigmatized behavior is not known. Certainly it seems that acceptance of masturbation among boys is greater than among girls. Various findings indicated that masturbation is a substitute for sexual intercourse for males, whereas for females it is a form of sexuality in its own right.

This different relevance of masturbation to adolescent sexuality was documented in reports on sexual fantasies (Laufer & Laufer, 1984). Women fantasize at a more personal–emotional level; men's fantasies are more anonymous. Katchadourian (1990) reported findings showing that erotic fantasizing is by far the most common sexual activity in adolescence. He suggested that these fantasies, beside providing pleasure, fulfill a number of different functions in the adolescent's erotic life: They are a substitute for the satisfaction of unattainable sexual needs or help the adolescent to learn about his or her sexual needs and preferences. According to Moore and Rosenthal (1993), sexual fantasies, accompanied by masturbation, allow the individual to rehearse sexual experiences; they also occur in anticipation of future sexual experiences. Thus, fantasizing, as rehearsal and as preparation for later realization of sexual activity is extremely important for adolescents. The importance of fantasies was also borne in the study of adolescent diaries: A significant percentage of the sexual experiences described by 15-year-old girls in their diaries was based on sexual fantasies (Seiffge-Krenke, 1993a).

***The Onset of Heterosexual Relationships: Dating.*** A close association between physical maturity and the onset of heterosexual contacts was reported in several studies (Bulcroft, 1991). The appearance of visible physical changes has a direct influence on how adolescents organize their leisure time (Hendry, Shucksmith, Love, & Glendinning, 1993). Adolescents become interested in new and more complex types of leisure activities involving members of the opposite gender.

In our culture, few young people in pre-adolescence date; by the time they reach adulthood, the overwhelming majority of them have dated or are dating on a regular basis. Dating is not synonymous with sexual intercourse or courtship. A *date* is a social engagement between young people with no commitment beyond the expectation that it is a pleasurable event for both (Dornbusch et al., 1981). Although pubertal development has a great bearing on when an adolescent begins to date, dating is highly regulated and constrained by social forces. Dornbusch et al. established that age explained far more variance in the onset of dating than did sexual development. The partial correlation coefficient between age and dating was .33 for males and .54 for females, whereas the partial correlation between sexual development (controlling for age) and dating was only .12 for males and .04 for females. According to this study, individual rates of physical maturation that deviated from the norms for that age had little impact on dating. Instead, it appeared that peer pressure to engage in dating activities determined the onset of dating in adolescence. In the United States, the median age when adolescents begin to date declined over time, from about 16 years old in 1930 to 13 years old in 1990. Several studies showed the robustness of a sequence of adolescent sexual behavior, which starts around 13 years old, with embracing and kissing, moving through petting or fondling breasts and sexual organs, and ending with intercourse (Moore & Rosenthal, 1993).

In a study of 836 15- to 18-year-old adolescents conducted by Miller, McCoy, and Olson (1986), the relation between early dating and sexual activity was examined. The authors found that early dating, especially early steady dating, was related to permissive sexual attitudes and early intercourse. Having a steady girlfriend or boyfriend may increase the likelihood of and pressure to engage in sexual activity. McCabe and Collins (1990) investigated how the sexual desires and behaviors of Australian 16- to 17-year-old adolescents changed as dating relationships deepened. There was a clear desire that sexual intimacy should increase from first date to going steady, whereby boys wanted more intimacy than girls did at all levels of dating. Roche (1986) reported similar findings for American adolescents. Thus, there is a strong association between dating experiences and adolescent sexual activities and behaviors. Early dating seems to be associated with more permissive attitudes as well as with early sexual experience.

***The First Experience With Sexual Intercourse.*** There is a strong association between physical maturity and experiencing sexual intercourse (Moore & Rosenthal, 1993). Although the age of first intercourse has decreased over the last 30 years, the close association of these phenomena has not changed at all. Early maturing adolescents begin to have sexual intercourse earlier, and late maturing adolescents begin later, each within an interval of approximately 3 years following physical maturation (Phinney, Jensen, Olsen, & Cundick, 1990). The processes involved in making the transition to nonvirginity was studied almost exclusively by North American investigators (cf. Jessor & Jessor, 1975; Strouse & Fabes, 1987). In Germany, few studies dealt with the psychological processes and variables determining the onset of heterosexual relationships; most investigated the effects of age and gender. In a replication of Sigusch and Schmidt's (1973) study on the heterosexual activity of adolescents, Clement, Schmidt, and Kruse (1984) found that 60% of the 18-year-old girls and 50% of the 18-year-old boys had experienced coitus around the middle of the 1980s. A comparison with Sigusch and Schmidt's findings from the 1970s showed that the percentage of sexually experienced 18-year-old males doubled, whereas the percentage of sexually experienced girls quadrupled. Schmid-Tannwald and Urdze (1983) found similar distributions. They reported that the percentage of sexually experienced adolescents rapidly increased between 14 and 18 years old. One out of thirty 14-year-old girls, 1 out of 10 15-year-olds, 1 out of 4 16-year-olds and every other 17-year-old girl had sexual intercourse. Schmid-Tannwald and Urdze also found that most adolescents regularly had sexual intercourse after the first coitus. One year after the first intercourse, every third girl and every fourth boy was still dating the partner with whom they had their first coital experience. However, as a more recent replication study by Schmidt, Klusmann, Zeitzschel, and Lange (1994) illustrated, the trend of having coitus at an earlier age does not seem to have persisted: The rates of heterosexual activity reported in the 1970s closely match those for the 1990s. Apparently, the risk of becoming infected with HIV and developing AIDS had a marked influence on the sexual activity of adolescents, as can be seen in the trend of delaying the onset of sexual activity. This may also explain why females are more active in heterosexual situations insofar as they take more initiative and show more control.

Studies of adolescent sexual behavior in the United States also found that the age of first intercourse steadily decreased until 1980, but this trend did not continue in the following 10 years (Gagnon et al., 1989). Following the sexual revolution of the 1960s, researchers began to document increases in sexual activities in both males and females. In addition, increasing proportions of adolescent females who had premarital sexual intercourse were noted. In two national surveys, Zelnik, Kantner, and Ford (1981) found that in 1971, 30% of all 15- to 19-year-old American women engaged in sexual intercourse; by 1976, the percentage rose to 41%. By 1979, 49% of all females and 56% of all males experienced sexual intercourse by 19 years old (Zelnik & Kantner, 1980). In the mid-1980s, 79% of all males and 63% of all females experienced intercourse by 19 years old. These percentages were higher for Blacks (92% of males and 77% of females by 19 years old) than for Whites (75% of males and 61% of females by 19 years of age) or Hispanics (79% of males and 59% of females by 19 years old; Hoffarth & Hayes, 1987).

These figures are similar to those available for Australian and British adolescents (Moore & Rosenthal, 1993). Indeed, the trend toward sexual intercourse at younger ages is present in most industrialized nations (Goldman & Goldman, 1988). In Sweden, for example, the mean age for first sexual intercourse dropped from 19 years old to 16 years old in the past 20 years. In the United States, Great Britain, Australia, and Germany, there has been a similar shift since 1970, especially among White females. However, as already mentioned, this trend has begun to reverse its direction. Since 1990, the age of initiation for intercourse increased.

Recent research on adolescent sexuality reveals many gender differences. Adolescent males' attitudes about premarital sex are more permissive than those of adolescent females; yet, males are less knowledgeable about contraception (Jemmott & Jemmott Ill, 1990). Females are more committed in their relationships with sexual partners and are less likely than males to have intercourse on a casual basis (Moore & Rosenthal, 1993). Mothers discuss topics related to sexual behaviors and contraception more with their daughters than with their sons (Scott-Jones & Turner, 1988). Research documented a strong relationship between attitudes about premarital sex and sexual behavior; that is, individuals who have more permissive attitudes are likely to engage in more intimate behaviors. An adolescent's sexual behavior is also influenced by how he or she perceives the attitudes of parents and peers. Adolescents who think their friends or parents approve of their sexual behavior are more likely to engage in sexual intercourse (Jessor & Jessor, 1977).

A number of studies analyzed the variables related to first intercourse, including age, gender, physical maturity, parental and peer relations, religion, race, and social class (Jessor & Jessor, 1975; Strouse & Fabes, 1987; Weddle et al., 1988). In one study of 814 sexually experienced females, chronological age and age of menarche were highly significant, as was race, religious affiliation, and household income (Bingham, Miller, & Adams, 1990). Treboux and Busch-Rossnagel (1990) conducted a LISREL analysis on social network influences on male and female high school students' sexual attitudes and behavior. They found that the transition to nonvirginity produced a greater change in the social environment of females than of males. In addition, parents were more influential for males, whereas friends were more important for females.

In reviewing the research on adolescent sexuality over the past decades, it becomes apparent that although such research has greatly expanded, it is still fraught with many shortcomings. Researchers continue to approach sex in adolescence as a nonnormative, if not deviant, activity (see, e.g., Jessor & Jessor, 1977). Accordingly, researchers following this perspective are most interested in identifying those factors related to the initiation of early sexual intercourse and the effective use of contraceptives. Indeed, the one area of adolescent sexuality that received most interest is the use of contraceptives. The literature is replete with evidence on the negative outcome of early sexuality in females. Moreover, researchers tended to study adolescent sexuality outside the social and developmental contexts in which it normally occurs (Weddle et al., 1988). Most important, little attention was devoted to determining the role of interpersonal relationships in the development of adolescent sexuality. Thus, most research focuses on the individual, and invariably, that individual is the adolescent female (Bolton & MacEachron, 1988).

The typical individual approach to research on adolescent sexuality has left a void in understanding the dynamics of sexuality. Is early sexual intercourse related to regular and frequent subsequent sexual activity? Who are the sexual partners? Is the initiation of sexual activity voluntary? Is it a pleasurable experience or one fraught with negative emotions? It seems that having had sexual intercourse once does not necessarily mean that adolescents maintain a high level of activity. For some adolescents, sexual intercourse is sporadic and rare (Moore & Rosenthal, 1993). How can this be explained? It is quite likely that the frequency of intercourse is related to the nature of the relationship with one's partner. The more committed the relationship is, the more frequent the sexual activity.

So far, little is known about the characteristics of the partner in heterosexual relationships, except for the fact that females report that their first sexual intercourse usually takes place with slightly older males. Some investigators found that the average age difference between male and female sexual partners is 3 years. As mentioned, female adolescents ascribe a high level of commitment to their partners, and designate affection and love as motives for intercourse more often than male adolescents, who emphasize relaxation and desire (Savin-Williams & Berndt, 1990). Neubauer (1990) analyzed the motives for taking up sexual intercourse in 14- to 18-year-old German adolescents. A factor analysis revealed three motives for beginning heterosexual relationships: curiosity (the adolescents wanted to know what sex was like), mutual affection (the adolescents were in love and wanted to belong to each other completely), and adult status (adolescents wanted to be like their friends and become an adult). These motives explain why, for a minority of young people, the initiation of sex is not voluntary (Moore & Rosenthal, 1993). Interestingly, Muehlenhard and Cook (1988) found that more males than females reported engaging in unwanted sexual intercourse. Fifty-two percent of males and 44% of females claimed they engaged in sexual intercourse because of peer pressure; 18% of males and 13% of females wanted to become more popular. Also, a discrepancy between males' and females' reports about who initiates sexual contact was observed (Anderson & Aymami, 1993). Nevertheless, for most girls and somewhat fewer boys, the act occurs in the context of an affectionate relationship. In spite of this, emotional reactions to the event vary. McCabe and Collins (1990) found that only one half of the girls enjoyed the experience, whereas 40% had negative reactions such as guilt, anxiety about pregnancy, and fear of discovery. Boys, on the other hand, felt quite differently, claiming feelings of excitement and satisfaction.

Where does sexual intercourse take place? There are often few alternatives. This situation of strong external limitations means that sexual intercourse often takes place spontaneously (i.e., when the opportunity of being alone arises). Interestingly, two thirds of Australian, British, German, and American adolescents engage in sexual intercourse where they are most likely to be caught in the act—at home (Gagnon et al., 1989; Moore & Rosenthal, 1993; Schmidt et al., 1994). This partly explains adolescents' negative reactions about sexual intercourse and why adolescents often do not use contraception. Indeed, as already mentioned, the use of contraception is one of the most frequently investigated issues related to adolescent sexuality, which again underlies the prevailing tendency among researchers to treat premarital sex as problem or risk behavior. What do adolescents actually know and think about birth control? Are they willing to use contraceptive devices? Do they use them in actual practice? These questions are addressed in the following section.

### Adolescents' Knowledge and Use of Contraception

As detailed in the previous section, sexual intercourse in adolescence usually occurs spontaneously and in situations for which little planning or preparation is possible (e.g., when the adolescents happen to be alone in the family home). The significance of these situation parameters, as well as psychological barriers, should be kept in mind in evaluating adolescents' use of contraception.

According to a study conducted by Brooks-Gunn and Furstenberg (1989), 50% of American adolescents did not use contraception during their first sexual intercourse. In 1973, Sigusch and Schmidt reported that 30% of German adolescents did not use birth control. At the beginning of the 1990s, these figures were essentially the same. Schmidt et al. (1994) found that 30% of the girls and 50% of the boys they studied used inadequate contraception or did not use any altogether. Only 25% of the American adolescents studied by Scott-Jones and Turner (1988) regularly used contraception. According to the study conducted by Morrison (1985), adolescents have negative attitudes about using birth control. Many female adolescents did not bother to use contraception because they were convinced that they could not become pregnant very easily. They believed that they were too young to become pregnant or that the low frequency of sexual intercourse would make conception unlikely. On the other hand, 15% to 25% of female adolescents in this study did not bother to use contraception, claiming that they would not mind becoming pregnant. Adolescents studied by Scott-Jones and Turner (1988) claimed that they did not know how to obtain contraception, which methods were reliable, or that they were too embarrassed to purchase them in public. Another frequently named reason for not using contraceptives was that birth control makes sex seem preplanned (Padilla & Baird, 1991). A decisive factor behind the nonuse of contraception is age, which covaries with infrequent yet spontaneous sexual activity. One fourth of the young women studied by Zelnik and Kantner (1979) reported that they did not use contraception when sexual intercourse unexpectedly took place.

These variables are intertwined with misperceptions of the risk for pregnancy due to adolescent egocentrism. In particular, the personal fable phenomenon (Elkind, 1967) in early adolescence is held responsible for the erroneous belief that the probability of becoming pregnant is low. A number of studies provided indirect support for the role of personal fable for adolescents who have sexual intercourse without using contraceptives. Arguments like "I felt that pregnancy would never happen to me" were frequently cited by adolescents in the studies by Arnett (1990) and Kalmuss (1986). The implications of these findings and those published by Morrison (1985) are that the personal fable hinders some adolescent girls in making realistic appraisals of their chances of becoming pregnant. Reluctance to use contraception may even be engendered by distorted perceptions of the partner's intentions. For example, Black adolescent females studied by Zabin, Astone, and Emerson (1993) explained that their ambivalence about using contraception was grounded on the (false) belief that their partners wanted them to conceive.

There is unanimous agreement in the literature that adequate knowledge of human reproduction and reproductive control marginally influences actual practices of birth control (Brooks-Gunn & Furstenberg, 1989; Davis & Harris, 1982; Morrison, 1985; Scott-Jones & Turner, 1988). Whereas some adolescents often act contrary to their better knowledge, others are simply uninformed or misinformed about reproductive processes. For example, a large percentage of American adolescents believed that a woman is most likely to conceive during menstruation and least likely during the middle of the menstrual cycle (Scott-Jones & Turner, 1988). Henshaw (1994) found that despite attendance in classes on human sexuality, adolescents were still misinformed about the relation between the phase of the menstrual cycle and increased likelihood for conception. Interestingly, the majority of the adolescents' mothers in this study were also unsure or misinformed about when the risk for conception was greatest during the menstrual cycle. A study of German adolescents (Schmidt et al., 1994) showed that despite having discussed the topic in classes on human sexuality, only one half of the girls and one fourth of the boys were correctly informed about the optimal date for conception. Nevertheless, girls are generally well-informed about maturation and reproduction, pregnancy, and contraception, a finding that was documented in both German and Anglo-American populations (Davis & Harris, 1982; Schmidt et al., 1994).

This is related to the prevailing attitude that reproductive control is a woman's responsibility. Girls not only have more knowledge about reproduction, contraception, and pregnancy than boys, but also are more interested in these topics. According to Davis and Harris (1982), most girls become informed about these topics through friends, school, books, and parents. In the study by Scott-Jones and Turner (1988), however, girls were usually informed about these topics by their parents, whereas boys learned about these topics through the mass media. In addition, there are indications that many adolescents consciously choose either parents or friends as conversational partners concerning topics related to sexuality. For example, Nathanson and Becker (1986) found that girls who spoke with their parents about these topics preferred not to discuss them with their friends and vice versa. One reason for this is related to diverging norms: An adolescent who is oriented to nonconformist peers cannot comply with his or her parents' conventional views. When parents talk about sexuality with their children, they are more likely to do so with their daughters than with their sons (Moore, Peterson, & Furstenberg, 1986). Schmid-Tannwald and Urdze (1983) analyzed the same issues in German adolescents and found that despite an overall high level of trust between adolescents and their parents, adolescents preferred to discuss these topics with their peers. Thus, it is not surprising that a third of the parents in this study were unaware of the fact that their son or daughter already experienced sexual intercourse. Nearly one fifth of the girls and one third of the boys complained that they had no one with whom they could openly talk about topics related to sex.

# 5

# The Links Between Stress and Health

In this chapter, research findings on stressors occurring during adolescence and their effects on health status are presented. A variety of salient stressors that the adolescent is most likely to be confronted with is described, and it is discussed how the accumulation of such stressors may exert negative effects on the adolescent's physical and psychological health. In addition, the question of whether adolescents today are subjected to more stress than in the past is addressed. The chapter begins with findings about the frequency of body complaints in adolescence, and makes apparent that a lack of illness does not necessarily imply well-being.

## TALKING WITH THE BODY: THE FREQUENCY OF BODY COMPLAINTS

Considering the mortality and morbidity rates presented in chapter 3, adolescents are a comparably healthy age group. Compared to children, they have a lay conception of illness that approximates adult conceptions. Nevertheless, they are not easily able to submit to the sick role. This is partly explained by the fact that adolescents have great difficulties in dealing with their bodies. Thus, although several studies reported high rates of somatic complaints in adolescents, many authors have noted that adolescents are often unable or unwilling to describe their symptoms precisely. In a study of body complaints in children from 8 to 15 years old, Brähler (1988) found five different areas of complaints: gastric complaints (e.g., stomachache, burping, stomach pain, or heartburn), cold symptoms (e.g., coughing, sore throat, or stuffy nose), pain (e.g., muscular aches in limbs or pain in the joints), exhaustion (e.g., morning tiredness, weariness, or daytime tiredness), and circulatory problems (e.g., feeling dizzy). Girls named more body complaints than boys, and adolescents reported more complaints than children. Interestingly, the frequency of body complaints named by adolescents was even higher than in adult samples. A comparison between the physical complaints reported by a standard sample of adults between 20 and 60 years old revealed that adolescents named more complaints than any of the adult age groups, even more than the oldest adults. In particular, the types of body complaints reported by adolescents indicated overall distress and nervousness.

In a more recent survey on health risks and medical and psychosocial care in Germany, Palentien and Hurrelmann (1995) found that adolescents suffered from a large number of body complaints that might be considered as psychosomatic (e.g., exhaustion, excessive tiredness, insomnia, headaches, indigestion, stomachaches, nausea, and circulatory problems). Twenty-eight percent of the physicians interviewed reported that adolescent patients showed signs of nervous strain. Greene, Walker, Hickson, and Thompson (1985) also reported that adolescents with recurrent somatic complaints were often encountered by general practitioners providing care for this group. In their survey of community health and medical centers in the United States, they found that adolescents from 11 to 18 years old, with a psychosomatic diagnosis, accounted for between 6% and 11% of all pediatric patients. Similarly, in their summary of research findings, Campo and Fritsch (1994) noted that despite the many reports of a high rate of somatization in adolescent patients, such medically unexplained physical symptoms received less systematic attention in the pediatric literature than in the adult medical literature. The most frequently cited complaints were abdominal pain, chest pain, and headaches. Although many of these patients were submitted to extensive medical tests, organic pathological causes were rarely found. It should be pointed out, however, that because the health complaints of adolescents tend to be more diffuse and do not appear to be very serious, they often are not taken seriously or disregarded by adults or medical professionals (see chap. 2, this volume).

What are mislabeled as "psychogenic" disorders or downplayed as "passing growing pains," may be the physical manifestations of adolescents' reactions to life changes and stressors as well as insecurities about their physical changes. For example, Greene et al. (1985) found that life stress was significantly higher in adolescents suffering from recurrent pain for which no organic etiology could be identified than in adolescents examined for routine checkups, acute illness, chronic illness, or pain with clinically diagnosed organic causes. In addition, the pubertal adolescent is acutely aware of the physical changes rapidly occurring in his or her body. With increasing age and advanced pubertal development, a stronger gender-specific differentiation in the types of symptoms reported becomes evident (Baum & Grunberg, 1991). Compared to male adolescents, females report a greater impairment of health; that is, they complain more about their health status and show more physical symptoms. Not only do they show higher rates of overall physical exhaustion, but they also complain more about physical changes in their bodies (e.g., gaining weight or skin and hair problems).

According to Hoehe (1988), female adolescents' somatic complaints increase around the time of menarche. This observation is closely related to the finding that female adolescents perceive physical changes in puberty much more negatively than do male adolescents (Brooks-Gunn, 1988). A direct link between physical maturation and somatic complaints is not characteristic for male adolescents. Nevertheless, it is unclear to what extent gender-specific differences in types and frequency of physical complaints are based on physiological differences, because female adolescents continue to suffer from a greater amount of somatic complaints from menarche well into the later stages of puberty. It is more likely that gender-specific role expectations about illness behavior play a role in determining which and how many complaints are actually reported. Thus, male adolescents are apt to mask or repress their physical ailments. Also, women tend to remain preoccupied with their physical well-being instead of distracting themselves through various activities (Nolen-Hoeksema, 1987), which might also account for the increased frequency of reported complaints in female adolescents.

These results indicate an increased vulnerability of adolescents to physical ailments, particularly among girls. Thus, although adolescents are seldom ill, their well-being is markedly impaired. As we see in the following sections, however, higher rates of somatic complaints in adolescents are not simply reduced to developmental changes occurring in puberty, but are also related to general societal and social stress factors that exert a direct influence on the adolescent's well-being.

## THE IMPACT OF STRESS ON HEALTH

At the end of the 19th century, inadequate personal hygiene, poor medical care, and harsh living conditions were the main factors behind the high morbidity and mortality rates of the time, especially among the poor (Freund & McGuire, 1991). Although living standards in many modern industrial societies improved since then, the citizens living in such societies are confronted with new and different kinds of burdens introduced by the progress of civilization, such as new patterns of societal interaction, changed cultural concerns, and ecological–environmental problems, that directly or indirectly affect their health. It is now generally accepted that somatic illness is precipitated by more than one causal factor and that a dynamic interplay among environmental, social, cognitive, and physiological factors may affect physical health. This contemporary approach toward explaining the etiology and modification of illnesses, as incorporated in theoretical concepts of psychosomatic medicine (Lask & Fosson, 1989), has been increasingly accepted by proponents of a more traditional, biologically oriented school of medicine. Moreover, considerable evidence accumulated, showing that the immunological response is modified by psychosocial stress (see, e.g., Baum & Grunberg, 1991).

Over the years, the belief that stress can lead to various illnesses or disorders, such as heart attack, gastric ulcers, or cancer, has been assimilated by the general population. In considering the multifactorial causes of many disorders, research in psychology primarily concentrates on understanding the links between different types of stressors and health problems. Three main areas of research can be distinguished: the relation between critical life events and the outbreak of illness (see, e.g., Dohrenwend & Dohrenwend, 1974, 1981), the relation between stressful life situations and working conditions and illness (see, e.g., Schwefel, Svensson, & Zöllner, 1987), and the relation between illness and everyday stress or daily hassles (DeLongis, Folkman, & Lazarus, 1988; Gruen, Folkman, & Lazarus, 1988).

There is quite a body of empirical evidence showing that several types of stressors are disturbing enough to affect normal biological and physiological functioning of the circulatory or immune systems, which, in the long term, is detrimental to overall health (Levi, 1981). An early explanation of the relation between stress and the etiology of physical illness was proposed by Selye (1946). He suggested that contact with internal and external stimuli that may threaten an organism's normal physiological functioning results in a nonspecific physiological activation (General Adaptation Syndrome). According to Selye, if the defensive processes in this syndrome (brought into play to deal with noxious stimuli) are prolonged, the organism may suffer from irreversible bodily damage, which in turn leads to disease. Accordingly, so-called "stress illnesses" are linked to an organism's inappropriate nervous or hormonal reactions to various demands; that is, the stress reaction continues beyond the actual confrontation with the stressful stimuli, leading to organ and tissue damage. Selye's model suggests the basic possibility that physical damage is caused by stress; nevertheless, its scope is limited to a stimulus–reaction paradigm that neglects the influence of psychological factors.

### Types of Stressors and Properties That Make Events Stressful

In recent years, there has been widespread interest in identifying the properties that make events stressful. In research on adults, most efforts focused on specific aspects of life events (e.g., their frequency, predictability, uncertainty, and control; Lazarus & Folkman, 1991). Predictability of an event allows individuals to prepare for it in some way, thereby reducing the aversiveness of the stressor. Likewise, control refers to the individual's options to control the event's outcome. It must be pointed out, however, that the frequency of events, as well as their predictability and control, are not uniform for all ages and differences in these event parameters may have important implications for health. Most of the studies on the impact of stress on health were conducted on adult populations, and only recently have research efforts concentrated on the implications of stress experienced in adolescents. In general, two different types of stressful events were analyzed; they differ in frequency, predictability, control, and negative impact on adolescent health. They are termed *nonnormative* and *normative stressors* and basically parallel the distinctions made by Lazarus and Folkman (1984) between critical life events and everyday hassles or between major events and daily events according to Compas, Malcarne, and Fondacaro (1988).

***Normative Stressors.*** The adolescent years are characterized by numerous biological, cognitive, and social changes. In our society, increased responsibilities, accessibility to adult rights, and school changes mark the transition to adulthood. All these events affect adolescents' definitions of themselves and their interactions with others. In particular, early adolescence (approximately 10 to 14 years old) is considered to be a difficult yet challenging phase due to pubertal developments, relational changes, and school transition (Paikoff & Brooks-Gunn, 1991). Most early adolescents enter a new school, and the strain associated with adjusting to new academic and social environments are potentiated by the biological developments occurring in puberty, such as changes in physical size and body concept or the emergence of sexual desires and anxieties about sexuality. As outlined in chapter 4, school changes are particularly stressful for girls. Due to their more rapid maturational development in puberty, physical changes are more likely to occur around the time they enter a new school. Owing to their slower development, boys are less likely to be confronted with both normative stressors simultaneously (Petersen & Leffert, 1992). Feelings of being different—not meeting the norm and having matured too quickly or not quickly enough—represent additional stressors that arise in the pubertal phase of development. In addition, parent–child relationships change (Hill & Holmbeck, 1986), and the adolescent's interactions with and acceptance by friends become increasingly important. In mid-adolescence, the adolescent's needs for peer acceptance are especially great, and the adolescent begins to spend more time with peers outside the home (Larson & Richards, 1991). Thus, stressors emerge in relation to these changes, that is, there are more disputes with parents about curfews, clothing, driving, and personal freedom (Smetana, Yau, & Hanson, 1991). Dating and the initiation of intimate, heterosexual relationships also occur in this phase and are accompanied by stressors such as fear of rejection or feelings of incompetence. In late adolescence, the increasing independence from parents can result in the adolescent's establishing an independent household (Cantor, Acker, & Cook-Flannagan, 1992). Graduation from high school is considered to be a significant juncture in the transition to adulthood (Aseltine & Gore, 1993). All of these events are normative in that they occur at about the same time for the majority of individuals in this age group and are associated with specific developmental tasking expectations of family, friends, and society. They are highly predictable, comparably frequent, and perceived as mildly stressful and controllable (Seiffge-Krenke, 1995).

***Non-Normative Stressors.*** In addition to these changes, other, nonnormative stressors or critical life events increase the likelihood of maladaptation. Nonnormative family stressors were studied intensively. Adolescents are more at risk of developing illness when the family situation is unstable or when there is serious marital discord (Dawson, 1991). In extreme cases, marital discord leads to divorce, a phenomenon that has increased in all Western industrialized societies over the years. The influence of parental divorce on a child's well-being is frequently studied (for a review, see Amato & Keith, 1991).

The chronicity of the stressors is also relevant. Often high levels of stress precede the event and persist long after it has occurred. Many of the nonnormative stressors experienced by adolescents are controlled or influenced by family situations and are chronic in nature. Ongoing, stressful family situations can, for example, produce more discrete life events, such as separation or divorce (Garmezy & Masten, 1994).

Psychiatric illness in one or both parents is another situation that is considered to be a chronic stressful life situation. Most studies on this kind of stressor focused on maternal dysfunction and its impact on child and adolescent health; little attention was devoted to paternal disorders (Phares & Compas, 1992). Additional sources of familial stress occur following the death of a relative, instances of child molestation or abuse, parental drug abuse or criminal activities, or chronic illness in the family (Hauser & Bowlds, 1990). According to the traditional understanding, these stressors are critical life events that are relatively infrequent, hardly predictable, and extremely burdensome. Because most of these events are hardly foreseeable and can seldom be controlled or influenced by the adolescents, anticipatory preparation for or coping with the event is extremely difficult. Consequently, the emergence of nonnormative events have more dramatic health consequences for adolescents than normative stressors (Masten, Neemann, & Andenas, 1994). On the other hand, due to the unusual timing and high stressfulness of nonnormative events, social support is greater and thus buffers the potentially damaging effects on health (see chap. 6, this volume).

***Number, Timing, and Synchronicity of Changes.*** Although normative stressors such as school change, physical maturation, and the onset of heterosexual relationships are expected, age appropriate, and moderately stressful, the accumulation of diverse stressors has deleterious effects. By definition, nonnormative stressors occur quite seldom; however, should they occur simultaneously or in rapid sequence with normative or developmentally related stressors, serious health damage can result. As for the accumulation of major stressors such as critical life events, Rutter, Graham, et al. (1976) found in their study of British adolescents that the risk of an unfavorable outcome exponentially increased with an increased number of stressors confronting adolescents. In this study, adolescents in families with major stressors did not show an increased risk for psychiatric illness as long as only one stressor was involved. When two stressors simultaneously occurred, the risk became four times as great. In other words, the stressors potentiate one another so that the combination of stressors is more than the sum of effects of individual stressors. Furthermore, additional stressors such as everyday hassles may appear in their wake. This link was confirmed by Lazarus and Folkman (1984), whose study on adult populations revealed a correlation of $r = .30$ between critical life events and everyday hassles. Thus, we must assume that the different types of stressors that occur in a developmental phase interact with one another in a yet unknown way to produce health-damaging effects.

Various authors have observed that the number of changes occurring in adolescence, compared with other developmental stages, is unusually high (Newcomb, Huba, & Bentler, 1981). Simmons, Burgeson, and Carlton-Ford (1987) pointed out that the sheer number of changes occurring during early adolescence exerts an impact on health. Research showed that girls are more likely than boys to experience more conflicting demands during this period. Simmons and Blyth (1987) demonstrated how the demands of popularity and achievement orientation produce emotional conflict in early adolescent girls. They found a linear relation between more changes and poor psychosocial outcomes.

In addition, the timing of events was found to influence health outcomes. A large body of work indicated that, when the timing of pubertal development deviates from normative expectations, problematic outcomes may be the result (Petersen & Ebata, 1987). Again, girls are more affected. Early maturing girls are more likely to develop a more negative body image and are also more likely to develop eating disorders (Brooks-Gunn & Warren, 1985). Unusual timing of physical maturation is also linked to depression in girls (see chap. 4, this volume).

Finally, the synchronicity of changes is another factor related to negative outcomes in health (Rice, Herman, & Petersen, 1993). Unusual timing of a normative event, like physical maturity, produces changes in relationships with parents and peers. In addition, the synchronous occurrence of a further normative event (e.g., the transition from primary to secondary school) also contributes to stress in youth, especially when the transition occurs during the time when pubertal development is most rapid. Although school change per se has few harmful effects on most adolescents, there are certain vulnerable subgroups. Because boys are less likely than girls to experience maximal pubertal growth at about the same time as the normative transition from primary to secondary school, the negative effects of synchronous school transition and pubertal changes on health are largely confined to girls. Thus, the gender differences in timing of puberty (in combination with the normative timing of the school transition) partly explains the findings of gender differences in body complaints and psychopathology (Baum & Grunberg, 1991).

There are fewer changes in late adolescence than in early or mid-adolescence, which probably accounts for the finding that the transition to adulthood does not present major adaptation problems (Aseltine & Gore, 1993). Although most researchers found that young adolescents have many conflicts with their parents (Smetana et al., 1991) and that the average youth shows a decline in school achievement (Petersen, Kennedy, & Sullivan, 1991), positive family relations are mobilized and achievement is improved as adolescents enter college or take full-time jobs (Hogan & Astone, 1986).

### Stress and the Development of Symptoms

Although a wide range of social and biological factors play a role in adolescent health problems, research indicating a consistent association between stressful events and psychological disorders in adults suggests that stress is an important factor in younger populations too. Stressful experiences occurring early in development contribute to psychological and physical symptoms and disrupt positive development. Furthermore, stressful events and psychological and physical symptoms may be reciprocally related, each contributing to the etiology and maintenance of the other. Thus, stressful events during adolescence set in motion a process in which stress, emotional or behavior problems, and body symptoms contribute to one another in a self-perpetuating cycle. In the following, the association between stress and the appearance of physical and psychological symptoms is analyzed.

***Stressful Events and Somatic Complaints.*** In spite of the potential importance of studying the health consequences of stressful events in adolescence, empirical research has only recently addressed this issue. Two different areas of research can be distinguished: studies investigating critical life events or major events and those investigating everyday stressors or minor events. Although most studies have focused on the association between different types of stressors and behavioral and emotional disorders, only a few studies have addressed the links between stress and physical disorders or body complaints. Greene et al. (1985) administered the Johnson and McCutcheon (1980) Life Event Checklist to 172 adolescents admitted for the first time to an outpatient clinic. The majority of subjects were either self-referred or referred by outside physicians. The diagnostic groups included routine physical examination or checkup; acute minor illness; abdominal pain, chest pain, or headache with clinically diagnosed organic cause; pain without identifiable organic cause; behavioral and emotional problems, including acting out and depression; and stable chronic illness not associated with major limitations (e.g., diabetes). Results showed that patients coming for routine examinations (or because of acute minor illness, stable chronic illness, or pain with established organic cause) reported comparably low scores of negative life events ($M$ ranged from 3.4 to 4.1), whereas the adolescents suffering from pain without identifiable organic causes and patients with emotional and behavioral problems reported much higher rates ($M$ = 13.2 and 22.5, respectively). However, a causal relation between high stress levels and recurrent pain or emotional or behavioral problems cannot be assumed, due to the cross-sectional nature of the study. Nevertheless, these findings were quite consistent with those obtained by Hodges, Kline, Barbero, and Flanery (1984), who reported a significant relation between life stress and recurrent pain (without organic cause) in adolescence.

In a prospective study, Padilla, Rohsenow, and Bergman (1976) explored the relation between life stress and accident frequency in a sample of 103 seventh-grade boys. Subjects were asked to complete the Coddington scale and were interviewed weekly over a 5-month period about the occurrence and severity of any accidents they experienced. Results showed that early adolescent boys who experienced higher levels of life-changes reported having significantly more accidents than did boys with low life change scores. Life stress was found to be a stronger predictor of accident frequency than an index of risk taking. Because accidents are a major cause of death among adolescents, this finding is particularly important. In a study that specifically dealt with accidental athletic injuries, Coddington and Troxell (1980) obtained life stress scores for the previous 12 months in 114 high school football players and followed these students to determine the frequencies of their athletic injuries during the subsequent football season. Adolescents who experienced critical life events such as parental illness, separation, divorce, and death in the family were found to be more likely to sustain significant athletic injuries than those who did not experience such events. These findings suggest that one effect of major stressors is the reduction of personal or parental vigilance that leads to ignoring relevant environmental cues that, if approximately processed, might have helped to prevent these accidents.

Several studies dealt with the association between chronic illness and critical life events. An especially high incidence of critical life events was found in children and adolescents afflicted with cancer (Eiser, 1990). In the first study designed by Green (1954), 31 of 33 pediatric patients with leukemia experienced major losses and separations 2 years preceding the onset of the illness. One half of these losses were reported to occur within 6 months before the onset of the disease. In another study, Johnson (1986) found that the mean score of critical life events in a group of adolescent cancer patients was more than double the mean found for the healthy control group. Some of the most frequently named events were marital separation or death of a close family member (52% in the cancer group compared to 16% in the control group), change in residence

(72% vs. 24%), and change in health of family members (60% vs. 24%). Although these findings cannot be construed as evidence of a causal relation between life stress and cancer, they impressively demonstrate the cumulation of stressful events in adolescents who must cope with a major event—chronic illness.

The studies presented so far primarily dealt with the association between life events and the onset of physical illness. Although this association was not confirmed for most other chronic illnesses, the impact of major stressors on the course of the illness was frequently demonstrated. Several studies of diabetic samples (see chap. 7, this volume) showed that critical life events are associated with difficulties in diabetic control, at least in patients with juvenile onset of diabetes. In the Brand, Johnson, and Johnson (1986) study, the relation between life stress and diabetic control was investigated in 141 adolescents attending a 2-week diabetes summer camp. Life-stress measures for 1 year preceding camp were obtained using the Johnson and McCutcheon (1980) Life Events Checklist, and a number of measures were generated reflecting diabetic control (e.g., blood and urine sugar levels, and Hemoglobin $A_1$ levels). In addition, adolescents' perceptions of control over their environments were assessed. The results suggested that life stress had a more adverse impact on adolescents who perceived themselves as having little control over their environments. In a more recent study of 120 diabetic adolescents, Ingersoll, Orr, Vance, and Golden (1992) found that those who reported more frequent negative life events were more likely to have poorer metabolic control. The correlation between negative life events and poor metabolic control amounted to $r = .25$. Taken together, the research findings suggest a relationship between cumulative life changes and adolescent health status. While the strongest association between life events and the onset of chronic illness was empirically verified in cancer patients, the negative impact of critical life events over the course of the chronic illness was found in several studies of patients with other chronic diseases (see also chap. 7, this volume). Although the physiological mechanisms of these associations were not clarified, it appears that not a single event, but rather the accumulation of several severe stressors results in impaired health, especially in individuals with low perceived control.

Research on other types of stressors is meager. Although studies on adult samples confirmed that minor events or everyday stressors negatively affect physical health (see Kohn, La Greniere, & Gurevich, 1991 for a summary), no study to date analyzed this relationship in adolescent samples. This is an important research gap because most adolescents encounter normative stressors and strains in adolescence and only some experience major life events. An accumulation of critical life events, in particular, events involving loss, is more common in adults.

***Stressful Events and Psychopathology.*** In attempting to understand the association between stressful events and emotional or behavioral problems, more research was devoted to examining different types of stressors, especially during recent years. Much like research with adults, early investigations of stressful events in adolescence emphasized the role of discrete, major life events like experiencing parental divorce, moving to a new home, or experiencing death of relatives, rather than the role of minor stressors such as doing chores, having parental restrictions, or getting bad grades in school. The majority of early studies in this area were cross-sectional in design and found a moderate association between major life events and a variety of types of psychological maladjustment (for reviews, see Compas, 1987; Johnson, 1986). Correlations between stressful events and emotional or behavior problems were typically found in the range of $r = .20$ to .40, thus paralleling results reported in studies of major life events in adults (see, e.g., Thoits, 1983). Although these early studies were useful in providing a foundation for research on adolescent stress, results obtained in cross-sectional studies cannot be used as evidence that stressful events are a risk factor for developing emotional or behavior problems. In order to establish a link between stress and psychopathology, a prospective longitudinal research design is required. However, longitudinal designs do not solve the problems of confounded measures or constructs (see Compas, 1987; Johnson, 1986).

In the first prospective study in this area, Gersten, Langner, Eisenberg, and Simcha-Fagan (1977) found that life events did not explain any of the variance in behavior problems after parental and family variables have been accounted for. Cohen, Burt, and Bjorck (1987) and Swearingen and Cohen (1985) also did not find an association between young adolescents' self-reports of major life events and self-reported anxiety or depression 5 months after controlling for initial levels of anxiety and depression. However, Cohen et al. (1987) found that self-reports of negative events at the second time point accounted for a small (5%) yet significant proportion of the variance in depression and anxiety, after controlling for initial self-reports of depression and anxiety obtained 5 months earlier. Siegel and Brown (1988) and Compas, Howell, Phares, Williams, and Giunta (1989) provided stronger support for the role of stress as a risk factor in young adolescents. Siegel and Brown (1988) examined the association of minor events or daily stressors with self-reported depressed mood and physical illness in a sample of early adolescent girls at two points in time 9 months apart. Stressful events at the first time predicted later depressed moods for the younger adolescents, and for the whole sample, stressful events predicted depression in interaction with positive events. Negative events predicted physical symptoms only in interaction with four positive events. That is, negative events were predictive of maladjustment only in the presence of low levels of positive events.

Generally, negative events are shown to have a stronger link to adjustment and health indicators than positive events. However, most studies focused on negative outcome indicators, so that the relative contributions of negative and positive events to health remain unknown. Moreover, the role of normative stressors was not given equal attention. One exception is the study by Compas, Howell, Phares, Williams, and Giunta (1989), which investigated the relations between both major stressful events and minor events or daily stressors on early adolescents' self-reports of internalizing and externalizing syndromes, as well as mothers' reports of their children's emotional and behavior problems, in two surveys separated by a 9-month time span. The association between self-reported stressful events and self-reports of emotional or behavior problems was significant at the second time point, with stress accounting for 11% of the variance in emotional and behavior problems after controlling for initial levels of problems. Furthermore, stressful events reported in the first assessment predicted emotional and behavior problems 9 months later, accounting for 2% of the variance, again controlling for initial emotional and behavior problems. Analysis of data at the second time point indicated that daily (but not major) stressors were predictive of emotional and behavior problems; a similar pattern emerged for the prediction of problems at the second time point. Stressful events predicted self-reports of both internalizing and externalizing problems, whereby the trend was stronger for internalizing problems.

In summary, prospective studies of the links between different types of stressors and symptomatology generated mixed findings. In some studies, the effects of minor events or normative stressors on psychological symptoms were stronger than the effects of major events or critical life events. The contribution of critical life events compared to minor stressors in predicting health outcome was more clear in studies focusing on a special type of psychopathology—adolescent depression. Compas, Orosan, and Grant (1993) reported that over 40 studies documented findings supporting the hypothesis that stressful events occurring in adolescence produce negative emotional states such as depressive mood or depression. Such a relationship was found to exist in studies during which stress was operationalized as accumulation of critical life events or nonnormative events (Cohen et al., 1987) as well as in those examining normative events or everyday hassles (Compas, Howell, Phares, Williams, & Ledoux, 1989).

One of the most well-known studies was conducted by Newcomb et al. (1981), who investigated the effects of 39 critical life events (such as death of a relative, divorce of parents, relocation of household) in 1,000 adolescents. These authors found that critical life events and depression were positively correlated ($r$ = .20). Subsequent studies established that the relation between critical life events and the appearance of depressive symptomatology is considerably weaker (between $r$ = .20 and $r$ = .30) than that between everyday stressors and depression (between $r$ = .50 and $r$ =. 60). Evidence to support this view was obtained in both clinical and nonclinical samples. In one of our own studies (Seiffge-Krenke, 1995), we investigated the relation between different stressors and depression in a nonclinical sample of 136 adolescents 12 to 17 years old and found that the correlation between depression and critical life events was quite low ($r$ = .19) In contrast, more commonly occurring stressors, such as arguments with the parents, bad grades, or breaking up with a boyfriend or a girlfriend, correlated quite strongly with depression ($r$ = .60). Thus, the contribution of non-normative stressors to explaining variance in depression was less than that of normative stressors. These findings encourage the view that development-related stress plays a predominant role in the etiology of depressive illnesses in adolescence. In this study, relationship stressors were perceived as the most stressful of all normative stressors.

Similarly, Siddique and D'Arcy (1984) examined the relations between perceived everyday stress in family, school, and peer group situations and measures of psychological well-being such as anxiety and depression. They found that family stress had the strongest negative health impact. Masten et al. (1994) further differentiated among negative, ambiguous, and chronic stressors and assessed adolescents' and their mothers' evaluations of these types of stressors. Based on the adolescents' evaluations, chronic negative stressors showed the highest impact on mental health problems ($r$ = .38) and externalizing ($r$ = .42) and internalizing symptoms ($r$ = .38). Correlations between mothers' reports of different types of stressors and adolescents' adjustment problems were also positive but not as high. These findings demonstrate the importance of distinguishing between types of stressors with respect to frequency, impact, and chronicity. Furthermore, future research efforts should take into account that the different types of stressors are not independent of one another, and thus are oriented to an integrated model of stress (see, e.g., Wagner, Compas, & Howell, 1988).

## CONTEXT EFFECTS: NEW CHALLENGES FOR HEALTH?

The different types of stressors and their effects on physical and psychological health having been described, this section discusses the question of whether adolescents today are subjected to more stress than in the past. The role of context and situational factors in stress and coping is critically important, especially because the living conditions and social environments of adolescents today have dramatically changed since the 1950s, 1960s, and 1970s.

### Historical Changes and Macrosocial Stressors

In all modern Western societies, there have been considerable changes in the tasks and demands with which the adolescent is confronted. These changes are partly related to the fulfillment of certain developmental tasks, and to conflicting demands inherent in these tasks. These changes are further complicated by others associated with modern-day living conditions, as reflected, for example, by the increasing numbers of single-parent families or stepfamilies, increasing rates of unemployment and economic hardship, and the continuous migration of families of rural or poorer background into societies with high Western standards.

***Changes in Various Developmental Tasks.*** The transition from childhood to adolescence changed in qualitative and quantitative aspects. First, the time span allowed for this transition varies depending on the specific tasks the adolescent is confronted with and on his or her physical maturity. For example, over the years, the age at which adolescents complete their education and professional training in schools, academies, or universities has steadily increased, so that adolescents today begin to enter the workforce much later than several decades ago. This trend resulted in the fact that most adolescents today do not begin to seek employment or start to earn their own living until they are in their early 20s. This extension of the phase of moratorium (Marcia, 1980), past adolescence and into adulthood, means that adolescents deal with a variety of other normative developmental tasks (Havighurst, 1972) such as the development of heterosexual relationships. Physical maturity is accelerated, and due to more liberal norms and values in most Western societies, adolescents are allowed to begin heterosexual relationships earlier than in the past decades (see chap. 4, this volume). Several decades ago, the time between physical maturation and the assumption of the adult role was relatively short, as is still the case in underdeveloped countries. Today, due to accelerated physical maturation, extended schooling and training, and the postponement of marriage, this time span varies from 10 years to 15 years. In this regard, it is important to acknowledge the early contributions of Blos (1954) and Keniston (1975), who pointed out the danger of the pathologically prolonged and protracted adolescence. On the other hand, it is possible for adolescents to experience heterosexual relationships earlier nowadays and to establish an independent household while being financially dependent on their parents. Especially for early maturing adolescents, there is a potential danger of developing "too much, too soon" (Galambos & Tilton-Weaver, 1996, p. 2). Potential health risks are thus likely to be associated with a pathologically prolonged, as well as a reduced, time span for adolescent development.

The adolescent's ability to deal with these developmental tasks is naturally impaired by the fact that such tasks are seldom explicitly defined and subject to change. In addition, in modern, democratic societies, there is a noticeable trend toward value pluralism, calling, on the one hand, for positive, tolerance-promoting values, and, on the other hand, leading to the disintegration of existing value systems. In the wake of this development, traditional cultural norms lose much of their social regulatory importance. Adolescents are left with a vaguely defined behavior codex or lack a framework from which they orient their actions and in which they solve their age-specific developmental tasks. Thus, adolescents are confronted with a complex problem-solving process whose outcome remains relatively open and undefined. On the one hand, this offers the adolescents greater possibilities of shaping their own personality; on the other hand, increased freedom becomes stressful, because an open and unstructured developmental process elicits various insecurities and irritations. In addition, adolescents often feel pressured to make hasty decisions whose long-term consequences are not predictable.

***Fears About the Future.*** Despite the achievements in technological and medical sectors, a secured material affluence, and a high standard of living, modern industrial and urban developments have made it difficult for adolescents to shape their futures. Environmental destruction, the threat of war, unstable economic developments, and AIDS are perceived by many adolescents as threatening. Such threats, however, are not perceived or experienced by all adolescents in the same manner. Thus, whereas adolescents in crisis areas and underdeveloped nations consider such problems to be existentially threatening, adolescents in more politically stable regions of the world, for example, in the Federal Republic of Germany, develop anticipatory fears.

This trend was indicated by two more recent, representative studies that investigated the fears about the future among adolescents in the Federal Republic of Germany (IJF, 1990). The adolescents participating in these studies felt threatened by increasing environmental destruction and the danger of a nuclear catastrophe (e.g., explosion of a nuclear reactor or nuclear war). According to a study conducted by the Institute for Research on Adolescence (Institut für Jugendforschung, 1990), that interviewed adolescents 14 to 17 years old, the most significant health problems were related to environmental pollution, drugs, and AIDS. It is worth mentioning that fears about potential health risks, (e.g., becoming infected with the AIDS virus) were highest among those adolescents who had the lowest probabilities of developing AIDS. This mismatch between risk and fear was termed *AIDS phobia*. Also, anticipatory fears of becoming unemployed were higher in the younger as compared to the older adolescents. The IJF study also showed a clear discrepancy between adolescents' general fears about the future and their individual expectations about the future. Despite their concern about ecological problems, adolescents were basically quite optimistic about their own futures. The differences observed between the degree of global threat and personal consequences are related to the abstract nature of the threat itself. Also, adolescents attempt to deal with a less discrete threat that is not under their direct control by disregarding it, preferring to remain optimistic about the future. In this regard, the findings of Klingman et al. (1991), obtained in a study of Israeli adolescents who were interviewed directly before and after the nuclear reactor catastrophe in Chernobyl, are interesting. After the tragedy occurred, adolescents showed less interest in dealing with the threat of nuclear reactor accidents, which the authors interpreted as a sign of intense denial or repression of the actual event.

***Living Under Dangerous and Insecure Conditions.*** The more diffuse global, social threats and fears represent important background variables for the adolescent's overall well-being and general expectations about the future. The stressful or health-damaging effects of these macrosocial stressors, however, can only be demonstrated in adolescents who are directly affected by these stressors. The strongest effects on the emotional and physical health of adolescents are observed in regions experiencing wartime conditions and chronic political conflicts: Everyday existence here is fraught with intensely traumatizing experiences. Since the early study by A. Freud and Burlingham (1943), there has been a growing body of research findings and clinical observations that indicate that youths growing up in wartime conditions and other forms of crises adapt in ways that produce developmental impairment, physical damage, and emotional trauma (Goleman, 1986; Rosenblatt, 1983). The ongoing conflict between Israel and Palestine is one such impressive example. In his summarizing essay, "Youth in Dangerous Environments: Coping With the Consequences," Garbarino (1990) reported on a study conducted by Punamaki (1987) of Israeli and Palestinian children living near the border between Israel and the West Bank, the so-called "Green Line." Not only the physical injuries resulting from violent confrontations, but also the constant stream of traumatizing events (such as death of or injury to relatives or acquaintances) were found to lead to serious emotional disorders and anxiety disorders among the Palestinian children and adolescents. Similarly, children and adolescents exposed to the stress of extreme violence develop mental health problems years after the experience (Goleman, 1986). For example, a follow-up study of Cambodian children who experienced the moral and psychological devastation of the Pol Pot regime in the 1970s revealed that 4 years after leaving Cambodia, 50% developed posttraumatic stress disorders (Garbarino, 1990).

***Immigration.*** The health status of adolescents is also adversely affected by less traumatizing stressors related to social and political conditions. Throughout the world, many families are encouraged or forced to leave their homes and emigrate to other countries. For example, the migration of people from Eastern to Western regions of Europe has persisted over the decades, so that today, most Western-European nations are multiethnic, multicultural societies comparable to those existing in the United States.

Mental health professionals frequently reported signs of distress in the immigrant child (see, e.g., Ashworth, 1982). In attempting to explain such problems, researchers focused on two main aspects of immigration. Immigration is viewed as a situation involving many possible stressors, such as loss of familiar surroundings, changes in lifestyle and climate, and discrimination. *Acculturation*, the psychosocial process of adapting to a new culture, involves many challenges such as learning new languages, observing the local norms of social interaction, and wrestling with new values. Jerusalem (1992) termed the strains experienced by adolescents who have emigrated from their countries of origin "acculturation stress" (p. 16). According to Jerusalem, *acculturation stress* is characterized by insecurity about residence status, unfavorable educational and employment opportunities, substandard living conditions, language difficulties, and low social acceptance. In his study of 305 German and 133 Turkish male adolescents, Jerusalem found that the psychosocial status of Turkish adolescents was clearly worse: These young men had lower self-esteem and were lonely and apprehensive. In addition, many of the Turkish adolescents had a poor command of German, and their lack of proficiency in this foreign language made their day-to-day lives very stressful.

This result confirms studies conducted in the United States, showing that immigrant children are more distressed than nonimmigrant children, showing greater problems associated with low self-esteem and nervousness, frequent physical illness, school difficulties, and juvenile delinquency. However, there are also reports that immigrant youths are not more distressed than nonimmigrant peers (for a summary, see Touliatos & Lindholm, 1980). The study conducted by Chin, Feldman, and Rosenthal (1992) of different samples of Chinese immigrant youths in the United States and Australia showed that parental behavior and support had a beneficial role in moderating the negative effects of stressors experienced by the immigrant youths. The acculturation of values is particularly stressful for youths because immigration from East to West typically implies a shift toward individuation and autonomy, which has not yet been experienced by the youths coming from more traditional countries (Feldman, Mont-Reynaud, & Rosenthal, 1992).

***Poverty.*** Poverty creates a potentially dangerous threat for adolescent development. Health conditions become clearly worse under conditions of poverty. Malnutrition, higher rates of illnesses, especially infectious ones, and low access to hospitals, in part due to lack of insurance further complicate this threat. It is frequently demonstrated that poor people are more often sick and suffer multiple conditions and complications compared to those who are well off (for a summary, see Freund & McGuire, 1991). Since the early studies by Elder (1974), the links between economic hardship in the family and childrens' emotional well-being have been well-established. Troubled relationships develop under these conditions and further contribute to the stressors of poverty. In a more recent study, Ge et al. (1992) were able to show that economic hardship had a direct effect on the quality of marital relationships, which, in turn, disrupted and undermined parent–child relationships. In a study of 451 families living in the rural midwest of the United States, they examined the negative impact of financial problems on early adolescents' symptoms of psychological distress. Parents' and adolescents' negative feelings about their relationships tended to increase adolescent psychological distress. The results, however, did not lend strong support to the hypothesis that economic pressure directly affects adolescents' well-being. The diminished quality of marital and parent–child relationships, however, represents a significant pathway by which economic hardship places adolescents at risk for psychological dysfunction.

It is well-known that poverty is linked with various health-detrimental behaviors. The data collected in the National Adolescent Student Health survey (NASH, 1989) in more than 11,000 eighth- and tenth-grade students nationwide indicated a relation between poverty and increased risk of substance use (i.e., alcohol, cigarettes, and drugs) or risk-taking behaviors (e.g., using a gun for any reason, or riding in a car whose driver is under the influence of alcohol or drugs). Moreover, an association between teenage parenthood and subsequent poverty was noted for several decades (Anderson Moore et al., 1993). Early childbearing is more common among women from disadvantaged backgrounds. Moreover, teenage childbearing increases the probability of poverty over and above the risk due to background factors (e.g., the highest grade completed in school, womens' earnings, or the number of children).

***Violence in Social Settings.*** Another stress factor concerns violence in the family, neighborhood, and, in particular, school. School size was recognized as a factor affecting adolescents' adjustment to the transition from primary to secondary school. In most instances, adolescents enter a larger and more complex school environment. In any case, new students are the novice group. In studies in the United States, Britain, and Australia, young adolescents making the transition to secondary school described themselves in deprecatory terms, which suggests their sense of insignificance, powerlessness, and alienation as newcomers to the high school environment (Cotterell, 1992). Moreover, students attending high schools often witness or are subjected to bullying, extortion, and threats with weapons by other schoolmates in and out of the classroom. Bullying and victim problems among pupils are not recent developments; they have been an issue of great concern in Scandinavia for almost 20 years (Olweus, 1978, 1990). Investigators in Sweden and Norway reported a strong increase in bullying over this time span. According to the Bergen studies conducted by Olweus, more than 83,000 high school students or 15% of the total in Norwegian schools were involved in bullying incidents: 3% were bullying about once a week or more, 9% were victims, and 2% were both bullies and victims (Olweus, 1990). In general, the percentage of students who were bullied decreased with higher grades, that is, the younger and weaker students were the most threatened. Moreover, a considerable amount of bullying was committed by older students. The consequences of bullying on victims' health are dramatic (e.g., body complaints, suicidal ideation, and attempted suicide) and led to various intervention programs in school.

Violence in the family was frequently linked to health problems in adolescents and is now recognized as a major social problem in the United States. Interspousal aggression was found to be highly associated with parent–child aggression (Straus, Gelles, & Steinmetz, 1980). Although witnessing interspousal aggression did not have direct effects on psychological and somatic health, parent–child aggression was found to be related to various health problems in children and adolescents (e.g., anxiety, withdrawal, conduct problems, and hyperactivity; see Jouriles, Barling, & O'Leary, 1987).

Over the last 10 years, literature on family violence has grown enormously (see Spatz Widom, 1989 for a summary). The cycle of violence was carefully examined, and there is much evidence indicating, that abused children and adolescents become abusers, and victims of violence become violent offenders. The acknowledgment of the existence of child and adolescent perpetrators of sexual abuse is relatively recent and followed several years after the recognition of adult sexual abuse in the United States and Great Britain (for a summary, see Vizard, Monck, & Misch, 1995).

***Unemployment.*** Unemployment is another macrosocial stress factor affecting many adolescents today. Since the 1970s, joblessness has increased and persisted to become a structural problem, especially affecting socially disadvantaged adolescents and, above all, young women. About 20% of young people in Western Europe are without jobs. In the Federal Republic of Germany, about 25% to 30% of all registered jobless individuals are under 25 years old (Klink & Kieselbach, 1990; Vonderach, 1989). The rate of unemployment among adolescents in England has reached levels above the average for Western Europe. Unemployment among young people in Spain is also very high—about 48% (Kieselbach & Svensson, 1988). Youth unemployment is currently considered to be one of the greatest social problems in the Western world. Despite its magnitude, little research is devoted to studying the effects of unemployment on young people's health. In many instances, it is often difficult to discern whether unemployment contributes to symptoms of illness or if it is a result of already impaired health. Nevertheless, a link between youth unemployment and psychological disorders was found both in cross-sectional (Patton & Noller, 1984) and longitudinal research studies (Finlay-Jones & Eckhardt, 1984).

Based on their longitudinal studies of Australian and British adolescents, Klink and Kieselbach (1990) concluded that "the experience of unemployment among adolescents is a causal factor behind emotional stress and psychiatric morbidity" (p. 28). However, no clear effects on somatic health were found (McPherson & Wayne, 1983). With increased duration of unemployment (and depending on the individual coping resources), adolescents may develop feelings of anger, fear, loneliness, and depression, which increase the likelihood that they become involved in social activities potentially damaging to their health (e.g., smoking, drinking alcoholic beverages, or experimenting with drugs). Diekstra (1990) linked the suicide rates for adolescents and young adults in the majority of Northwest and Central European countries with the increase in unemployment in these same countries. Only a small percentage of unemployed young people commit or attempt suicide. In a 5-year, follow-up study of 1,083 Swedish adolescents, Hammarström (1990) investigated the effects of unemployment on health, thereby attempting to determine the mechanisms by which such effects are mediated. Compared to adolescents who were working, studying, or participating in an occupational training program, the unemployed adolescents showed significantly increased rates of psychological symptoms and alcohol consumption. Subsequent LISREL analyses demonstrated a causal relation among these two symptoms and unemployment. Serious illness (such as diabetes) was also analyzed, but the results did not suggest any causal relation between serious physical illness and unemployment. As in the case of other macrosocial stressors, there is no monocausal relation between unemployment and impaired health. Nevertheless, there is enough evidence to suggest that unemployment is a stressor that increases the adolescent's risk for impaired health or at least for engaging in activities that are deleterious to health.

### Is There More Stress Today?

We just discussed how in recent years changed living conditions introduced some new kinds of stressors. Can one thus conclude that life today is more stressful for most adolescents than it was in the past? The conditions of rising adolescent unemployment, higher rates of divorce, and a continued migration of families to Western industrial nations do indeed indicate that adolescents today are growing up in living conditions that are quite different from those in the past. Over the past 20 years, there has been an alarming increase in adolescent suicide (Holinger & Offer, 1982), adolescent drug and alcohol use (Novacek, Raskin, & Hogan, 1991), and adolescent depression (Allgood-Merten, Lewinsohn, & Hops, 1990). Although there are a variety of reasons for these increases, it is suggested that higher rates in morbidity and mortality, compared to the rates a few decades ago, are a direct result of increased stress.

To this date, no studies were conducted to determine if and how adolescents' perceptions of stress caused by critical life events or nonnormative stressors changed over the last decades. The high rates of youth unemployment and parental divorce, as well as changes in familial structure, indicate that the event parameters changed for a few critical life events, which, compared to several decades ago, are occurring very often (Seiffge-Krenke, 1995). However, this does not mean that these events are perceived as less stressful.

In contrast, there is a good body of information concerning how normative stressors have been perceived by adolescents with different cultural and socioeconomic backgrounds over the years. In the existing literature on adolescence spanning 20 years, several sources of stress were reported. Normative stressors emanating from the family, school, and peer group are considered to be of particular relevance (Compas et al., 1993; Siddique & D'Arcy, 1984; Stern & Zevon, 1990). Most studies found that female adolescents tend to perceive greater stress in most domains; in particular, they worry more about disagreements with parents, acceptance by peers, relationships with the opposite gender, and their academic performance (Burke & Weir, 1978; Frydenberg & Lewis, 1993; Siddique & D'Arcy, 1984). Such basic gender differences, as well as the types of normative events considered as most stressful, were also reported by European investigators. For example, in several studies of over 3,000 adolescents from different European countries, we analyzed everyday stress, such as problems in school, disputes with parents and friends, conflicts in relationships with the opposite gender, future-oriented problems, and so forth by means of the Problem Questionnaire (Seiffge-Krenke, 1995). A cross-cultural analysis revealed that future-oriented problems uniformly ranked first, followed by problems with parents and problems with friends. In some samples, school-related problems were even more stressful than problems with parents or friends. In all studies, such future-oriented problems were related to personal fears and worries (e.g., fear of unemployment or being unsure about the choice of future occupation) or general apprehensions about increasing environmental pollution and possible threat of war. The item with the highest mean value in all samples was Item 13: "The increasing destruction of the environment makes me afraid."

Figure 5.1 presents the results for a German sample of 1,028 adolescents aged 12 to 20 years. In this sample, future-related problems, identity problems, and relationship stressors ranked highest. In another study (Jansen, 1992), adolescents residing in regions of former East

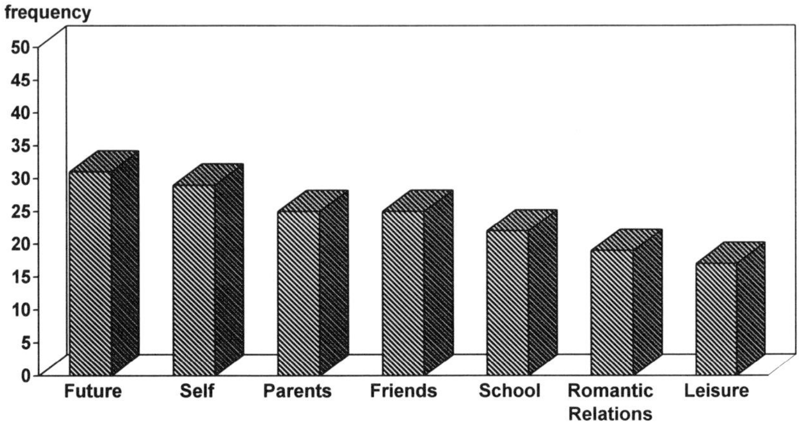


FIG. 5.1. Ranking of stressful problems named by 1,028 adolescents.

Germany after the opening of the borders showed an exponential increase in the frequency with which they reported future-oriented problems. This normative stressor was virtually unknown to them before the unification of East and West Germany. What is surprising is that these kinds of worries about the future were found to exist in earlier studies in the United States and the Netherlands using comparable instruments (see, e.g., McKay, 1977; Mönks, 1968; Remmers, 1962; Remmers & Shimberg, 1954). It is thus interesting to note that these fears about the future seemed to be present in adolescents coming from quite different cultural backgrounds, although the living conditions for adolescents have changed over the past 30 to 40 years. The findings converge in showing that young people are very much concerned about their own futures and the general development of society. Political and future events were also quoted spontaneously in interviews we have conducted more recently (Seiffge-Krenke, 1995). Although adolescents differ according to what they perceive as stressful, the marked continuity in basic rankings of normative stressors is remarkable and suggests a universality of stress perception over time and across nations. That is, despite increases or changes in macrostressors, the basic concern about the normative stressors of this developmental phase remained the same.

This is a remarkable finding that was identified in other domains, too (e.g., in sexual attitudes; Moore & Rosenthal, 1993 and in types of conflict between parents and adolescents; Montemayor, 1986). Since the early Middletown study in 1929, such conflicts have been strikingly similar (Hill & Holmbeck, 1986; Lynd & Lynd, 1929). As Hill and Holmbeck ironically noted, “parents and adolescents have quarreled for decades about mundane issues like hair, garbage, dishes, and galoshes” (1986, p. 158). Not only have the topics remained more or less constant, but also the frequency of parent–adolescent conflict has not increased significantly over the decades. The major concerns in this developmental phase have not changed much. Similarly, the sequence of what is perceived as most stressful basically remained the same for decades.

In examining these findings, it becomes clear that despite the enormous technological, medical, and social advances that were made in industrialized nations, such as the United States and Germany, the amount of stress in adolescents' lives today has not decreased or increased. It simply changed qualitatively. Thus, although adolescents today are less threatened by insufficient material security or poor health care, they are confronted with various psychological and social stress factors that adversely affect their well-being. In addition, macrosocial stress factors, which for the most part are not under the individual's control, greatly determine the adolescent's developmental context. Taking the research findings presented in this chapter together, the discrepancies are remarkable. While adolescents are comparably healthy, their well-being is considerably impaired and their body complaints are frequent. Moreover, there are indications of a universality in the perception of normative stress; that is, the sequence of everyday problems that are perceived as stressful generally remained the same over the past decades. This surprising result stands in contrast to findings indicating changing life conditions for adolescents living in Western industrialized nations. The fearful anticipations about the future that adolescents have shown over decades are related to these changes. The enormous importance of macrosocial stressors for adolescents is very clear, and it is obvious that adolescents are more sensitive than other age groups to these macrosocial changes.

# 6

# Social Support and Coping Style as Risk and Protective Factors

One implication of the results presented in the preceding chapter is that stressful experiences alone are insufficient to explain negative health outcome. In discussing this issue, a brief description of the concepts of social support and coping and a summary of findings regarding the buffering effect of social support are provided. In addition, findings on developmental patterns of coping during adolescence are reviewed. Although some coping strategies serve protective functions by reducing a stressor's negative effects, others exacerbate the effects of stress and thus represent additional risk factors. Therefore, in the last section of this chapter, the function of avoidant coping for specific clinical groups in dealing with stressful situations is illustrated. To this end, we draw on data collected during comprehensive studies on stress and coping in adolescence. These findings help show how dysfunctional coping styles also have important implications for seeking social support.

## FACTORS MEDIATING THE EFFECTS OF STRESS ON HEALTH

Over the last decades, few areas of research appeared as promising as that on social support, social support networks, and health. Hundreds of studies conducted with adults suggest that social support enhances both physical and psychological well-being and buffers the negative effects of life stress. In contrast, research only recently began to address the question of whether supportive relationships with parents, friends, teachers, and significant others affect the adolescents' health. Problems of definition and measurement made it especially difficult to conduct this research. As such, this chapter begins with a selective review of the social support literature as it relates to the assessment and conceptualization of support. In addition, different models that attempt to conceptualize the relation between stress and social support are presented.

### Social Support

Social support was hailed an important mediating variable in the relation between psychosocial stress and psychological and somatic symptoms (Thoits, 1982). In spite of a large body of research pointing to the importance of social support in managing stress and maintaining personal well-being, a number of fundamental conceptual and methodological problems were neglected. A variety of theoretical concepts and numerous methodological approaches make the results very difficult to compare. In the brief overview that follows, we attempt to clarify this theoretical disparity.

***The Concept of Social Support.*** Procidano and Heller (1983) distinguished between social network and perceived social support. The social network is described according to aspects of a more structural nature (such as size, depth, and complexity) as well as its functional characteristics (e.g., providing information, emotional support, and instrumental aid). Perceived support is, in contrast, the amount to which an individual believes that his or her needs for information, assistance, and feedback are met. Thus, perceived support represents an important factor in the individual appraisal of a stressful situation and subsequent coping. In their taxonomy of social relationships, similar to that provided by Procidano and Heller (1983), Lazarus and Folkman (1991) distinguished between emotional support (e.g., showing empathy and understanding) and instrumental support (e.g., giving advice). A more developmentally related differentiation was provided by Cotterell (1992), who described different types of support and network structures from which children and adolescents obtain support. According to this approach, a description of social network entails the consideration of the different sources of support available to and used by different age groups. Social network structure can also be described in terms of different provider systems (e.g., relatives [especially parents], friends, and nonrelated adults).

The social exchanges between an adolescent and these different support groups are likely to differ. Cauce and Strebnik (1989) distinguished three main network structures through which support is channeled to adolescents: formal structures of support (including school personnel) and two informal structures of support (family and friends). As individuals grow older, the relative importance of these support providers changes. Family support is more important during childhood; friends and other nonkin agents become more significant sources of support during adolescence (see also chap. 2, this volume). Having friends and being included in the peer group are among adolescent's most important concerns. Not surprisingly, the business of building peer relations consumes a great deal of time. Larson and Richards (1991) found that adolescents spend noticeably less free time with their parents and prefer to engage in activities with these close friends and peers. However, being with the crowd does not guarantee psychological well-being; it is having a secure relationship with intimate peers that is a protective factor in times of stress. Claes (1992) found that emotional adjustment was related to the number of intimate friends and heterosexual partners, and not to the number of acquaintances in an adolescents' social network. In addition, it is useful to describe social support according to so-called "objective variables" (such as size and depth) and "subjective variables" (perceived support), because both aspects strongly deviate from one another. In a study analyzing the use of social support groups for adolescent diabetics, Marrero et al. (1982) found that perceived support was very important. The participants often reported that they were able to carry over the skills and insights learned in the group to their daily lives. The support value of the group for the diabetic adolescents was also reflected by the very high degree of participation.

In this respect, it is important to address the problem of confounding between social support and symptomatology. To the extent that measures of social support and symptoms overlap in content and method, the association between these variables is spuriously high. The problem of confounded measures is especially serious when investigating the relation between social support and psychological symptoms, in particular depression. Statements intended to describe or measure satisfaction with available support, may in fact be viewed as constituting a measure of the individual's pessimism. Most existing social support studies employed depression as a main indicator of psychological outcome. For example, among the 57 studies reviewed by Cohen and Wills (1985), 44 studies used a self-report depression measure as a dependent variable. It is therefore important to consider whether the social support construct, and in particular satisfaction with social support, represents clusters of depressive symptoms. A multitrait–multimethod approach, according to which several aspects of social support are assessed using different methods such as interviews and questionnaires (e.g., Barrera,

1981; Slavin & Compas, 1989), is necessary. In their study, Slavin and Compas (1989) were able to demonstrate moderate convergent validity between more quantitative social support variables (e.g., available network, or utilized network) and depression with coefficients ranging from –.34 to –.51 in a sample of late adolescents. The correlations between satisfaction with support and depression ranged from –.29 to –.58.

***Stress, Social Support, and the Buffering Hypothesis.*** This distinction between availability of social support and perceived support is also relevant when analyzing the relation between stress management and adaptation. Cohen and Wills (1985) presented two conceptual models of stress and support—the main effect model and the buffer model. The concept of the *buffer model* focuses on the perceived availability of social resources. According to this model, social support intervenes between stressful events and stress reactions by reducing or preventing a stress appraisal. That is, the perception that others can and will provide necessary resources redefines the potential for harm posed by a situation. In contrast, the *main effect model* expects that social support results in a positive outcome, irrespective of the stress level at hand. Numerous studies indicate that people with spouses, friends, and family members who provide psychological and material resources enjoy better health than those with fewer supportive social contacts (see the reviews by Leavy, 1983; Thoits, 1982). A generalized beneficial effect of social support could occur because large social networks provide persons with regular positive experiences, a sense of predictability and stability in their life situation, and a recognition of self-worth. Integration in a social network also helps an individual avoid negative experiences that otherwise increase the probability of psychological and physical disorders. This kind of social network support also is related to physical illness outcomes through emotionally induced effects on neuroendocrine or immune system functioning (Jemmott & Locke, 1984) or through influence on health-related behavior patterns such as cigarette smoking, consumption of alcoholic beverages, or seeking medical care (Krantz, Grunberg, & Baum, 1985).

In an extreme version, the main effect model postulates that merely an increase in social support results in an increase in well-being, irrespective of the previous level of support. Although a single stressful event in itself does not place great demands on the coping abilities of most persons, when multiple stressors accumulate, persist, and strain the coping capacities of the individual, the potential for serious disorders increases. Feelings of helplessness arise because of the perceived inability to cope with events that demand an effective response. Social support alleviates the impact of stress appraisal by providing a solution of the problem, reducing the perceived importance of the problem, or stabilizing the neuroendocrine system, so that people are less reactive to perceived stress or apply facilitating healthful behavior (House, 1981).

Cohen and Wills (1985) named four support resources that operate as stress buffers: *emotional support* (information that indicates caring and acceptance), *informational support* (help in defining, understanding, and coping with stressful events), *social companionship* (spending time with others in leisure and recreational activities), and *instrumental support* (the provision of financial aid, material resources, and needed services). Although support functions can be conceptually distinguished, they are not usually independent of one another in natural settings. As outlined in the preceding section, the function of social support varies with age. In adolescence, social companionship is particularly important. This dimension has also been referred to as *belongingness*. It reduces stress by fulfilling a need for affiliation and contact with others, by helping to distract persons from worrying about problems, or by facilitating positive affective moods.

Despite the fact that the respective influence of parents and peers changes in adolescence, the stress-reducing influence of peers and friends was not studied in depth, compared to the large body of research focusing on the family as a significant source of support for adolescents coping with stress (Seiffge-Krenke, 1995). Burke and Weir (1978) examined adolescents' psychological health in relation to adolescents' satisfaction with help provided by parents and peers. Although adolescents were more likely to turn to peers for help, satisfaction with parental assistance was more strongly related to their psychological health and well-being than was satisfaction with help from peers. Similarly, in a study on depression (Seiffge-Krenke, 1995), it also became clear that different sources of social support were correlated differently with depression. Substantial negative correlations between depression and family cohesion ($r = -.42$) were found, whereas the correlations between adolescent depression and companionship with friends were lower ($r = -.18$). This indicates that despite the adolescents' increasing independence from the family, parents' support is more strongly related to psychological health than support by friends. Other investigators, too, demonstrated the importance of experiencing satisfactory relationships with others (i.e., receiving positive emotional support from and having little conflict with mothers, friends, siblings, and heterosexual partners) for overall positive adaptation in adolescence (Furman & Epstein, 1990).

Several studies in the past tried to find empirical evidence for the main effect or the buffering interaction effect models presented by

Cohen and Wills (1985). In a sample of 120 healthy adolescents 12 to 18 years old with psychological, behavior, and physical problems, Daniels and Moos (1990) found that social resources, such as good quality of relationship with parents and peers, were directly linked to better adolescent functioning and health. For example, more social resources from siblings and friends were related to less depression and anxiety; more resources from parents and friends were associated with fewer behavior problems. It was, however, typical of especially highly stressed youths to be unable to establish supportive relationships with parents, siblings, teachers, or friends. Compas, Slavin, Wagner, and Vanatta (1986) tested the buffering hypothesis (i.e., the significant interaction effect for social support and life events in relation to psychological outcome). Psychological dysfunction was expected to be relatively unaffected by level of social support when stress was low. In a study of 243 adolescents (mean age was 17.9 years), Compas and his colleagues (Compas et al., 1986) found that perceived social support was associated with symptomatology. More specifically, lower levels of satisfaction with social support were significantly related to symptoms of depression, somatization, and anxiety. The number of individuals available as sources of support was not related to the amount of physical or psychological symptoms. A significant relation was found between satisfaction with social support and psychological and somatic symptoms (independent of perceived negative events), with satisfaction with support and negative events explaining equal proportions of the variance in symptoms. Both variables combined accounted for only 12% of variance in symptoms.

In comparison, in the Daniels and Moos study (1990), negative events, ongoing stressors, and social resources combined accounted for an average of almost 35% of the variance in the outcome criteria. In the study of Compas and his coworkers, satisfaction with social support and negative life events did not interact in their relationship with psychological dysfunction. That is, the notion that social support increases in importance as negative events increase was not supported. This is consistent with data presented by Barrera (1981) relating satisfaction with support to symptomatology in pregnant adolescents. Neither network size, the interaction with negative events, nor satisfaction with social support were related to symptomatology.

In the study of Varni, Rubenfeld, Talbot, and Setoguchi (1989), the main effect and the buffering models were tested on a sample of early adolescents having congenital or acquired limb deficiencies. They found that classmates', parents', and teachers' social support were all significant predictors of depressive symptomatology, thus supporting the main effect model. Friends' support did not show a main effect. No buffering effect was found for the social support measures. Thus, higher levels of support provided by classmates, parents, and teachers under the conditions of chronic stress and daily stressors were associated with lower levels of depressive symptomatology. From this perspective, social support is perceived as a protective factor. Alternatively, low levels of social support are viewed as risk factor. Burt, Cohen, and Bjorck (1988) tested the main effect model and the buffer model on a sample of nonclinical adolescents. They found significant main effects of positive family climate (e.g., high cohesion) on depression. A stress-buffering effect of positive family climate on depression, as reported by Murch and Cohen (1989), was not observed.

Although the results of several studies support the main model of parental support, we found substantial evidence to support the interaction model, with parents and peers serving as stress buffers against depressive symptoms in a sample of 136 adolescents aged 13 to 17 years (Seiffge-Krenke, 1995). Taken together, relationships with parents and friends showed a buffer effect. The effect was much more pronounced in association with perceived family cohesion. Family cohesion also showed a significant main effect on depressive symptomatology. Thus, a high level of family cohesion, in general and under the conditions imposed by daily stress, was associated with lower levels of symptomatology. Relationships with peers, however, did not have beneficial effects, irrespective of whether the adolescents were under stress. Moreover, the buffer effect here was somewhat less than for perceived family cohesion. In contrast, Vernberg (1990) upheld the interaction model in predicting depression, but only for peer support.

In summary, the results relating various types of stressors and their effects on physical and psychological symptoms demonstrate a strong main effect of parental support, pointing to the protective function of supporting and cohesive family relations. In addition, this protective or stress-buffering effect was confirmed under conditions of high stress. Thus, for parental support, a buffering and a main effect were substantiated in research, suggesting that the two effects are not mutually exclusive. Concerning support from peers and friends, few studies to date have analyzed the protective function of friends, and the results are much more mixed.

### Coping Style

Research reported so far indicates that the experience of very stressful events or of cumulative changes in the lives of adolescents may be associated with health problems and physical illness; however, the correlations have not exceeded $r = .30$. Although studies including various types of stressors showed that minor stressors explain more variance in psychological symptoms than critical life events (see chap. 5, this volume), a substantial proportion of variance remains unaccounted for. One implication of studies of adolescent stress and physical and psychological symptoms is that stressful experiences alone are insufficient in explaining negative health outcomes during adolescence. Coping processes that are used in response to stress are important in understanding physical or psychological health.

***Conceptualization of Coping.*** According to the model developed by Rice et al. (1993), both external resources (such as parental and peer support) and internal resources (such as intelligence, perceived control, and adaptive coping responses) are thought to moderate the effects of different types of stressors on adolescent health. Lazarus and Launier (1978) understood *stress* to be created by any event in which an environmental or internal demand (or both) tax or exceed an individual's adaptive resources, and *coping* was defined as a process of managing these external or internal demands. Lazarus and Folkman (1991) pointed out that the coping process has three key features: the individual's action, the specific context of coping, and how an individual's actions change as the stressful encounter unfolds. In addition, they characterize coping as a process of continuous appraisals and reappraisals of a changing person–environment relationship. The reappraisal of what is happening in turn influences subsequent coping efforts. The coping process is thus continuously mediated by cognitive reappraisals. The entire coping process can occur in a few moments or hours, or it may continue over weeks or even years.

In the past, several conceptualizations of coping were developed using adolescent samples. In their overview of theoretical contributions to coping research, Tolor and Fehon (1987) distinguished between two broad categories of coping styles: problem-focused or emotion-focused coping and approach or avoidance. The classification of coping styles, according to approach or avoidance behaviors, is also found in the studies on adults (see Kobasa, 1982; Pearlin & Schooler, 1978; Vaillant, 1977). This classification is based on the conviction that avoidant coping and poor adjustment are correlated with one another. The Lazarus group preferred to highlight the functions of coping by making the distinction between coping that is problem-focused (i.e., directed at altering the problem that causes the distress) and coping that is emotion-focused (i.e., directed at regulating emotional responses; Folkman & Lazarus, 1985; Lazarus & Folkman, 1991).

Similar types of coping responses were identified in adolescents. In their study of adolescents, Ebata and Moos (1994) favored the approach–avoidance model. They differentiated between approach-oriented strategies—that included cognitive attempts to understand or change ways of thinking about the stress and behavioral attempts to deal with the stressors—and avoidance strategies which included cognitive attempts to deny and minimize stress. Although coping is typically understood as a reaction to a present or past stressor, it also occurs prior to a confrontation with the stressor (i.e., as anticipatory coping). We examined these two kinds of coping activities in our own research on the role of daily stressors in the lives of adolescents. Anticipatory coping was assessed in a large representative sample using the Coping Across Situations Questionnaire (CASQ), and coping after an event had taken place was examined by process-oriented interviews in small groups (for more details see Seiffge-Krenke, 1995). Major events were included according to their actual occurrence in the adolescents' lives. We found that action blockade or passivity was much more prominent in coping immediately after an event happened than in anticipatory coping. Anticipatory coping was analyzed in a large sample including 2,176 German adolescents (12 to 20 years old) and 1,000 adolescents from Finland, Israel, and the United States. In these cross-cultural samples, two functional coping styles (active coping and internal coping) and one dysfunctional coping style (withdrawal) emerged (Seiffge-Krenke, 1992; Seiffge-Krenke & Shulman, 1990). *Functional coping styles* include active problem solving and support seeking, as well as reflections about possible solutions; *dysfunctional coping* is characterized by a failure to solve the problem at hand immediately. Thus, a distinction between an active approach of tackling problems versus problem avoidance and withdrawal was found in most studies of adolescents.

***Coping Styles That Promote Health.*** In analyzing how adolescents cope with normative demands and minor stressors, we found that in all cross-cultural samples the two functional modes of coping (e.g., active support seeking and internal reflection of possible solutions) were most frequently employed, whereas defenses, such as denial or withdrawal, were applied to a lesser extent (Seiffge-Krenke, 1995). More precisely, the proportion of functional to dysfunctional coping modes was approximately 4 to 1, a ratio that has been found in diverse cross-cultural samples, too. Thus, the normative demands typical of this age group were approached in an adaptive way. Our subjects presented themselves as competent copers, well able to deal with problems arising in different fields such as school, parents, peers, and romantic relations. This generally positive and adaptive way of dealing with minor stressors was confirmed with the two different methods used. Apart from the greater emphasis on active support seeking in anticipatory coping and the less active, more internal approach in coping immediately after the stressor occurred, the similarities in coping styles measured by these two methods were impressive. This basically active approach in tackling stressful events was reported by other investigators as well. In the studies conducted by Compas, Malcarne, and Fondacaro (1988) and Tolor and Fehon (1987), problem-focused strategies, such as taking action or seeking information, were the most frequently reported strategies found in adolescent samples. In a more recent study using the CASQ in an American sample, Herman-Stahl, Stemmler, and Petersen (1995) reported two basic coping modes: approach-oriented coping and avoidant coping. This two-dimensional model was found using confirmatory factor analysis of the CASQ. Approach-oriented coping was related to psychological health, with approach copers reporting the fewest symptoms of depression.

Although developmental changes in responses to stressors are expected, the effects of age on coping have not been thoroughly investigated. This situation resulted, in part, from sampling procedures according to which adolescents were only represented as a subsample of a larger sample with a huge age span (see McCrae, 1982) or in mixed samples of adolescents and young adults (see Folkman & Lazarus, 1985). Several studies show that older adolescents use more emotion-focused coping or avoidant coping than younger adolescents (Compas, Malcarne, & Fondacaro, 1988; Hanson, Cigrang, Harris, & Carle, 1989). Other studies produced conflicting results (see, e.g., Blanchard-Fields & Irion, 1988; Stark, Spirito, Williams, & Guevremont, 1989; Stern & Zevon, 1990). In particular, no consistent age-related changes in problem-focused coping were found to take place from childhood through adolescence. Compas et al. (1993) argued that the use of problem-focused coping skills does not increase from middle childhood through adolescence because such skills have already been acquired and used at an earlier stage, whereas learning processes related to emotion-focused coping still continue through adolescence.

Our own studies show that mid-adolescence seems to be a turning point in the use of certain coping strategies (Seiffge-Krenke, 1995). It is well known that, compared to children, adolescents are more involved and intimate with peers and friends, turning to them for support formerly provided by the family (see chap. 2, this volume). We observed that after the age of 15 years, adolescents tried more frequently to obtain support from peers and friends when they had problems, and they increasingly discussed everyday stressors with people who were in a similar situation. Should the problem involve interpersonal conflict, they were more likely to speak openly about the problem with the concerned individual. These developmental changes in the use of social support were intertwined with changes in social and cognitive development leading to increased cognitive complexity and social maturity. After the age of 15 years, adolescents increasingly adopted the perspective of significant others, so that they were more willing to make compromises or yield to the wishes of others. Also, they reflected more about possible solutions to their problems, thus cultivating a variety of coping options. The link between the level of social–cognitive maturity and functional coping style also becomes obvious when comparing factor structures in early adolescent and mid-adolescent samples (Kavšek & Seiffge-Krenke, 1996). Whereas two basic coping modes—approach and avoidance—can be established for the younger adolescents (11–15 years old), for the older adolescents (16–19 years old), the approach dimension was differentiated into a behavioral and cognitive component, whereas the avoidance dimension remained the same.

***Gender Differences in Coping.*** Although the overall pattern of coping seems to be basically functional and approach-oriented both in male and female adolescents, gender differences were reported with respect to certain coping strategies. Several studies found differences between males and females in help-seeking behavior. For example, girls are more likely to seek social support than boys (Patterson & McCubbin, 1987; Seiffge-Krenke, 1992, 1995; Seiffge-Krenke & Shulman, 1990; Stark et al., 1989). This is consistent with findings in adults (Billings & Moos, 1981; Stone & Neale, 1984). In addition, females more frequently discuss a problem or event with others and try to approach the person concerned. Female adolescents rely more heavily on social networks (e.g., they discussed problems more freely with the person concerned, talked them over, and asked for help and assistance). These trends are in line with research on adults indicating a general tendency among females to rely more heavily on social networks than males (Haan, 1974) or to seek help in extrafamilial settings (Belle, 1987).

What was striking in our research, however, were the gender differences both in active coping and in withdrawal: females had higher scores in both coping styles (Seiffge-Krenke, 1993b, 1995). A trend for females to name more coping strategies than boys was also reported (Compas, Forsythe, & Wagner, 1988), indicating that females make greater efforts to deal with stressors. These gender differences in coping styles were frequently linked to the emergence of psychopathology in adolescence.

Several authors referred to the co-occurrence of increased rates of depressive symptoms in females and the development of rumination (Compas et al., 1993; Nolen-Hoeksema, 1991; Rice et al., 1993). The strong gender differences found in adolescents' coping styles points to an early onset of these differences (Frydenberg & Lewis, 1993; Seiffge-Krenke, 1995); however, direct tests of this developmental hypothesis have not yet been carried out. Also, the links between gender differences in coping styles and differences in physical health were not explored in depth. The strong gender differences in reported physical complaints (see chap. 5, this volume) point to a similar link.

***Coping and Resiliency.*** Research on health psychology of adolescents has profited from findings generated in the fields of developmental psychopathology. Protective factors (see chap. 1, this volume) such as invulnerability or resiliency were found in studies on children and adolescents exposed to various risk factors and cumulative stressors. Our understanding of the reasons why some children are not damaged by deprivation and highly stressful living conditions increased during the last decades. It was demonstrated that resilient adolescents are able to continue a relatively healthy emotional development despite serious stressors and unfavorable life situations (Garmezy et al., 1984; Rutter, 1987; Werner & Smith, 1982).

Many recent studies of the relations among stress, social support, and general adaptation were borne from previous research projects, such as the study conducted by Werner and Smith in the 1950s on children from Kauai, Rutter, Graham, et al.'s (1976) study in Great Britain or the two studies on adolescents conducted in the 1960s: the Berkeley Study conducted by Haan (1977) and the Menniger Coping Project led by Murphy and Moriarty (1986). The common denominator of these early studies was the finding that resilient adolescents (i.e., adolescents who remained relatively healthy and showed an overall good adaptation, despite many and disrupting stressors) came from families with relatively intact parent–child relationships. In addition, interpersonal relationships in these families were close and cohesive, the adolescent's attempts to achieve autonomy were not thwarted, and rules and limits in the family were clearly defined. Troubled, vulnerable adolescents showed signs of accumulated stress and lacked social support systems. Above all, resilient adolescents were competent in their choice of and identification with resilient models of social support. The coping capacities of resilient adolescents showed two particularly outstanding qualitites: First, most studies found that resilient children and adolescents dealt with the life stressors in a competent and active way, that is, they acted and did not just react; second, in cases of major disturbances in parent–child relationships, the presence of alternative caregivers in the household (such as grandparents) and the child's or adolescent's ability to seek alternative sources of support, which might serve as a refuge from stressful events (Rutter, 1987) or help in actively dealing with the stressors (Werner & Smith, 1982), increased resiliency.

In summary, research on coping styles in adolescence provided us with important insight into the ways of dealing with different types of stressors as well as developmental changes, according to age and gender. However, further research is needed to understand the exact nature of the links between coping and physical and psychological symptoms. The individual coping response is important not only for dealing with immediate stressors, but also for the nature of one's social support. Ineffective coping responses lead to poor interpersonal relationships, thereby reducing available coping resources (Rice et al., 1993). For example, an adolescent who copes through inappropriate demonstrations of anger or excessive emotion becomes unpopular with friends. Therefore, the manner in which an adolescent copes with different types of stressors not only influences his or her adaptation during a particular transition, but also partly determines the personal and social resources that will be available in subsequent transition periods.

## HIGHLY STRESSED ADOLESCENTS: PECULIARITIES IN COPING STYLES AND SUPPORT SEEKING

In the following, the possible links among stress, coping, and relationships are discussed, based on results obtained in studies of several clinically referred samples as well as samples suffering from high stress but not yet referred to psychological treatment. Although the effect of active support seeking and problem-focused coping in reducing the impact of different types of stressors is typical of normal samples, these same mechanisms are rarely observed in clinical samples. In fact, what constitutes a protective factor in normal samples becomes a risk factor in clinical samples; that is, active support seeking and problem-focused coping exacerbate the effects of stress.

Compas, Hinden, and Gerhardt (1995) identified four different trajectories for adolescent development. One subgroup of adolescents showed stable adaptive functioning, the second showed maladaptive functioning. The third group of adolescents was characterized by a temporary pattern of deviance that is limited to the adolescent years. Finally, other adolescents were recovering from childhood problems and showed improved development during adolescent years. *Stable adaptive functioning* is typically seen in adolescents who traverse adolescence in relatively low-risk environments. *Stable maladaptive functioning* is found in the developmental trajectories of individuals who enter adolescence with a history of problems or disorders and who are exposed to chronic stress and adversity in the absence of social or personal resources that mitigate against these risks.

An additional group of adolescents should be added to this list, namely, highly stressed adolescents who have not yet been referred to medical or psychological treatment. Research on this group would greatly contribute to our understanding of the mechanisms involved in the development of psychological disorders. In a study of adolescents suffering from high stress, but not yet referred for medical examination or psychological treatment, we found that coping style and seeking support were characterized by a highly ambivalent pattern of approach and avoidance. We selected 43 adolescents with high rates of minor stressors and 43 adolescents with low rates of minor stressors from a representative sample of German adolescents 12 to 20 years old (see Seiffge-Krenke, 1995). Normative stress was measured using the Problem Questionnaire (Seiffge-Krenke, 1995), which assesses the stressfulness of 64 items covering normative everyday problems. Although the highly stressed adolescents included in the study did not show any evidence of health problems, they reported a great many problems with parents, same-sex friends, partners in romantic relations, as well as feelings of depression, boredom, anxiety, or nervousness. In contrast, low-stressed adolescents reported very low rates of relationship and identity stressors. Age and gender were evenly distributed in both groups.

What was striking in analyzing coping behavior in these groups, by means of the CASQ (Seiffge-Krenke, 1995), was that active coping and withdrawal were evenly balanced in the highly stressed group, whereas low-stressed adolescents showed a clear preference for active coping. Withdrawal or dysfunctional coping was very low in low-stressed adolescents and amounted to 15%. In contrast, highly stressed adolescents frequently employed withdrawal or avoidant coping for many different problem domains. However, they did not differ from their less stressed peers with respect to the use of active coping. Nevertheless, closer inspection revealed that they restricted their support seeking to more neutral sources such as books and magazines. Moreover, the willingness to accept offers of professional help was different between the two groups. Table 6.1 shows significant differences between the highly stressed and low-stressed adolescents in their respective attitudes to-

TABLE 6.1
Differences in Attitudes Toward Psychotherapy Between Highly Stressed ($n$ = 23) and Low-Stressed ($n$ = 42) Adolescents

| | *Stress* | | | | | |
|---|---|---|---|---|---|---|
| | *High* ($n$ = 43) | | *Low* ($n$ = 42) | | | |
| *Scale* | *M* | *SD* | *M* | *SD* | *F* | *p* |
| 1. Scepticism toward psychotherapy | 39.9 | 7.0 | 32.4 | 5.6 | 1.1 | .27 |
| 2. Readiness to accept help | 64.1 | 12.0 | 59.7 | 10.9 | 1.8 | .07 |
| 3. Need for privacy | 29.9 | 7.1 | 22.9 | 5.7 | 4.8 | .001 |
| 4. Attitudes toward mental illness | 25.5 | 6.4 | 24.8 | 9.2 | .63 | .71 |

ward psychotherapy as assessed by the Schmitz Psychotherapy Questionnaire (1981). Highly stressed adolescents were only slightly more willing to seek professional help compared to their less-stressed peers, but their need for privacy was much higher. Their subjective sense of suffering and their disinclination to talk about it were equally balanced. Thus, they were caught up in a dilemma between approach and avoidance in their coping strategies in general and in their help-seeking behavior in particular.

## AVOIDANT COPING: A COMMON COPING STYLE IN CLINICAL SAMPLES

Whereas effective coping decreases the effects of stress, ineffective coping exacerbates the effects of stress on health. *Avoidant coping* was identified as a risk factor in several studies. Holahan and Moos (1987) and Nolen-Hoeksema (1987) posited avoidant coping as a risk factor in their studies of risk, resistance, and stress in adult samples. Similarly, in adolescent samples it was established that the ways in which adolescents cope with stressful events account for the adverse effects of stress. Ebata and Moos (1994) explored the relation between coping and distress in three groups of adolescents suffering from rheumatic disease, conduct disorder, and depression, respectively, as well as in one group of healthy adolescents, which served as the control group. They reported that adolescents suffering from depressive moods and conduct disorders relied more on avoidant coping and that depressed adolescents used significantly less approach-oriented coping than any of the other groups. In examining the links between coping and well-being, Ebata and Moos found that approach-oriented coping (i.e., attempts to act on or modify stressors through cognitive or overt behavior) was linked with more positive adjustment, whereas avoidant coping (i.e., attempts to escape from or avoid stressors, or deny their existence) was generally associated with poorer adaptation.

Compas, Malcarne, and Fondacaro (1988) and Petersen (1993) found similar associations between problem-focused coping and positive mental health and emotional-focused coping and poor psychological adjustment. In a more recent study applying the CASQ on a sample of 603 adolescents in Grades 6 to 11, Herman-Stahl et al. (1995) found that approach copers reported the fewest symptoms of depression, whereas avoidant copers reported the most. This finding of a basic distinction between a more active coping approach in nonconspicuous samples and avoidance in clinical samples was also made in our own research using the CASQ. We observed that healthy adolescents employed avoidant coping or withdrawal very rarely (for more details, see Seiffge-Krenke, 1995). Avoidant coping or withdrawal was far more prominent in all studies conducted on clinical samples (Seiffge-Krenke, 1989). For example, the withdrawal rates found in a study of 46 psychiatric patients were nearly twice as high as those for the healthy control group of 289 adolescents. Figure 6.1 illustrates the results obtained with the CASQ on this sample of adolescent patients that were referred to a psychiatric outpatient clinic, but were not yet receiving treatment.

The rates for withdrawal in response to self-related stressors were especially high (amounting to 45% of the coping response), as were the

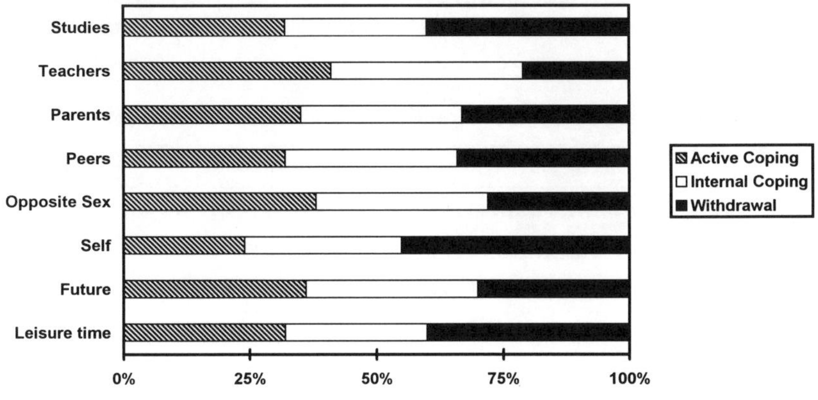


FIG. 6.1. Active coping, internal coping, and withdrawal in 46 clinically referred adolescents.

withdrawal rates for minor stressors related to leisure time, school, and parents. Furthermore, withdrawal proved especially effective for discriminating between different clinical groups (Seiffge-Krenke, 1989). Adolescents with high stress who were not referred to counseling ($n$ = 43), adolescents in psychotherapy—diagnosed as suffering from depression or from problems in interpersonal relationships—($n$ = 37), and adolescent drug abusers ($n$ = 28) were adequately identified by their tendency to withdraw. In trying to separate these different groups, we calculated a canonical discriminant function including the three scales of the CASQ for assessing coping behavior, the self-concept dimensions of the Offer Self-Image Questionnaire (OSIQ; Offer & Offer, 1969), the Schmitz Questionnaire (1981), assessing attitudes to psychotherapy, and the variables of age, gender, and SES. As is shown in Table 6.2, *avoidant coping* or withdrawal made the largest contribution to group discrimination, followed by self-concept dimensions.

In comparing the withdrawal rates for these groups, it was found that the depressed adolescents showed the highest rates and the drug abusers showed the lowest rates. In several follow-up studies, we were able to confirm that adolescents in clinical samples showed greater amounts of avoidant coping than healthy controls. In most of these studies, adolescents with internalizing disorders (e.g., depression) exhibited the highest withdrawal rates; adolescents with externalizing disorders, (e.g., drug abusing or delinquent) showed the lowest withdrawal rates, although they were still significantly higher than those for the healthy control groups. Moreover, a close association between behavioral and emotional dysfunction and dysfunctional coping styles (like withdrawal) was established. In a study of fifty-two 12- to 17-year-old adolescents identified as depressed according to the clinical cutting point (e.g., scores at or above the 82nd percentile, $T > 60$, using parents' ratings on the

TABLE 6.2
Separating Different Clinical Groups by Discriminant Analysis

| *Level* | *Variable* | *Wilks Lambda* | *Significance* |
|---|---|---|---|
| 1 | CASQ Scale 3: Withdrawal | .84 | .0001 |
| 2 | OSIQ Scale 1: Positive self-esteem | .79 | .001 |
| 3 | OSIQ Scale 3: Confidence in one's own abilities | .67 | .001 |
| 4 | Gender | .60 | .001 |
| 5 | Schmitz Scale 1: Skeptical toward psychotherapy | .55 | .001 |

CBCL), the correlation between the internalizing score and withdrawal amounted to $r = .71, p < .001$ for females and $r = .44, p = .05$ for males.

In another study on 120 adolescents with various problems seeking help in a counseling center, we administered the adolescent self-report of symptomatology (YSR) and the CASQ. Again, the association between behavioral and emotional problems and avoidant coping was substantial. The correlations between the YSR total score and withdrawal amounted to $r = .52, p < .001$ for females and $r = .42, p = .05$ for males. In summary, it was established that withdrawal or avoidant coping was a predominant coping mode in adolescents with poor psychological adjustment. The very high withdrawal rates in depressed adolescents were outstanding. Interestingly, Herman-Stahl et al. (1995) also used the CASQ to find that subjects who changed over time from approach to avoidant coping (e.g., withdrawal) showed a significant increase in depressive symptoms, whereas subjects who switched from avoidant to approach coping (e.g., active coping and internal coping) displayed a significant decrease in depression over time.

The work of Nolen-Hoeksema and her colleagues (Nolen-Hoeksema, 1987, 1991; Nolen-Hoeksema & Girgus, 1995) contributed substantially to our understanding of dysfunctional coping styles and symptomatology. Nolen-Hoeksema (1991) suggested that different coping styles are fostered by gender-specific socialization processes. The male stereotype of being active and ignoring moods leads to an increase in distracting response to depressive mood. The female stereotype of emotionality and inactivity leads depressed females to ruminate instead of distracting themselves from their depressive mood. Rumination was found to maintain and increase depressed mood, whereas distraction alleviates depressive mood.

In fact, female adults are twice as likely as male adults to suffer from depression. These gender differences exist for major depressive disorders and for less severe forms of depression. In contrast, among prepubescent children, there is a slight tendency for males to show more depression than females (Nolen-Hoeksema, Girgus, & Seligman, 1991). It appears that this switch in gender differences for depression occurs some time in mid- to late adolescence, although the precise timing is unclear. In a longitudinal study on 197 school children, Nolen-Hoeksema and her colleagues found that boys consistently reported more depressive symptoms than girls and also exhibited more unfavorable coping styles, such as a pessimistic explanatory style for negative events (Nolen-Hoeksema et al., 1991). Thus, an association between depressive symptoms and a dysfunctional coping style (even before adolescence) was established.

As was outlined in the first section of this chapter, during the adolescent years gender differences between males' and females' coping behaviors dramatically increase. One such difference is a more ambivalent coping style (more active and more avoidant) in females. Further studies using longitudinal samples are necessary to clarify the links between psychological dysfunction and a dysfunctional coping style such as avoidant coping or withdrawal. In addition, the coping styles of adolescents with externalizing syndromes warrants further investigation. There is some evidence that delinquent adolescents not only show elevated withdrawal rates, but also show less internal coping compared to nonconspicuous controls (Lösel, Bliesener, & Köferl, 1989). This suggests a deficit in the capacity for internal reflection about possible solutions, which is important in designing intervention strategies.

A further question to be dealt with more extensively in further research concerns the adaptive and maladaptive aspects of avoidant coping. In our distinction between functional coping modes (i.e., active coping and internal coping) and dysfunctional coping modes (i.e., withdrawal), *dysfunctional* refers to the aspect that the problem is not *immediately* solved (Seiffge-Krenke, 1995). Nevertheless, withdrawal is a meaningful way of coping with situations of extreme stress. Several authors discussed how withdrawal serves as a protective function when an individual is overly strained by aversive events (Suls & Fletcher, 1985). In addition, withdrawal is an appropriate response in all situations where direct action is inhibited by external barriers. This aspect was especially stressed by Lazarus and Launier (1978). Moreover, one must consider the point in time at which coping is evaluated, whether the stressful situation can in fact be controlled, and the degree of correspondence between the coping style and the demands of the stressful situation (Roth & Cohen, 1986).

Denial, avoidance, and distraction are sometimes seen as less effective forms of coping, because they deal with symptoms rather than causes of the problem. Yet, as Hauser and Bowlds (1990) showed, in certain circumstances these reactions lead to a positive outcome by helping to establish an emotional equilibrium. How does one determine when avoidant coping is adaptive? Avoidant coping cannot simply be labeled as inherently good or bad; rather, the specific context has to be considered. A strategy that is effective for one problem or person might not work for another. The effectiveness of a given response also varies over time. A coping style that is at first beneficial can become maladaptive if used continuously.

Indeed, in their meta-analysis, Suls and Fletcher (1985) demonstrated that although avoidance was associated with a more adaptive outcome in the short term, its beneficial effect waned with time. The findings on clinically disturbed adolescents point to a similar situation: Irrespective of the problem at hand, these adolescents rather uniformly used withdrawal as a predominant coping style. It is possible that these adolescents lack the ability to adequately discriminate between types of stressors and characteristics of stressful events, which, in turn, leads to maladaptive functioning. The capacity to adopt a different coping style, according to the demands of various stressful situations, is thus a prerequisite of adaptive coping.

## DEFICITS IN SOCIAL SUPPORT AND NETWORK STRUCTURE OF DISTRESSED ADOLESCENTS

Social relationships are among the most complex of human activities and can be both a source of stress and satisfaction. As already outlined in chapter 5, many everyday stressors in adolescence concern relationships with parents, friends, and romantic partners. In addition, several major stressors are related to loss and emotional damage in close relationships. Lazarus (1985) argued against upholding the solely positive perspective of close relationships. Accordingly, he warned that sayings, such as “A friend is the best medicine,” trivialize the multiple and often contradictory functions of social support. In the following sections, some of the pitfalls in social support network structures and obstacles in using social support are outlined.

### Decreasing Support When Dealing With Chronic Stressors

Several studies reported that despite an abundance of social support, families with chronically ill adolescents are more often socially isolated (Eiser, 1992). Also, there is some evidence to suggest that the size of support networks declines over time. In a study of 35 adolescents with cancer and their families, Kazak and Meadows (1989) found that their social support networks became smaller over time. It is likely that although others are well prepared to be helpful in the initial stage of the disease, their concern or ability to help declines the longer the disease persists. This phenomenon occurs in cases of other chronic stressors: coping with unemployment (Hammarström, 1990), parental divorce (Farber, Felner, & Primavera, 1985), and early motherhood (Coletta, Hadler, & Gregg, 1981). Studies of unemployed adolescents and adolescent mothers showed that these youths have few friends and become increasingly dependent on the family (Codega, Pasley, & Kreutzer,

1990). Additional research is needed to clarify how adolescents perceive the importance of different support networks and, in particular, the rewards and costs involved. Too much support might lead to dependency on others and hinder the adolescents' attempts to cope with a stressor and develop autonomy (Seiffge-Krenke, 1997c). In contrast, a lack of social support might increase the burden of a major stressor or be perceived as an additional stress factor. So, one is left with the question "How does one decide how much support is appropriate for healthy functioning?"

### Deficits in Relationships and in the Capacity to Elicit Support

Other issues concern the way adolescents with health problems perceive their social support system and make use of it. It is well-known that adolescents with a history of chronically depressed mood and a history of chronic stress in the family show efforts to orient themselves away from the family and become more socially active with peers (Compas et al., 1993). An example of the highly stressed adolescents' tendency to withdraw from the stressful situation in general and from social relationships in particular is provided in the preceding section. For several years, it has been acknowledged that a child's lack of friends or experiencing difficulties in the peer group is perceived by parents as a strong indicator that their child is emotionally or behaviorally disturbed (Achenbach, 1991b). Moreover, an analysis of disturbed adolescents' friendships revealed that these youths have atypical views of friendship and unrealistic expectations of people they know (LeGaipa & Wood, 1981). For example, one expects that an adolescent who is anxious or feeling upset will seek support from a parent or close friend. Instead, these investigators found that when communication with friends was strained, the disturbed adolescents sought the company of nonrelated adults, including teachers and neighbors. Reliance on teachers for social support was very low in the healthy control group. LeGaipa and Wood also described the difficulties experienced by normally adjusted adolescents when relating to unhappy or depressed peers, noting that their subsequent interactions were characterized by uncertainty, awkwardness, hesitancy, and tension. This observation emphasizes that a fundamental aspect of exchange between friends in adolescence is reciprocity. Similarly, in exploring the relation between social skills and healthy social functioning, Johnson (1991) argued that individuals free of negative psychological symptoms were more likely to attract or maintain positive social relations than were individuals who exhibit such symptoms. In a longitudinal analysis, he found that strong social ties were most likely to be damaged by psychological stress; that is, network members in close relationships with the adolescents were most likely to be burdened by demands for support.

Cotterell (1994) analyzed the social network structure of distressed and normally adjusted youths attending the same school. Four kinds of social support—emotional, practical, advice, and companionship—and their related social networks were described and compared. Cotterell found that distressed adolescents had distorted views of how such social networks usually function. Conspicuous was the lack of discriminatory power found in the distressed group, which led them to perceive any attention from significant others as social support. The adolescents in the distressed group reported that a significantly greater portion of their social network relationships were very close; they also cited a larger number of members in their networks who provided them with much support. These adolescents had problems in distinguishing between friends and acquaintances or between formal and informal support providers (e.g., family members). During the interviews, the distressed adolescents cited "friends" giving high levels of support although these "friends" has discontinued the friendship a few days prior to the interview. Some also claimed that recently acquired friends and teachers provided high levels of support. However, further inquiry revealed that these assessments were overstated. It appeared as if these adolescents were assessing their needs for support rather than the actual support they were receiving. Such misperceptions were related to their insecure attachment histories. According to Sroufe and Fleeson (1986), a stable perception of support originates in early childhood. During this time, the child's experiences with support lead to the development of working models of the self, significant others, and the ways others relate to the self. Secure attachment experiences in childhood foster the capacity to experience emotional intimacy and to give and receive support in adolescence.

### Obstacles in Soliciting Alternative Sources of Support

There is no doubt that adolescents differ in their desire or need for support, in their skills in soliciting support from others, and in their perceptions of the availability of supportive others. Research on resiliency demonstrated that the ability to solicit social support from others is crucial. Garmezy's (1983) review of the research findings on resiliency led him to identify three general protective factors that distinguish stress-resistant youths from those adversely affected by stress: advantageous personality dispositions (e.g., social responsiveness), cohesive and supportive family environments, and the presence of external sources of support. The latter appears to be the least documented and understood. One example of these external sources of support is found in a supportive personal relationship with an adult (e.g., a relative or another individual with whom the adolescent closely identifies).

In a study of adolescents whose parents had major affective disturbances, Beardslee and Podorefsky (1988) found that one half of the adolescents who showed healthy functioning reported turning to someone outside the family during episodes of acute parental illness; some of them named adults. These authors observed that the resilient adolescents' outside commitments and relationships allowed them to distance themselves from their parents' illness. Farber et al. (1985) also found that disengagement from the family contributed to an adolescent's resilience in the wake of parental divorce. Thus, it appears that distressed adolescents benefit from increasing and deepening their associations with supportive adult figures. However, several obstacles inhibit the development of close personal relationships between adolescents and adults with whom they interact outside the home.

First, many of the adults who come into regular contact with adolescents occupy formal roles such as teacher, athletic coach, or job supervisor. Adults in these positions must observe rather strict rules of conduct in their interactions with adolescents. Furthermore, these adults receive parental or institutional sanctions to mete out rewards and punishment.

A second obstacle to the formation of more personal relationships between adolescents and adults is related to the typical structure of such interaction. For most adult–adolescent activities, large groups of adolescents are instructed or led by adults, leaving few opportunities for one-to-one dialogue. This accounts for the finding that adolescents consider adults to be among the least desired individuals who can provide help and support (Greenberger & Steinberg, 1981). In addition, adolescents show a low willingness to disclose personal information to adults (see chap. 2, this volume). Despite these constraints on the development of personal relationships with adults, nonrelated adults are significant figures in adolescents' social networks. For example, in a study of 2,800 adolescents in the seventh to tenth grades, Blyth, Hill, and Thiel (1982) found that roughly 10% of all significant adults were not relatives and most of these adults were of the same gender as the respondent. Approximately one half of nonrelated adults were seen in the school and 60% were seen in home settings. Similarly, Gottlieb and Sylvestre (1994) found that all the respondents in their study reported that they had regular contact with adults whom they knew on a regular basis. Most of the respondents identified at least one older person to whom they had turned in a time of stress. Although few adolescents reported disclosing personal information to older relatives, such as grandparents, aunts, or uncles, they valued the comfort, acceptance, and security they experienced in their relationships with them. Adults chosen as trusted partners were those who communicated a more personal interest in the adolescent or revealed information about themselves that the adolescent considered to be more private and personal in nature. For the adolescent, this represented a tacit acknowledgment that the adult considered the adolescent mature and trustworthy enough to be privy to such information, which, in turn, encouraged the adolescent to divulge self-related information.

### Relationships That May Increase Health Risks

While adolescents struggle to disengage themselves from their parents, they become more involved with their peers. This sometimes include engaging in high-risk activities that adversely affect health and adjustment. A growing number of studies investigated parent and peer effects on smoking, drinking, and marijuana use among adolescents (see chap. 3, this volume). In most of these studies, differences in value systems between parents and peers were found to account for the negative effects of peer interaction on health. Parents tend to be concerned about the long-term consequences of their adolescent child's health-deterrent behaviors and often encourage positive health behavior such as eating nutritious foods and exercising. In contrast, adolescents and their peers tend to strive for enjoyment of the present without showing much concern about the future or the long-term consequences of their behaviors. Much evidence accumulated that peer-oriented social activities are associated with poorer health behavior over time. Indeed, peer relations and social activities provide much pleasure and offer valuable learning experiences, nevertheless, the adolescent is more tempted to engage in dangerous behaviors—driving recklessly, experimenting with alcohol or drugs, and so forth. Much impulsive, risk-taking behavior occurs in the context of adolescent social activities, either as a central goal of adolescent social activity or as an outgrowth of initially more benign activities.

Whereas the relative influence of parents on adolescent health behavior diminishes with age, the influence of peers increases. Certain parental behaviors interact or buffer the effects of the adolescent's value orientation. Kandel (1986) showed that peer influence tends to increase alcohol and marijuana use, whereas parental influence tends to inhibit such substance abuse. Similarly, an adolescent's smoking behavior is encouraged when peers also smoke (Fiore, 1992). In a longitudinal study of parental and peer effects on adolescents' health behavior, Hansell and Mechanic (1990) found strong and consistent support for the hypothesis that a high level of social activities with peers was associated with more negative health behavior, such as drug and alcohol use, and smoking, over time. In contrast, parent-oriented activities were associated with more positive health behavior such as use of seat belts, participation in athletic activities, and eating breakfast. Should adolescent alcohol and drug users come from families in which parents themselves use a variety of drugs including alcohol and psychoactive drugs, parental influence works synergistically with and potentiates peer influence. The highest rate of adolescent drug use (70%) in the sample studied by Kandel (1986) was found when both parents and peers reinforced each other's influence on the adolescent; the lowest rate (12%) was found when neither used drugs. Although parents and peers both have independent effects on an adolescent's health behavior, the peers' influence was much greater on all activities, including those associated with risks to health.

## LACK OF SOCIAL SUPPORT, DYSFUNCTIONAL COPING, AND SYMPTOMATOLOGY: A VICIOUS CIRCLE

In chapter 5, we discussed the findings on sources of risk in biological, psychological, and social domains. Different types of stressors and the number, timing, and synchronicity of such stressors were outlined. In addition, changes in living conditions due to increasing violence, poverty, unemployment, or migration rates that might also be associated with increased health risks were discussed. Although an awareness of risk factors assists in identifying individuals that are more likely to develop health problems, it cannot explain how or why problems develop. For this reason, research must turn to the search for the processes and mechanisms that may lead to negative health outcomes.

In this chapter, we began by focusing on stress, coping, and social support as fundamental aspects of adolescent functioning in normal samples. Different types of stressors that adolescents are confronted with were outlined as well as the ways adolescents cope with these demands. Social support as a stress buffer was also examined. Thus, the focus was on social support and coping as protective factors in mediating the effects of normative and nonnormative stressors. In addition, the links between stress, coping, and relationships were examined in several samples of clinically referred adolescents as well as in samples of adolescents who were suffering from high stress but were not yet referred for psychological treatment. It became apparent that stress and internal resources (such as coping), as well as external resources (such as social support), must be conceptualized differently when dealing with clinical populations. The active support seeking and problem-focused coping typical of normal samples was shown to reduce the impact of different types of stressors; this mechanism is rarely observed in clinical samples. What constitutes a protective factor in normal samples (the way of coping and using social support) becomes a risk factor in clinical samples, that is, the effects of stress are exacerbated.

Most individuals complete adolescence without developing major psychological or physical problems. Many studies paint a rather rosy picture of positive development during this age span. In fact, the prevalence rates for psychopathology are not higher compared to other age groups (Earls, 1986). However, some adolescents' developmental trajectories include health problems; some are transient and others become chronic conditions. Adolescents belonging to this group show specific characteristics. Most of them have experienced an accumulation of major stressors. In addition, with increasing number of stressors, the coping style changes from a predominantly active approach to avoidant coping or withdrawal. Thus, a lack in discriminatory power, as well as a rather inflexible application of a certain coping mode, is characteristic of this group. Also, deficits in social support and network structure contribute to maladaptive functioning.

A few statistics illustrate how dramatic these changes can be. Johnson (1986) reported a mean score of 9.26 critical life events in psychiatric samples as compared to 2.13 in nonconspicuous samples. As outlined in chapter 5, these nonnormative events are qualitatively different from normative stressors and greatly disrupt the adolescent. As detailed in the previous sections, up to one half of the coping responses in these clinical samples entailed avoidant coping or withdrawal, which was applied indiscriminantly in dealing with different types of stressors. Moreover, lack of social support and severe disruption in close relationships were characteristic of most adolescents in these clinical samples. For example, emotional neglect, abuse, and own deviant behavior were found in parents of delinquent adolescents (Farrington, 1989), which makes it questionable whether they can support and supervise their children in an adequate way. Similarly, a particular family pathology was found in other clinical samples. Depressed adolescents described their parents as being hostile, authoritarian, rejecting, and affectionless. In prospective samples, fathers' rejection and mothers' psychological control were found to be the most powerful predictors of adolescents' depressive symptoms (Baron & McGillivray, 1989).

It would be adaptive for an adolescent who experiences negative family relationships to be able to compensate for the missing support by turning to friends, other relatives, or non-related adults. However, the specific attachment history of these adolescents persists in other relationship patterns (e.g., if support in the immediate family is low, support by other family members and friends is likely to be low, too). Studies on antisocial and aggressive behavior further illustrate an intergenerational transmission of negative behaviors through imitation and learning processes in the family, which has led to the violence-begets-violence hypothesis (Spatz Widom, 1989). Also, adolescents who have negative relationships with parents and friends can miss out on learning specific social skills. The inability to make appropriate assessments about the function and closeness of different social network members seen in clinically referred adolescents was outlined earlier. Their deficits in relationships and in using social support are related to their dysfunctional coping style. The efforts to find a substitute for a particular relationship deficiency are weakened by a dysfunctional coping style and deficits in social relations. Thus, the accumulation of stressors, a dysfunctional coping style, and deficits in relationships create a vicious circle, which contributes to increased symptomatology. However, it is clear that compensatory processes are extremely difficult to realize for adolescents in clinical samples, especially if this vicious circle existed for some time (East & Rook, 1992; Stocker, 1994).

In summary, adolescents that manage to successfully master these stressors emerge with increased abilities and resources, whereas others who cannot cope with these stressors in an adaptive manner develop new or increased problem behaviors and relationship deficits. In examining the chain or sequence that unfolds as a result of cumulative stress, a cumulative deficit in both coping style and seeking, as well as using social support, became obvious. These findings are clear in their implications for prevention and intervention (see chaps. 8 and 9, this volume).

# 7

# The Challenge of Coping With Chronic Illness

Whereas normative stressors are usually dealt with without manifest abnormalities, the first appearance of a serious incurable chronic illness could become a nonnormative stressor that possibly overtaxes an adolescents' coping abilities. This chapter provides a brief overview of the current state of research on coping with illness in adolescence. Then, the focus shifts to how the afflicted adolescent makes use of assistance provided by social and medical support systems, in which manner an adolescent's further development is affected by the illness, and what kinds of long-term consequences are involved. In particular, the effect of the chronic illness on psychological health is analyzed. Research findings obtained in the Bonn longitudinal study of diabetic adolescents and their families (Seiffge-Krenke et al., 1996) are presented to illustrate these salient issues.

## CURRENT STATE OF RESEARCH: AN OVERVIEW

As detailed in chapter 3, adolescents assume a middle position in the morbidity rates and seldom become physically ill. Adolescents do not spontaneously talk about problems related to health and illness, perhaps because they are so very concerned with their physical development and want to be as normal as possible. One should not forget, of course, that at least 10% of all families in Germany care for a chronically ill adolescent; comparable overviews in the United States and Great Britain reported rates of 7% to 12% (Eiser, 1992; Gortmaker, Walker, Weitzman, & Sobol, 1990).

Various authors described the enormous psychological consequences of the onset of a chronic illness in adolescence and spoke of an interruption of previous development, described, for example, by Jamison, Lewis, and Burish (1986) as "developmental breakdown" (p. 611). They emphasized that adolescents are not able to appropriately cope with these additional, illness-related stressors (Ben-Sira, 1984). Other studies, in contrast, demonstrated that the general adaptation shown by adolescents with chronic illness is impressive and passes without major psychopathology (Garrison & McQuiston, 1989; Gortmaker, Perrin, Weitzman, Halmer, & Sobol, 1993). Before discussing these controversies, we first look at the current state of research and main issues concerning questions about coping with illness in adolescence.

An analysis of research findings on adolescent coping shows that despite the low incidence of illnesses in this developmental period, there is a considerable body of research on issues related to coping with illness (Seiffge-Krenke, 1995). Coping with illness is one of the most frequently studied topics on adolescent coping, accounting for about 24% of all studies in this area. Another analysis revealed that interest both in theoretical–conceptual studies and empirical studies has increased over the years; however, adolescents are typically studied as a subgroup of a larger group of individuals within a broader age span (Seiffge-Krenke & Brath, 1990). *Adolescence* was clearly defined as the age span of 12 to 18 years in only 30% of the 249 publications analyzed. This reflects the tendency to select mixed groups with a broad age span and not differentiate further within the phase of adolescence.

Early research especially focused on rarely occurring illnesses that are extremely burdensome, cannot be treated adequately, and are often terminal or associated with serious, permanent handicaps. Over the years, the volume of research on chronic illness has increased, and attention has been directed to other types of chronic illnesses that are less threatening, for which adequate therapy is available, and which, in general, can be easily self-managed. This includes diabetes and, especially more recently, a few cancer-related illnesses that were once inexorably fatal, but due to improved diagnostic and therapeutic methods, have become chronic, if not burdensome conditions. In addition, illnesses with high mortality rates, some of which are associated with critical, occasionally life-threatening phases (e.g., acute kidney failure, dialytic shock, acute asthma attacks, diabetic coma, and hypoglycemic shock) were also studied.

Early studies on coping with illness showed considerable methodological weaknesses related to definitions, operationalizations, and data collection. In our analysis, we found that 42% of the studies employed a very broad definition of coping (i.e., as used in the sense of general adaptation; Seiffge-Krenke & Brath, 1990). In 27% of the studies, a very narrow scope was used (e.g., coping was equated with compliance or adherence to the medical regimen), and only 31% employed a definition that included both functional and dysfunctional ways of dealing with the illness (e.g., coping or defense). Also surprising were restrictions in methods depending on the ages of patients studied. In children, coping was predominantly investigated at the family level; in adolescents, the focal point was almost exclusively on individual coping, and family coping was assessed only in 14% of all studies.

Most studies were based on samples of individuals suffering from similar types of illnesses or belonging to the more undifferentiated group of "chronically ill," without including control groups. Because most of the illness types studied were quite rare, most studies were based on small samples (from individual case studies to $N = 50$). In addition, most studies were cross-sectional and did not include control groups: Only 12% of the studies included a healthy control group, 10% included a control group consisting of patients with another type of illness. Longitudinal studies were rare and amounted to 8% of all studies analyzed.

According to a more recent meta-analysis of 85 studies published between 1990 and 1995 (Hanl, 1995), these basic conceptual and methodological problems still persist. Over 75% of the studies were based on samples with mixed age groups (i.e., children and adolescents). Up to 40% of the more recent studies on coping with illness included a control group: Only 11% made use of a longitudinal research design. Furthermore, it should be pointed out that most investigators studied illnesses that had shown increased rates of prevalence in recent years. Such illnesses are those that show a moderately severe course and for which adequate medical treatment is available. Among these illnesses, diabetes was the most frequently investigated: According to Hanl's analysis, 62% of all empirical studies published between 1990 and 1995 included samples of diabetic patients.

## FACTORS THAT INFLUENCE COPING PROCESSES AND COPING RESOURCES

We now turn our attention to the process of coping with illness in adolescence. More specifically, we review findings on the developmental, social, life-history, and illness-specific factors that play a role in shaping a person's coping resources and abilities.

Developmental factors were largely neglected in research on coping with chronic illness in adolescence. Although the influence of age on coping behavior was well-documented in studies on healthy adolescents (see chapter 5, this volume), only a few investigators have taken this into account in research on adolescents afflicted with serious illnesses. For instance, it was reported that 13- to 17-year-old pediatric cancer patients make more frequent use of cognitive coping mechanisms than 7- to 12-year-olds (Eiser, 1990), and that 13- to 15-year-old diabetic patients show less adherence to physicians' instructions compared to younger patients (Jacobson et al., 1986). Such findings indicate that compliance worsen despite increased age and that increased cognitive understanding does not inevitably result in improved coping with illness (Joy, 1987). Various authors reported that patient maladaptation increases with age (Hurtig, Koepke, & Park, 1989; Kager & Holden, 1992), which suggests that ill adolescents perceive their illness to be more burdensome as they get older.

Several authors reported gender differences in coping with physical impairments and chronic illness. Male adolescents appear to have greater difficulty in coping with decreased physical strength and mobility (Hofmann & Becker, 1973), whereas female adolescents suffer more from the changes that make them physically unattractive (Zeltzer, Kellerman, Ellenberg, Dash, & Rigler, 1980). Some studies show that females adapt more positively to some illnesses, for example, to diabetes (Niemcryk, Spears, Travis, & Gray, 1990) and cancer (Sanger, Copeland, & Davidson, 1991), whereas other studies have not established an association between gender and adaptation to the illness (Safyer, Hauser, Jacobson, & Bliss, 1993; Smith, Mauseth, Palmer, Pecoraro, & Wenet, 1991). Gender differences were also found with respect to the coexistence of physical and psychological diseases. The findings of Rodin, Daneman, Johnson, Kenshole, and Garfinkel (1985) indicated a comorbidity between diabetes mellitus and eating disorders (i.e., anorexia nervosa, bulimia) in female adolescents, whereas Rovet, Ehrlich, and Hoppe (1988) reported that male diabetic children and adolescents are particularly at risk for developing behavioral disorders.

The constant burdens imposed by a chronic illness deplete the adolescent's personal resources and abilities to cope if he or she is unable to tap resources of social support, in particular, those provided by the family. The family, however, is not only a social resource. Instead, the individual family members, the family as a unit, and members of the adolescent's extended social environment are all affected by and react to the illness. According to the classic study conducted by Minuchin and colleagues (Minuchin et al., 1978), unclear role definitions and lack of problem-solving competence in the family particularly impair the adolescent patient's ability to cope with the illness. In addition, increased conflicts in the family appear to negatively influence psychosocial adjustment to chronic physical illness (Hanson, De Guire, Schinkel, Henggeler, & Burghen, 1992; Patterson, Budd, Goetz, & Warwick, 1993; Wertlieb, Hauser, & Jacobson, 1986). In contrast, families experiencing little conflict and exhibiting high levels of cohesion and organization, as well as open expression of feelings, contribute to successful coping with the illness (Anderson, Auslander, Jung, Miller, & Santiago, 1990; Marteau, Bloch, & Baum, 1987; Wysocki, 1993).

Outside the family, the adolescent's most important social interactions are those involving peers and close friends. The affliction with a serious chronic illness (due to hospital stays and operations), often makes it impossible for the adolescent to continue regular school attendance and maintain school performance. Nevertheless, the adolescent often compensates for the gaps in educational continuity by exercising an uncommon self-discipline and by relinquishing leisure activities. In the long run, the increasing deterioration of health, coupled with overt, often unattractive, changes in physical appearance, as well as the necessity of being subjected to prolonged medical procedures, lead to a solidification of the patient role and decisive loss of social status. In 1980, Johnson pointed to the enormous consequences of chronic illness for friendship relationships, but since then this factor has been neglected in most studies. In one of the few studies on this topic, Wallander, Varni, Babani, Banis, and Wilcox (1988) reported feelings of social isolation and problems with friends in chronically ill adolescents.

Evidence has accumulated showing that everyday stressors and critical life events are strongly associated with the adaptation to the illness (e.g., Brand et al., 1986; Hanson, Henggeler, & Burghen, 1987; Smith et al., 1991), whereas other studies did not find an association between stressful events and adaptation to the illness (Gilbert, 1992). Delamater, Kurtz, Bubb, White, and Santiago (1987) demonstrated that coping mechanisms play an important role in mediating such relationships. The findings from this study showed that adolescent diabetics with good, satisfactory, and poor metabolic control did not differ with respect to perceived stress, but they exhibited different coping strategies. Adolescents with poor metabolic control resorted considerably more often to wishful thinking and avoidance, yet sought help more often.

Despite the enormous variation in coping competencies and life circumstances, chronically ill adolescents exhibit great similarities in their styles of coping. Cognitive coping and problem-focused coping represent the most common approaches (see Eiser, 1990). However, illness-specific coping behavior is also seen. For example, patients suffering from different forms of asthma, as well as children and adolescents with hypopituitarism, show difficulties in dealing with frustrating situations (Drotar, Owens, & Gotthold, 1980; Perrin, 1985). Such findings suggest that both non-illness-related, as well as illness-specific, burdens have an effect on the coping process.

However, more studies focused on defense reactions as compared to coping with illness. Several authors reported that adolescents suffering from chronic physical illness show defense mechanisms like denial and rationalization (e.g., Jacobson et al., 1986). The nearly universal use of denial among adolescents trying to cope with chronic illness was documented in many other studies and was observed to exist at the interpersonal level (e.g., in the collaboration among patient, family, and physician; Erlich, 1987; Reiser, 1987).

Additionally, important aspects of coping are related to severity, as well as to visible signs, of the illness. Research on these aspects generated quite heterogenous findings. Several studies showed that the greater the degree of emotional maladaptation, the more grave the illness is (O'Malley, Koocher, Foster, & Slavin, 1979). Other studies comparing patients suffering from different types of illness also showed that the extent of emotional maladjustment appears connected with the severity of the illness; likewise, improvement of physical health is associated with improved status of emotional health (Orr, Weller, Satterwhite, & Pless, 1984). Equally important for coping with the illness is the extent to which the illness affects physical appearance: The presence of an overt stigma (e.g., dermatological reactions, bodily disfigurations, or amputated limbs), are not uncommonly associated with intense insecurity and behavioral disorders.

Coping with chronic illness in adolescence is also influenced by developmental processes. A 14-year-old adolescent is affected in a completely different manner by a critical life event, such as a serious chronic illness, than a 24-year-old adult, who has already solved most of the developmental tasks still confronting the adolescent. In fact, empirical investigations showed that the mastery of important developmental tasks is delayed or impeded (see, for a summary, Seiffge-Krenke, 1997b). Not only is the achievement of age-specific developmental tasks delayed, impaired, or rendered impossible by illness, but additional problems associated with the specific developmental dynamics of this age group also arise (see chap. 2, this volume). For adolescents, frequent daydreaming, a decreased willingness to disclose personal information to parents, a general tendency to distance oneself from adults, and an increased orientation toward the peer group further complicate the situation. Participation in peer activities and risk-taking behaviors can have deleterious consequences for the adolescent's prognosis, treatment, and compliance.

## A WINDOW ON HEALTH HAZARDS: COPING WITH JUVENILE DIABETES

In the following, we examine the stressors and challenges of coping with chronic illness by considering one illness in particular. Juvenile diabetes (also called Type I diabetes or insulin-dependent diabetes mellitus, IDDM) is a complex disorder of metabolism that is primarily a result of a relative or complete lack of insulin secretion by the beta cells of the pancreas or of defects of the insulin receptors, resulting in excessive amounts of glucose in the blood and urine, excessive thirst, and weight loss, and in some cases leading to such complications as infections and gangrene of the limbs or blindness. It is one of the most frequently occurring and widespread illnesses in childhood and adolescence (see chap. 3, this volume) and has recently received more attention in research (see previous section).

A number of psychosocial variables suspected of influencing metabolic control and compliance in the diabetic patient were studied. Such variables include knowledge and attitudes about the illness, biographically important events, age, competence in coping with the illness, as well as the social support system. Most studies showed relationships between these variables and the quality of metabolic control; however, these studies were based on correlative analyses. Such studies were criticized by LaGreca (1988, p. 140) as being based on a "shotgun approach," that is, attempts to establish univariate relations between an assortment of variables and metabolic control. This methodological approach is inadequate, considering the complex nature of the illness process and coping with the illness. In order to best accommodate for the various problems involved in coping with illness, a longitudinal perspective must be included. Not only must developmental aspects be considered, but also the interactions between the afflicted individual and his or her family (e.g., parental influence on the coping process of their ill children). Unfortunately, the changes introduced by the illness in the lives of afflicted adolescents, their parents, and siblings were hardly investigated.

In the following, we present some results of the Bonn longitudinal study on coping with chronic illness in adolescence (Seiffge-Krenke et al., 1996), which sets coping with illness in the developmental context. An important aspect of this research involved identifying the specific health hazards related to this disease. Furthermore, we observed how diabetic adolescents and their families cope with this illness, in order to determine which coping strategies adolescents choose in the various phases of the illness and what kind of assistance is offered by medical support systems (physicians) and social support systems (friends and family). We were also interested in learning to which extent the adolescent's personal resources (such as self-concept or competence in coping) might affect how he or she deals with this burden. Another issue of interest in this study was related to the changes in the family dynamics introduced by a family member being afflicted by serious chronic illness. The onset of a chronic illness around the time when adolescents are normally beginning to distance themselves from the parents might result in a delay in mastering certain developmental tasks. Therefore, a further aim of the study was to describe the adolescent's adaptation to the illness, especially in relation to developmental progression and psychological health.

Due to the low incidence of the disease, adolescent diabetics were recruited from a total of 17 hospitals in Germany. Every effort was made to achieve a close parallelization with healthy adolescents. We were particularly interested in studying as many adolescents as possible who had only recently been diagnosed with the disease. A total of 109 12- to 16-year-old diabetic adolescents, as well as 108 healthy peers and their families, participated in the study. The majority of families in our sample were intact, with both parents married or living together. Eighty-four percent of the diabetic adolescents came from intact families; 76% of the healthy adolescents' families were intact. The numbers of siblings in the families with healthy and diabetic adolescents were comparable—1.4 and 1.3, respectively. The diabetic adolescents' physicians also participated in the study. The longitudinal study began in 1991 and ended in 1995. Each of the annual waves of the investigation included extensive questionnaires as well as interviews with the adolescents, their parents, and the physicians. Adaptation to the illness was measured according to three criteria: the realization of developmental tasks typical of this age group, the frequency of behavioral and emotional problems, and the status of metabolic control. Levels of glycosylated hemoglobin ($HbA_1$) served as a measure of metabolic control. In the following sections, the results of this study are integrated with the findings obtained by other investigators, according to the relevant topic.

### Stressful Events, Coping, and Defense

Some studies in the past attempted to demonstrate that an increase of serious problems or critical life events is responsible for the etiology and pathogenesis of insulin-dependent diabetes (e.g., Hinkle & Wolf, 1952; Robinson & Fuller, 1985; Stein & Charles, 1975). Although the causal relation between critical life events and the onset of IDDM is questionable, several studies substantiated the significance of stressful events for metabolic control and prognosis of the disease (Barglow et al., 1983; Brand et al., 1986; Chase & Jackson, 1981; Hanson et al., 1987). Additional differentiations are necessary, including number, stressfulness, and controllability of perceived events. Brand et al. (1986), for example, referred to the relationship between life stress and measures of diabetic control for negative events, but not for positive life changes. Delamater et al. (1987), in contrast, found no relation between everyday hassles and metabolic control. Stabler et al. (1987) reported that stressors not only exert direct physiological effects (e.g., increased levels of fear may raise blood sugar levels), but also have an effect on the self-management of diabetes (e.g., by affecting diet, athletic activity, or other health-related behaviors), which, in turn, affects the adjustment to diabetes. Furthermore, acute stress alters blood sugar levels, increases the concentration of free fatty acids, and leads to later damage in the form of coronary heart disease.

As detailed in chapter 5, all adolescents are subjected to a variety of stressors that are part of their development. We agree with Riegel (1976), who considers such stressors as having a development-stimulating function. In our longitudinal study, we therefore used an integrative stress approach, that encompassed both normative, daily events (i.e., mildly stressful everyday problems such as bad grades or quarrels with parents) as well as non-normative, major events (i.e., highly stressful or critical life events like parental divorce, relocation of the family household, or a sibling leaving the family home). Being diagnosed with diabetes as a critical life event differs qualitatively from normative stressors in that it has a discrete onset, affects only a small percentage of adolescents, and leads to a major transformation of the adolescent's and his or her family's previous lifestyles. In light of such major effects on the family system and the often subtle restructuring of family roles and relational patterns that takes place in response to having a chronically ill family member, we were interested in learning how both the adolescent and the concerned family members perceived the burden introduced by the illness.

In our longitudinal study, we thus investigated how diabetic adolescents and their parents perceived everyday burdens and critical life events over the course of 4 years and compared this information with that obtained from healthy adolescents and their parents. The mean number of critical life events occurring up to 2 years before onset of the illness reported by diabetic adolescents was not greater than that of healthy adolescents. However, diabetic adolescents reported an unusually low number of everyday problems compared to healthy adolescents. There was also a striking difference between healthy and ill adolescents in how they subjectively dealt with their burdens and problems. According to the results of the CASQ (Seiffge-Krenke, 1995), which assesses coping skills in various problem domains (such as future, school, family, friends, heterosexual relationships, and self), chronically ill adolescents differed from healthy adolescents in that they were less inclined to actively exploit social resources and also devoted significantly less thought to the problems concerning them. Altogether, it was rather surprising that afflicted adolescents reported fewer everyday problems and were less active in attempting to solve their problems than their healthy counterparts. These basic differences were observed throughout the whole course of the study. An analysis of the data obtained in the fourth survey in 1994 revealed that the discrepancies in stress perception and coping strategies were even greater than in 1991. However, poor metabolic control was associated with a high number of everyday stressors and a less active approach in solving these problems. An analysis of the interrelations between everyday problems and coping with the diabetics' $HbA_1$ values at the first survey showed that self-related problems were highly correlated with metabolic control ($r = .45$, $p = .05$). In addition, active coping ($r = -.36$, $p = .05$), as well as internal coping ($r = -.25$, $p = .05$), were significantly negatively associated with metabolic control. This suggests that poor adaptation is accompanied by many everyday problems and deficient coping abilities.

In addition, we examined to what extent illness-specific coping styles were associated with the status of metabolic adjustment. According to Marrero et al. (1982), adolescent diabetics who undertake problem-focused coping attempts rather than emotionally focused ones show a worse metabolic control than patients who resort to using both of these modalities in a balanced manner. However, other authors (see, e.g., Delamater et al., 1987) found no significant differences between adolescents with good and poor metabolic control with respect to the use of problem-focused coping. Their results showed that poorly adapted diabetics engaged in considerably more wishful thinking and avoidance, yet were also more active in seeking support. We developed a method of assessing individual coping with illness (FKJDI, Seiffge-Krenke, Moormann, Nilles, & Suckow, 1991), which we used to examine coping styles in dealing with nine illness-specific problems (e.g., hospital stays, metabolic disturbances, blood tests, injections, diet, and long-term damage to health). The results showed that the diabetics reported high levels of

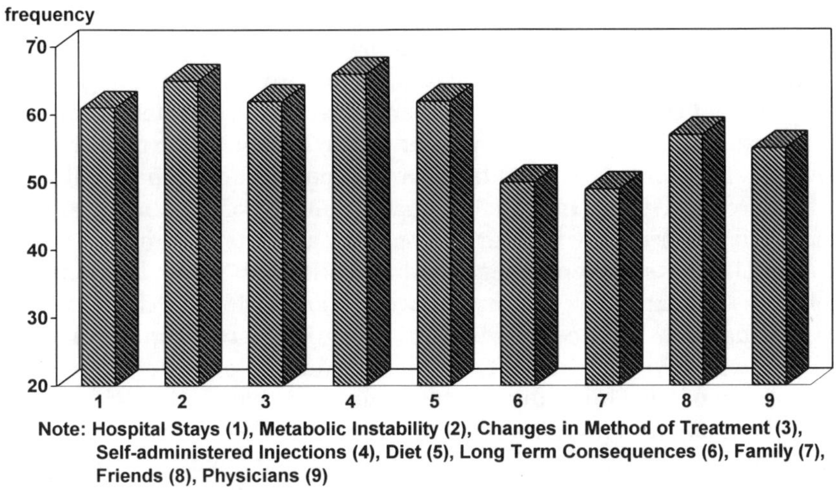


FIG. 7.1. Adolescent diabetics' evaluations of the stressfulness of nine illness-specific stressors ($n$ = 108).

stress in the first survey with respect to most of the illness-specific stressors (see Fig. 7.1). The perception of high stressfulness in these areas remained constant throughout the study—the impact of these stressors did not change much over time.

Furthermore, the diabetic adolescents showed hardly any differentiations in their coping styles in dealing with any of these problems. All nine illness-specific problems elicited many cognitive coping attempts, which reflected the importance of cognitive control in these patients. Similar to the pattern observed in coping with everyday stressors, the diabetic adolescents were reluctant to use social resources in dealing with illness-specific stressors. The adolescents with poor metabolic control were especially less able to accept the support of parents, friends, and physicians and thought they had to deal with these problems themselves. Accordingly, they blamed themselves when imbalances in their metabolic control occurred. Diabetes-related problems augmented their decreased feelings of self-esteem so that they were reluctant to say they were diabetic. Denial, avoidance, and secrecy were relatively prominent modes of dealing with the illness, especially in the group of poorly adapted diabetics. The strong withdrawal from social relations and the difficulty in accepting help was alarming. The poorly adapted diabetics' coping styles were considered prototypical of what we have observed as a general trend among the ill adolescents; that is, most of them preferred to deal with their problems on their own. This basic approach did not change during the course of our study.

Although diabetic adolescents tended to deny the burdens imposed by everyday problems, but strongly emphasized the burdens related to the illness, the ill adolescents' parents were overly concerned about all the problems facing their children. In particular, the mothers felt much more burdened than the adolescents themselves. In the interviews conducted separately with the adolescents and their parents, the diabetic adolescents' parents described considerably more burdens and problems—such as the constant preoccupation with their child's illness, the feeling of being responsible for everything, the time-consuming organization involved in visits to doctors and in planning meals, the supervision of the child outside the home, and so on—than the adolescents themselves. The diabetic adolescents' mothers articulated many of the burdens that were reported by other parents caring for chronically ill children, such as constant monitoring of the afflicted child (Hauser, DiPlacido, Jacobson, Willett, & Cole, 1993), the feeling of being left alone by the husband to deal with the problems (Cook, 1984), chronic overconcern with the sick child, the unfulfilled need to rest and relax (Cole & Reiss, 1993), and fears about later damage to their child's health (Ahmed & Ahmed, 1985). Whereas in our interviews, the parents appeared quite desperate and often mentioned that they would like to receive professional help in order to deal with the emotional strain, the adolescents presented themselves as being "very normal." They not only named significantly fewer illness-specific burdens, but also fewer everyday problems and worries than their parents.

The course of a chronic illness is characterized by several phases related to dealing with the first diagnosis, hospitalization for initial treatment, and corresponding curative procedures. Several investigators pointed out that, above all, the first phase of the illness is full of crises, but with time, the individual becomes increasingly better able to cope with the disease (see, e.g., Kovacs et al., 1985). In the initial phase, defense mechanisms such as denial and trivialization were frequently found (Jacobson et al., 1986; Kovacs & Feinberg, 1982), which corresponds to our observations of the importance of denial and secrecy shown by the diabetic adolescents. In a few families, increased defense-related behaviors among all family members was observed in the initial phase. The following case vignettes illustrate this phenomenon.

> Case A: This patient was a 13-year-old female adolescent with recent onset of the disease. The first signs of the illness were ignored by the family for a long time. Specific inquiry revealed that for over 6 months before the diagnosis was made, the patient consumed over 6 liters of mineral water

per day, without the family being overly concerned or having consulted a physician (the patient's mother was a nurse). It was the patient's older brother, 18 years old, who insisted on consulting a physician. The brother was responsible for purchasing the family's bottled water and finally refused to carry any more heavy cases. Despite the fact that the patient's mother was a nurse, and thus would be expected to possess at least basic knowledge of medical problems, this family exhibited extraordinary denial with respect to the possibility that the daughter might be diabetic.

Another family showed an enormous increase in defense behavior shortly after diagnosis:

Case B: This 14-year-old female patient was ill for only a few weeks before she participated in the first interview in my investigation. At that time, the family communicated very openly and expressed fear and worry about dealing with the disease. The adolescent was also easy to approach in the individual interview. A few months later, the interviewer called on the family to conduct another interview, but this time was received very grimly. The family made it clear that they had nothing to say that had not been already said and did not know what the interviewer "still wanted from them." Also, the afflicted daughter appeared unusually withdrawn. The interviewer became concerned that the family might discontinue their cooperation with the research project team.

In another case, the family was completely oblivious to their diabetic son's emotional strain, whereas he clearly felt helpless and troubled:

Case C: The patient was a 12-year-old boy who was only recently diagnosed with the disease. His mother also recently remarried. The new family included his stepfather and a 4-year-old stepsister. The mother, energetic, eloquent, and a dominating personality in the family, was very positive in her assessment of her son's ability to cope with the illness. She claimed that her son had no problems with the illness and dealt with the illness excellently. She was particularly proud of his self-sufficiency, which she always encouraged. The woman appeared cheerful and optimistic and did not foresee any difficulties. On careful examination, it became apparent that the boy's perspective stood in glaring contrast to his mother's. He was deeply unhappy, lonely, and terribly anguished by fears of dying. He was alone all day long, because his parents just opened a tax advisory business and his stepsister was cared for outside the home. He suffered from the constant fear of falling into a coma and dying without anyone being there to rescue him. This emotional burden was intensified by the difficult family situation: There was an intense rivalry between the stepfather and the boy over the mother. In addition, the boy did not have a single friend, and he did not have any contact with a peer group.

This family showed an impressive splitting in affect in the initial phase of the illness. On the one hand, the mother was cheerful and carefree. However, due to her complete denial, she was unable to perceive how troubled her son actually was. Instead, she praised his self-reliance, which in reality was only feigned. On the other hand, in the interviews, we found the adolescent patient to be afraid, depressed, and perhaps even suicidal. The family's denial of the seriousness of the illness was so intense that even 8 months after the onset of the disease, there was still no physician who supervised the patient's metabolic control.

In these and other cases, a splitting in the defense reactions between parents and afflicted adolescent was observed in the initial phase. Some families also showed an increased number of defense strategies, some of which existed before the diagnosis of diabetes. This not only impaired the awareness of the symptoms and postponed the necessary treatment, but also influenced coping with the disease. Whereas the coping styles of parents and adolescents in families with healthy adolescents were highly correlated when dealing with everyday stressors ($r$ = .62), in families caring for a chronically ill adolescent coping styles used to deal with everyday stressors as well as illness-specific stressors diverged. In particular, the diabetics' mothers showed ambivalent coping responses, reflecting both activity and pessimism, and the fathers of diabetics showed a continuous decrease in active problem solving over the 4 years. Thus, parents of diabetics in this study did not provide efficient coping models for their afflicted children.

### Illness-Related Knowledge, Attitudes, and Compliance

The preceding section vividly illustrates the danger or threat imposed by the illness and the way adolescents and their families react in the initial phase. One may be justified in asking if knowledge about the illness, its causes, and prognosis, helps in dealing with the threat of a chronic illness. Knowledge about the causes of diabetes, the therapeutic management and self-care, as well as attitudes about the illness, were frequently cited as essential prerequisites for compliance and metabolic control (Johnson, 1980, 1984). Yet, a substantial association between degree of knowledge about the disease and the status of metabolic control was not found in most studies. Roth, Borkenstein, and Otto (1987) reported, for example, a correlation of $r$ = –.16, which was confirmed in our investigation ($r$ = .11) using the same instrument. Among the 11 scales of a questionnaire developed by Roth et al. (1987) assessing diabetes-specific knowledge, only one scale ("physiology and causes of diabetes mellitus") differentiated between good and poorly adapted adolescents with juvenile diabetes, whereas poorly adapted adolescents showed lower values. A comparison of means reported by Roth, Neuper, and Borkenstein (1988) showed that subjects were well-informed about the illness, having achieved scores found in adolescents who had participated in a teaching camp for diabetics. Also, no differences in the level of knowledge between males and females or among the different age groups were found. This high level of diabetes-specific knowledge was observed throughout our study. The comparably high ages (12 to 16 years old) of our patients most likely account for the advanced cognitive level, the increased extent of knowledge about the illness, and the high amount of self-management in our group. Ninety-seven percent of the adolescents in our study performed their own insulin injections and reported that they were involved in the planning of their diets.

Knowledge about diabetes thus appears to be a necessary, but not sufficient, condition in itself for achieving good metabolic control. At first sight, it is surprising that knowledge about the illness is not significantly correlated or is even negatively correlated with the status of metabolic control. In fact, Hamburg and Inoff (1985) reported a high level of knowledge about diabetes, but unsatisfactory metabolic control.

In addition, attitudes about the illness do not show fundamental relations with the level of metabolic control, as several studies showed. In our study, we used the Diabetic Adjustment Scale designed by Sullivan (1979). The results showed that the diabetics in the sample were not only autonomous, but exhibited high compliance at the beginning of the study. Nearly all of the adolescents (93%) were committed to doing all they could so that the treatment would be successful, and nearly as many (87%) adhered to the requirements of the diabetes treatment regimen. It was interesting to discover, however, that at least 31% claimed that they sometimes thought it was good to have hypoglycemia. This finding indicates a willingness to take on risks or an interest in new experiences. A comparison between the diabetics with good and poor metabolic control revealed highly significant differences: Adolescents with poor metabolic control more frequently reported that when they were doing well, they forgot to inject themselves with insulin and lied more often about the results of their urine glucose tests. In addition, they thought they were less attractive, that their bodies had too many bruises and hardenings around the sites where they injected insulin, and they found it difficult to find a boyfriend or girlfriend. These feelings probably made them less inclined to adhere to the physician's instructions.

Compared to illness-specific knowledge, which did not change much over time, compliance with the medical regimen clearly worsened over the course of 4 years in diabetic adolescents, irrespective of metabolic control. At the end of our study, less diabetics thought it was necessary to strictly follow the physician's instructions (first wave: 78%, fourth wave: 51%), and their commitment to following the treatment also decreased significantly (first wave: 93%, fourth wave: 72%). Apparently, theoretical knowledge and adequate understanding of the illness are necessary, but not sufficient, conditions for coping with illness. The worsening of glycemic levels during adolescence due to hormonal changes has an impact. The diabetic may experience that despite good compliance, an optimal value of $HbA_1$ is not obtained and thus he or she becomes less encouraged to adhere to the regimen. In addition, age-specific activities, such as snacking, eating out at fast-food restaurants, experimenting with alcoholic beverages, increased mobility, and risk-taking behaviors, represent considerable temptations for the afflicted adolescent. Often, the adolescent's only option is to withdraw socially or to seek companionship with other afflicted adolescents. In our study, a paradoxical finding emerged in the group of poorly adapted diabetics. These children showed adequate knowledge and positive attitudes toward the illness, but also forgot about physician's instructions or falsified results of blood or urine tests. In addition, they had problems with integration in the peer group. Such findings again emphasize that developmental factors are more relevant to maintaining good metabolic control than cognitive factors.

### Internal Resources: Health Status, Body Image, Self-Concept, and Perceived Developmental Progression

Studies of chronically ill adolescents typically neglected internal resources such as self-concept, personality variables, and overall health, and concentrated too much on identifying and describing the social resources that buffer the effects of stress (Jamison et al., 1986). For a long time, studies on diabetic adolescents only focused on a certain aspect of internal resources. Hence, corresponding to studies carried out on adult diabetics, much research concentrated on understanding the diabetic personality (Dunn & Turtle, 1981), thereby attempting to define personality variables that might be typical of the diabetic adolescent. Little consideration was devoted to examining the roles of other important internal resources such as self-concept. This is surprising because it is known that self-concept assumes a central role in the developmental process of identity restructuring during adolescence (Dusek & Flaherty, 1981) and reference to its protective function in coping with illness was made early on (Badura, 1971; Pearlin & Schooler, 1978).

In our study, an analysis of results obtained with the Offer Self-Image Questionnaire (OSIQ) revealed age and sex differences similar to those initially reported by Offer (1984), which were frequently replicated in the literature. Thus, for example, girls in the sample showed a lower self-esteem than boys. In general, the self-concepts of the diabetic adolescents were very similar to those of healthy adolescents. However, adaptation to the illness had an influence on self-concept. Poorly adapted diabetics were found to have a generally less positive self-concept. This finding matches those of other studies in which a lower self-esteem was found in chronically ill adolescents, compared to healthy adolescents (Bulman & Wortman, 1977; Pearlin & Schooler, 1978). Consequently, poorly adapted diabetics have limited internal resources to buffer the effects of stress. One consequence of a more negative self-concept could be that poorly adapted diabetic adolescents are more inhibited about making use of the social support systems available to them. This problem was identified in the analysis of their coping behavior and is discussed in the next section.

With respect to health status and body image, the results are divergent. On the one hand, the diabetic adolescents are prone to exhibit a façade of normality. The analysis of data on health-related complaints, for example, revealed that the diabetic adolescents described their overall health status as being better than in the healthy control group. Only 30% of the diabetic adolescents mentioned physical complaints, compared to 53% of the healthy adolescents. The most common complaint was pain, above all, in the head region, followed by cold and flu symptoms, uneasiness, and stomachaches. When asked whether they or other family members suffered from other chronic illnesses, both the healthy and diabetic adolescents reported the same rates. About 13% reported having a chronic illness such as asthma or allergies, and 25% reported that other family members suffered from a chronic illness. Thus, in summary, the diabetic adolescents reported the same amount of health problems, such as additional chronic illnesses, but a lower number of physical complaints.

Despite this overall good health status, diabetic adolescents showed a more negative body image. For example, in the semistructured interviews, nearly all afflicted adolescents displayed evidence of marked problems in accepting their bodies. Many diabetics also said that they perceived a strong threat to their physical identity, caused by the daily self-injury of injections and the related lesions, hardenings, and bruises.

The experience of one's own body as being deformed and damaged often caused the adolescents to feel so ashamed that they avoided participating in certain activities with their peers, such as visits to the swimming pool. The results of an analysis of the semantic differential, as presented in Fig. 7.2, showed that diabetic adolescents experienced their bodies as being less healthy, less interesting, less mature, and less flexible. A longitudinal analysis of body concept showed that diabetics were able to develop a more positive body image and integrate physical maturity into the body concept. Yet, differences were still evident up to the third survey.

A relation between poor metabolic control (elevated $HbA_1$ values) and negative body image was already evident at the beginning of our study, when we first administered the semantic differential. Patients with poor metabolic control defined their bodies as being more ugly ($r = -.33$), weak ($r = -.25$), plump ($r = -.23$), unkempt ($r = -.34$) and childlike ($r = -.26$), compared to diabetics with good metabolic control. Obviously, poor metabolic control is associated with an even more negative perception of the body.

The results clearly illustrated that the diabetic adolescents felt quite healthy (i.e., they named low physical complaints). But they were very sensitive about having the stigma of a defective body. The perception of being more childlike could indicate delayed maturational processes; however, this was not confirmed by our comparison of the average ages of physical maturation in both groups. Despite an enormous delay of 2

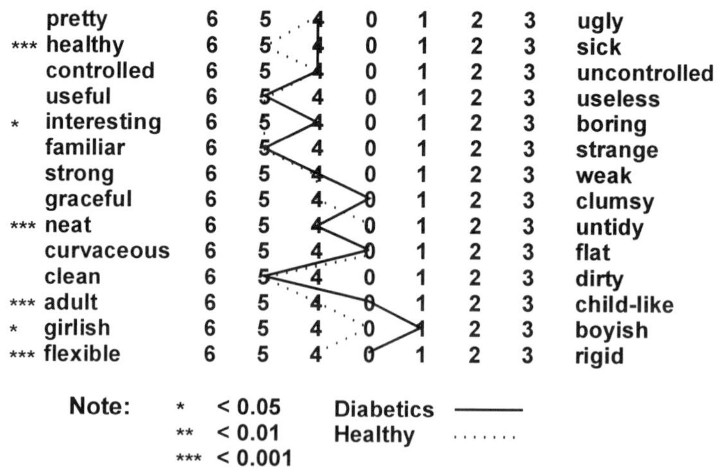


FIG. 7.2. The body image of diabetic ($n$ = 108) as compared to healthy adolescents ($n$ = 107).

to 3 years, diabetics were able to adequately perceive and integrate their physical changes into their body concept.

Another important aspect concerns the adolescents' overall psychosocial development. In our longitudinal study, we examined how well adolescents mastered several developmental tasks, as defined by Havighurst (1953), such as dealing with physical maturity, autonomy from parents, peer group integration, beginning heterosexual relationships, and the development of occupational competence. Healthy adolescents showed a greater desire to master the tasks related to achieving increased autonomy from their parents and developing close friendships and heterosexual relationships than their diabetic counterparts. In addition, they approached these tasks more actively and were more successful in realizing them (Seiffge-Krenke, 1997b). In particular, female diabetic adolescents showed less desire to master (and were less successful in mastering) developmental tasks leading to increased autonomy from their parents and increased orientation to same- and opposite-sex peers than their healthy peers. Thus, it can be speculated that achieving independence and autonomy is generally more difficult for female adolescents than for males (Gilligan, 1982), especially for chronically ill females. Interestingly (and convergent with the diabetics' body concept), diabetic adolescents described a lower developmental status with respect to their physical maturity, compared to healthy adolescents. The longitudinal analysis revealed, however, that diabetics were able to make up for most delays by the end of the study. All in all, the group of diabetics showed a remarkable developmental progression over the course of 4 years. For example, they achieved the levels attained by the healthy adolescents for most tasks. After 4 years, a lower developmental status in diabetics was observed in only two tasks: the onset of heterosexual relations and the development of an individual lifestyle. It appeared likely that the normal process of mastering these tasks was negatively influenced by being forced to comply with the restrictions associated with a strict medical regimen.

### Family Relations and Coping With Illness

The onset of juvenile diabetes in our sample had typically occurred at a time when the adolescents were beginning to distance themselves from their parents; yet, the parents were still considerably involved in the management of the illness. Thus, a great deal of cooperation and control in the family was required, which placed great demands on all family members. The results presented so far confirm that the parents felt extremely burdened by this situation. Thus, it is not surprising that some researchers found adjustment problems among parents of chronically ill children (Crain, Susman, & Weil, 1986) and high rates of family conflicts, which, in turn, contributed to a worsening of metabolic control in the adolescent (Koski & Kumento, 1975). The reciprocal nature of the adjustment process in the context of the family was first described by Hauser and Solomon (1985). On the one hand, familial patterns of coping with chronic illness influence the afflicted adolescent; on the other hand, the illness represents a source of first acute, then chronic, stress in the family. Several studies in the past (see, e.g., Delbridge, 1975; Koski, 1969; White, Kolman, Wexler, Polin, & Winter, 1984) established links among pathological familial relationships, an unfavorable course of illness, and poor compliance. Other studies confirmed the central importance of the family climate and family interaction for the successful treatment of diabetes. For example, in a study of 10- to 20-year-old diabetics, Shouval, Ber, and Galatzer (1982) observed that compliance with the therapeutic regimen was enhanced in families that were emotionally supportive and in which the family members were not pressured to strictly obey rules. According to Anderson, Miller, Auslander, and Santiago (1981), parents of well-adapted diabetics encouraged their children more often to be more self-reliant and to be open in expressing their feelings than parents of children with poor metabolic control.

The family climates of adolescents who showed good metabolic control were cohesive and seldom showed conflict (Hanson & Henggeler, 1984; Hauser, 1992; Marteau et al., 1987). In a study conducted by Hauser and Solomon (1985), significant correlations were found between good diabetic adjustment and a family climate characterized by an emphasis on self-reliance, orientation to active recreational pursuits, and a high level of organization. According to Wertlieb et al. (1986), diabetic adolescents show fewer behavior problems when their families engage in high levels of active leisure time activities, are well-organized, and share responsibility. Taken together, the most favorable family climate shows cohesion and solidarity, is clearly organized and well-structured, is less strained by conflict, encourages various social activities and leisure time pursuits, and helps the children to achieve age-typical independence and self-reliance.

In our longitudinal study, we found definite changes in the family climate (as measured by the Family Environment Scale [FES] Moos & Moos, 1981) in families caring for diabetic adolescents, compared to the families with healthy adolescents. As is seen in Fig. 7.3, the family climate in families with diabetic adolescents was characterized by a more rigid family structure, organization and control of the family activities, and a strong achievement-orientation.

This characterization of the family climate from the adolescents' perspectives corresponds well to the parents' assessments. In contrast, families with healthy adolescents claimed that the family members were closer to one another, conflicts were dealt with more openly, and family members enjoyed a greater amount of autonomy; thus, altogether indicating the presence of a family climate that promoted development. Thus, our diabetic families corresponded to the achievement-oriented family type according to Billings and Moos (1982), characterized by a high level of organization, control, and achievement orientation, as well as a decreased emphasis on family members' independence. This achievement-oriented family climate appears to be characteristic of families with diabetic adolescents, regardless of metabolic control. Except for the fact that the members of families with a diabetic adolescent showing good metabolic control reported a better quality of interpersonal relationships, no differences were found with respect to other family dimensions. This indicates that although cohesion and unity in these families are strong, the adolescent still experiences more control and less autonomy than does the diabetic adolescent with poor metabolic control. The lowered external orientation of all families with diabetic children also has negative consequences for the development of the adolescent. Patterson, McCubbin, and Warwick (1990) stressed that intellectual and recreational activities are very important for coping with chronic illness, because they provide opportunities for the family

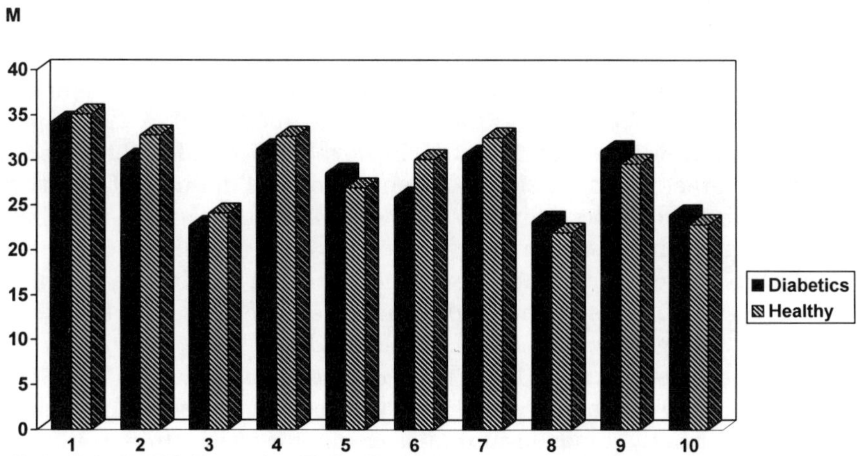


Note: Cohesion (1), Expression (2), Conflict (3), Independence (4), Achievement Orientation (5), Intellect.-cult. Orientation (6), Active/Recreational Emphasis (7), Moral/Religious Emphasis (8), Organization (9), Control (10)

FIG. 7.3. Differences in perceived family climate in families with diabetic ($n$ = 107).

members to relax and enjoy some diversion from daily stress and thus are resource promoting.

Although the observed changes in the family climate represent functional coping behaviors elicited by being confronted with caring for a diabetic child, especially in the initial phase of the illness, in the long run, they can lead to an overly rigid family structure that is detrimental to the development of all family members. This danger was evident among the diabetic adolescents in our sample, who showed slower developmental progression and more limited autonomy than their healthy peers. Also, an analysis over time revealed that the achievement-oriented family climate did not change over the 4 years of our investigation. This implies a potentially inhibitory influence on development in all diabetics, irrespective of their metabolic control.

Having outlined these general changes in family climate of families caring for a diabetic adolescent, we may now focus on the specific modes of familial coping, with respect to coping with general family stressors and coping with the chronic illness.

An analysis of family coping with everyday problems measured by the Family Crisis-Oriented Personal Evaluation Scales (F-COPES; McCubbin & Patterson, 1982) revealed that the diabetic adolescents' mothers were more inclined to passively accept the difficulties in their families, as compared to the healthy adolescents' mothers. Only mothers of well-adapted adolescents showed more efforts to encourage the family to accept outside assistance than did the mothers of adolescents with poor metabolic control. The fathers of well-adapted and poorly adapted diabetic adolescents did not differ with respect to how they coped with familial difficulties. In addition, major differences were found in illness-specific coping efforts among the parents (as measured by the Coping Health Inventory for Parents [CHIP] developed by McCubbin et al., 1983). Whereas the diabetic adolescents' mothers did not differentiate their coping efforts according to their child's gender, age, or metabolic control, the fathers were more involved with their afflicted daughters than sons. For example, they were more active in helping their daughters to seek social support and to maintain self-esteem, emotional stability, and good compliance. These findings lend support to the gender-role intensification hypothesis developed by Shulman and Seiffge-Krenke (1997), who observed that the roles of mothers and fathers were more strictly divided in families caring for a sick child, compared to families with healthy children.

In summarizing the results presented so far, it becomes apparent that, compared to the diabetic adolescents themselves, the parents reported a greater number of stressors and perceived themselves to be more burdened by the illness. Mothers and fathers dealt with the illness differently, whereby especially the fathers showed differences in their coping behaviors depending on their child's gender, but did not differ from their spouses with respect to perceptions of family climate. Although the very rigid, achievement-oriented family climate observed in families caring for a diabetic adolescent may be essential for achieving good metabolic control in the initial phase of the illness, it remains unclear what the long-term effects of this family climate on the adolescents are. In particular, this family climate hinders the achievement of age-specific developmental tasks, which is a grave consequence indeed. As already mentioned, diabetic adolescents make up for most of their setbacks in several developmental tasks over the years, but a certain delay in individuality and approaching members of the opposite gender were still noticeable by the end of the study.

An analysis of communication patterns among family members in the diabetic family also substantiated this concern. In our study, we requested the families to complete the Family Interaction Task (FIT; Condon, Cooper, & Grotevant, 1984), which required the entire family to solve a problem together. On two occasions, in 1991 and 1993, the family sat together and planned a joint vacation. Already the first measurement revealed that in the families with diabetic adolescents, the individual contributions made to discussion were shorter and argumentation was more defensive. In contrast, the members of families with healthy adolescents not only engaged in more conversation, but also attempted to integrate the various contributions made to the discussion. Following Hauser's (1992) theory, diabetic families showed communication patterns characteristic of constraining interaction (i.e., an interactional pattern likely to bridle development). In contrast, communication in healthy families resembled enabling interaction, which promotes development. Two years later, communication was still limited: The individual family members made fewer contributions and the diabetic adolescents tended to give in to the others' suggestions. The diabetic adolescents' mothers' indirect suggestions were striking. The communication skills in families with healthy adolescents, in contrast, were more balanced, and the discussion was more lively and controversial.

### Relationships With Friends and Romantic Partners

As just outlined, we found various differences between the coping efforts exhibited by the fathers and mothers of diabetic adolescents. Whereas Etzwiler and Sines (1962) pointed out early on that the distribution of responsibility for the care and supervision of an ill child is often dependent on family role, surprisingly little research has been conducted since then about the differential influence of individual family members—in particular, fathers and siblings—on the diabetic child and his or her ability to cope with the illness. This holds true for other, nonfamily-related sources of support such as friends, schoolmates, or teachers. As Simonds (1977) showed, the diabetic child has problems in interacting with these individuals; nevertheless, they are important sources of support outside of the family (LaGreca, 1992; Marrero et al., 1982; Powers, Dill, Hauser, Noam, & Jacobson, 1985; Warren-Boulton, Anderson, Schwartz, & Drexler, 1981). Although the integration in the peer group facilitates age-typical development, compliance problems emerge, because the adolescent is more likely to engage in activities adverse to his or her health. This represents a dilemma insofar as the social support provided by friends entails not only stress-reducing, but also stress-inducing functions. While the family's role in providing support for the adolescent suffering from chronic illness received much attention, the roles of friends and the functions of friendships as sources of social support were hardly examined.

In our research project, much time was devoted to this important aspect. By employing standardized tests and interviews, we examined the roles of friends and romantic partners, as well as trying to understand the nature of typical conflicts with same-sex and opposite-sex peers. We found that diabetic and healthy adolescents possessed a rather extensive network of friends. Seventy percent of the diabetics and 75% of the healthy adolescents had three or more friends. It should be mentioned, however, that nearly 30% of the diabetic adolescents apparently had no friends at all, in comparison to 12% of the healthy adolescents. In order to assess the quality of friendships and relationships with romantic partners, the Network of Relationship Inventory (NRI) was administered (Furman & Buhrmester, 1985). Despite the existence of a fairly large social network, the quality of friendships in diabetic adolescents (compared to healthy peers) was poorer, characterized by less affection, less admiration, and less intimacy. In addition, the power structure of their friendships was less balanced. Less closeness and intimacy, as well as the asymmetric distribution of power between friends, indicate that characteristics of more mature friendships typical of this age group, such as reciprocity, cohesion, and intimacy (Buhrmester & Furman, 1987) were not yet realized. Furthermore, the interview data revealed that the majority of diabetic adolescents appeared unable to talk about conflicts arising in their friendships or about the ways such conflicts might be resolved. Although diabetics made gains in intimacy in friendship relations over time, their scores remained lower than the scores reported by healthy agemates (Seiffge-Krenke, 1997a). It, therefore, can be speculated that diabetic adolescents do not easily identify with healthy friends and this hesitation contributes to their lower level of friendship intimacy. This may be related to the fact that although affliction with diabetes is not overtly apparent, it nevertheless, greatly dominates the diabetic's daily life and leads to a feeling of being different. A similar result was found with respect to romantic relations: Diabetics started having sexual relations later and were less sexually active. More important, they reported less intimacy in their romantic relations (as measured by the NRI), when compared to healthy agemates. Instead, to chronically ill adolescents, instrumental aid was important in romantic relations (Seiffge-Krenke, 1997a).

In summary, the data on familial support systems and friendships in the diabetic adolescent showed that despite the apparent intactness and large scope of the diabetic adolescent's social network, the adolescents lowered emotional closeness to parents, friends, and romantic partners. They experienced high functionality, rigid structure, and relatively lower autonomy in their families. In addition, romantic relationships seemed to serve different functions for diabetic and healthy adolescents. These basic differences in the qualities of relationships with parents, friends, and romantic partners hardly changed over time.

### The Physician–Patient Relationship

In attempting to identify which resources adolescents actually exploit in coping with chronic illness, not only the social support system, but also the medical support system must be considered. In this regard, the relationship between patient and physician is critically important for compliance and coping with illness. Adult patients with chronic illness rank trust in their physician as being especially beneficial in helping them to cope with their illness (Freund & McGuire, 1991). However, as was already discussed in chapter 2, it cannot be assumed that such findings obtained in adults are applicable to the adolescent, who, due to the normal separation processes occurring in the parent–child relationship, becomes an "unmotivated patient" (Rogers, 1970). In contrast to the general tendency among healthy adolescents to avoid doctors (frequently reported in the literature), the chronically ill adolescents in our study maintained surprisingly good relationships with their attending physicians. In fact, in interviews, diabetic adolescents reported that they often discussed their problems and worries with their physicians, sometimes more often than with their parents.

According to the reports of adolescent diabetics, positive relationships with the physician were characterized by the following attributes:

1. When they knew the physician well.
2. When the physician was informed about their individual life situation.
3. When they were able to talk openly with the physician.
4. When they were not afraid of being negatively sanctioned if they deviated from the therapeutic regimen.
5. When the physician took the time to explain things in detail and so that they understood.
6. When they felt that the physician's recommendations helped them.

The physician's professional competence was highly regarded. Only a small portion of the diabetic adolescents reported very poor relationships with their physicians. These adolescents most likely suffered from the high turnover of physicians in hospitals. Indeed, this situation was consistently criticized by diabetic adolescents in our sample. Slightly less than half of the adolescents reported that they experienced continuity in their healthcare provider relationships. In fact, 41% of the diabetics sought care in another hospital at least once, and 10% changed hospitals or specialists several times.

The importance of the patient–physician relationship was also confirmed by the results of the questionnaire on coping with illness (FKJDI; Seiffge-Krenke et al., 1991). Over 70% of the diabetic adolescents named faith in physicians as being extremely important in helping them to cope with illness-specific problems like hospital stays, instability of metabolic control, and metabolic crises, blood samples, injections, diet, long-term damage to health, and future difficulties. It is interesting to note that over 50% of the diabetic adolescents felt that faith in their doctors exerted a positive influence on their interactions with the family, friends, and peers, which suggests that the physician was also able to offer them competent psychological advice. There were no significant differences between the adolescents with good and poor metabolic control with respect to their relationships with their doctors. However, a significantly greater number of diabetics with poor metabolic control reacted to problems with physicians and healthcare personnel by exhibiting withdrawal or by adopting the attitude that they had to solve the problems on their own. This illustrates how difficult it is to establish trust in the relationship between physician and adolescent at risk.

### Psychosocial Consequences of the Illness

The influence of the age of onset of diabetes for later adjustment to the illness was repeatedly documented; however, the evidence was contradictory with respect to its protective or damaging effects (see, e.g., Greydanus & Hofmann, 1979). Ryan, Vega, and Drash (1985) called attention to the fact that early onset of the illness (which is frequently accompanied by metabolic instability) increases the likelihood of neuropsychological changes and corresponding cognitive deficits, which, in turn, impair coping with illness. Rovet et al. (1988) reported such changes, in particular, those resulting in visual–spatial deficits.

In our sample of 109 diabetic adolescents, 10% were ill for less than 1 year, 22% were ill for 1 to 2 years, 22% were ill for 3 to 5 years, and 46% were ill for more than 5 years. The average duration of illness (5.4 years) was thus comparably short. At the beginning of this study, nearly one half ($n = 49$) of these diabetic adolescents had good metabolic control ($HbA_1 < 7.5$), 32 had satisfactory metabolic control ($HbA_1 = 7.5$ to 9.5), and only 16 had poor metabolic control ($HbA_1 > 9.5$). Thus, overall, the adolescents were well-adapted. The gender differences were negligible. A differentiation, according to age, revealed an interesting finding: Whereas good metabolic adjustment predominated in early adolescence (12 to 13 years old), in mid-adolescence (14 to 15 years old) overall metabolic adjustment was poor, and around 16 years old, the distribution of good and poor metabolic adjustment was balanced. This corresponds to the reports of physicians and parents, who claimed that more compliance problems occurred in mid-adolescence.

This cross-sectional finding was validated by the analysis of the longitudinal course of the $HbA_1$. In the first survey, when the diabetic adolescents had a mean age of 13.9 years, nearly one half of the sample showed good metabolic control. During the second and third years (mean ages = 15.1 and 16.2 years, respectively), metabolic control clearly worsened, and in the fourth year of our investigation (mean age = 17.1 years), the $HbA_1$ values decreased again, reflecting improved metabolic adaptation. The status of metabolic control was also dependent on the duration of illness: The adolescents afflicted with the illness for 1 to 2 years showed the best initial metabolic control, which increasingly worsened with the duration of the illness. This suggests that the adolescents strictly adhered to the therapeutic regimen after the onset of the illness, but over time, they became more lax in following physician's recommendations. It should be noted that after about 2 years of being afflicted with diabetes, a labile postremission phase sets in. This phase is characterized by the complete loss of pancreatic B-cells, which can result in considerable metabolic disturbances.

Because the sample showed a comparably short duration of illness, the long-term consequences of the illness described by parents and physicians supervising the afflicted adolescents were correspondingly few. As a rule, the parents named considerably more concerns about the future with respect to possible damage to health such as retinopathies, nephropathies and neuropathies than did the adolescents themselves.

It was frequently reported that the various strains related to treatment of diabetes and the continued impairment of normal developmental progression in children and adolescents represent increased risks for psychological maladjustment (see Wilkinson, 1987 for a summary). In several studies, increased fears and depressive symptoms, major behavioral problems, and an impaired self-concept were found (Sullivan, 1978; Swift, Seidman, & Stein, 1967). For many children and adolescents, the onset of a serious illness and the resulting identity and status problems create a vicious circle between feelings of inferiority and social withdrawal. If they are unsuccessful in dismantling negative attitudes about their own bodies and regaining their self-esteem, the illness typically follows a negative course, and ego development is delayed (Hauser, Borman, Jacobson, Powers, & Noam, 1991) The consequences of the enormous emotional strain are reflected in an increased prevalence of emotional and psychiatric disturbances seen in chronically ill children and adolescents. Wilkinson (1987), for example, reported that the incidence of psychiatric disorders in chronically ill adolescents is two to three times greater than in healthy control groups. Other studies, however, found that the incidence of psychiatric disturbances among diabetic samples hardly differed from those found in healthy peers (Simonds, 1977). In addition, compared with peers afflicted with other types of illnesses, diabetic adolescents showed the lowest incidence of psychiatric disturbances (Zeltzer, LeBaron, & Zeltzer, 1984). For the majority of the afflicted adolescents, most of these psychiatric disorders were related to initial stress reactions, and the symptomatology receded in a few months after diagnosis (Kovacs et al., 1985). Feelings of being different and a damaged self-concept due to the illness appear to normalize at the very latest by adulthood.

As just reported, in our longitudinal study, a more negative body image and a negative self-concept was found, especially among the poorly adapted adolescents. These deficits were less striking among the well-adapted adolescents, whose values were more similar to those found in healthy controls. In order to assess behavior and emotional problems, we also administered the YSR (Achenbach, 1991d) to the adolescents and the Child Behavior Checklist (CBCL; Achenbach 1991a) to the parents. The afflicted adolescents described themselves as being less burdened by symptoms, a result that was confirmed by the assessments made by both parents. Healthy girls, for example, had higher values than diabetic girls in six of the seven YSR scales—somatic complaints, depression, unpopular, aggression, delinquency, and thought disorder; healthy boys described themselves as being more delinquent and behaviorally disturbed than diabetic boys. This greater burden of symptoms perceived by the healthy adolescents was confirmed by parental assessments. It appears as if the desires to be "normal" and "just like the others," which were repeatedly articulated by the diabetic adolescents in the interviews, were so strong that the adolescents did not acknowledge the burden of symptoms or even deny problems. This is consistent with the findings already reported, that considerably fewer diabetic adolescents reported bodily complaints than did healthy adolescents, and diabetics also named fewer everyday stressors than did healthy peers. Only the diabetic males with poor metabolic control reported higher symptomatology, in particular, higher depressive mood, increased body complaints, and higher social withdrawal. Their parents also described their sons as being more physically burdened, more schizoid, and depressive.

Although the presence of intense defense formations at the beginning of the illness was repeatedly documented (see, e.g., Erlich, 1987; Jacobson et al., 1986), it was surprising that diabetic adolescents showed fewer behavioral and emotional problems than did physically healthy adolescents. This discrepancy was described by the adolescents themselves and their parents throughout the study. In addition, adolescents who were ill for over 5 years did not perceive the burden of symptoms to be greater or less than the recently diagnosed adolescents or than those who were ill for 1 to 2 years. The various defense mechanisms exhibited by families were already described earlier. In some families, however, it is more obvious how the illness potentiates a neurotic family development. The following case report is an example of how the outbreak of the illness was used to intensify incestuous relationships. Other cases concerning the problem of boundaries between mothers and afflicted adolescents are described in Seiffge-Krenke (1997c):

> Case D: When the interviewer called on the patient's family to conduct the scheduled interview, she was coldly received by the patient's mother, who was dressed in black. The interviewer's initial suspicion that something was wrong with the patient's mother was later confirmed, when she learned the patient's mother was epileptic. Her 13-year-old daughter, who was ill with diabetes for over 1 year, made a precocious impression and appeared very flattered by being visited. The mother made several intrusive interruptions during the individual interview with the daughter, by

claiming, for example, that she had to clean up and by placing cake directly before her diabetic daughter, commenting that the cake was intended for the interviewer only. The patient herself reported that she got along better with her father than with her mother. The alleged closeness of father–daughter relationship was confirmed on the father's appearance: The daughter virtually blossomed. In contrast, as soon as her mother appeared, the daughter assumed a tense posture. During the subsequent interview with the whole family, the father clearly dominated, whereas the mother's contributions were lethargic and complicated, and she was frequently interrupted by her husband and daughter. The father confirmed that his daughter came to him and not to his wife to talk about all her problems. He mentioned that his daughter was very involved with the topic of sexuality. In this connection, the mother noted that since the onset of the illness, her daughter started to sleep with her father in the parents' bed, whereas she herself slept in her daughter's room. The mother appeared weak and submissive; however, many of her contributions to the discussion were differentiated and thoughtful. She often felt helplessly subjected to her daughter's aggression. The father reported that the mother suffered from epilepsy and thus was often so forgetful that he felt it necessary to do everything himself. The mother protested, saying that she certainly was able to take care of things. The interviewer had the impression that the daughter assuredly and sovereignly assumed control over her parents, and that she was now the "queen" of the family. Obviously, diabetes potentiated the development of a pre-existing and strongly incestuous father–daughter relationship from which the mother was increasingly excluded.

# 8

# Health Care-Seeking Behavior in Adolescence

There is a difference between an adolescent's awareness of illness and seeking medical or psychosocial treatment. This chapter focuses on theory and data concerning the motives and reasons that play a role in determining why adolescents do or do not use health services, especially those offering psychotherapy or psychological counseling. In analyzing some of the components of adolescent aversion to physicians and other health care providers, emphasis is placed on considering the general developmental dynamics particular to adolescence. As will be seen, the reasons why adolescents do or do not seek and accept medical or psychosocial care are strongly linked to their general reservations about accepting help from adults. In addition, the concrete expectations parents have about help offered by physicians, psychologists, and other health care professionals is discussed.

## ILLNESS BEHAVIOR AND THE RELATIONSHIP BETWEEN PHYSICIAN AND PATIENT

There were frequent reports in the literature that adolescents lack an awareness of how urgently they require medical or psychosocial care (e.g., Golombek, 1969; Rinsley, 1980). Also, it was reported that adolescents as a group show a marked tendency to avoid physicians and institutions providing health care, are uncooperative with health care providers, and show low compliance (Garrison & McQuiston, 1989). Adolescent patients in general and hospitalized adolescents in particular are described as being less collaborative and more antagonistic toward psychotherapy than adults (O'Malley, 1990). As a first approach toward explaining why adolescents accept or reject a health care provider's offers to help, an understanding of the nature of the patient–provider relationship is useful. Unfortunately, little work was done to examine the nature of the relationships between adolescents and health care professionals. This is surprising, because the quality of the relationship between the patient and health care professional affects the extent to which health care services are utilized. Furthermore, the quality of the encounter between patient and provider modifies patient behavior (i.e., subsequent adherence to medical recommendations and active collaboration in psychotherapy). In addition, the relationship between adolescent and health care provider is affected by the patient's motivations for seeking care. In the case of the adolescent patient, this factor becomes highly important.

### Utilization of Medical and Psychotherapeutic Services: Explanatory Models

A patient afflicted with a physical illness involving pain and discomfort is usually grateful for medical treatment that alleviates such complaints. The patient is also likely to accept psychosocial counseling offered by a psychotherapist. However, only a small proportion of illnesses begin with pain, and even healthy patients need to consult a physician in the absence of symptoms, for example, when preventative checkups are necessary. Moreover, health and illness are different yet not necessarily distinct states of being; that is, they belong to a continuum extending from unlimited well-being to life-threatening conditions.

The model of health care processes proposed by Lehtinen, Ville, and Väisänen (1978) describes the individual steps of the decision-making process involved in seeking and utilizing health care services, including psychotherapy. According to this model, two distinct phases are identifiable in this process: a phase in which the awareness of the illness becomes consciously or unconsciously organized (Steps 1 to 4), followed by a phase in which the patient makes a decision to seek medical treatment or other professional health assistance (Steps 5 to 7). Altogether, the following decision-making steps are involved:

1. The patient does not perceive disturbance to well-being.
2. The patient is bothered by or suffers from disturbance.
3. The patient describes himself as being sick (self-diagnosis).
4. The patient consciously or unconsciously organizes a state of being ill (associated with lay concepts of etiology).
5. The patient recognizes that medical treatment is necessary and is willing to accept help from professionals instead of relying on self-treatment.

6. The patient consults a physician and does not engage in *lay referral*—does not discuss health disturbances with or seek advice from nonprofessionals (e.g., family, neighbors, or friends).
7. The patient chooses a certain physician according to ideas about methods of treatment.

The level of perceiving symptoms and interpreting them as such is considered as the first step. People differ in their sensitivity to physical symptoms or according to how they define various symptoms as serious or important. For example, perception of illness varies depending on SES, whereby low-income individuals show a higher tolerance of symptoms and a lower knowledge about health care (Freund & McGuire, 1991). There is also evidence of cultural differences in the way bodily symptoms are perceived, interpreted, and presented. For example, Zola (1966) found that depending on their cultural background, many individuals postponed consulting a physician despite bodily discomfort, especially when the patient thought the symptom was unusual or somehow threatening. When such patients stated that they needed medical treatment, this was usually related to social pressure; that is, the health disturbance required the legitimization or approval of other persons in the environment prior to the individual's seeking medical treatment or acting on symptoms. These individuals thus were compelled to describe themselves as being "sick" and took the appropriate actions. Illness behavior was similarly described by Lederer (1967), who defined a *patient* as "a person with an illness" (p. 248). According to this author, illness is composed of the following four stages:

1. The transitional period between health and illness.
2. Dealing with the diagnosis and therapy.
3. Accepting the illness.
4. Recovery and convalescence.

When people become sick, they observe certain unpleasant manifestations or experience painful sensations. They are unable to carry out normal, routine activities and are easily tired. When symptoms involve important parts of the body, the illness becomes more threatening. However, according to the model proposed by Lehtinen et al. (1978), this threat is not necessarily sufficient impetus for the individual to consult a physician and can, in cases of symptoms related to a hereditary predisposition to illness, result in the tendency to postpone seeking medical treatment or consulting a physician. As the illness progresses, the individual then seeks a physician's diagnosis and recommendations for therapy. Lederer (1967) stressed that most patients are apprehensive or have mixed feelings about seeking treatment because they expect great limitations to be placed on their day-to-day lives. After accepting the illness, the individual is set in a social setting that corresponds to his or her illness. Lederer recognized the regression during the acute phase of the illness as having important curative influence (i.e., in this phase the patient is concerned with self-preservation and self-protection in a way that resembles a child). In the recovery phase, when the pathogenic process has been checked, the regressive process must be concluded, and the patient must re-enter the adult world.

In the process of dealing with institutions providing health care services, the individual is not only ascribed the status of a patient, but is also treated differently according to SES. As early as 1958, Hollingshead and Redlich established that health care providers showed differential treatment in the care depending on SES of their patients. In their analysis of "who becomes sick, injured, or dies," Freund and McGuire (1991, p. 31) noted that social class was one of the most useful indicators of health care-seeking behavior and illness (e.g., lower SES was associated with higher rates of morbidity and mortality). In addition, health care-seeking behavior and utilization of medical services were consistently related to socioeconomic dimensions.

### Why People Avoid Physicians: Patient Types

Many ill people postpone consulting a physician, sometimes until a point when little can be done to treat the illness or disease. This tendency to avoid physicians is often related to the severity of the illness. It is a common misconception that health care-seeking behavior is largely a process of obtaining professional medical care. Most health-enhancing or preventive health care measures are nonmedical, and most ailments are never brought to a physician's attention (Zola, 1983). An analysis of health behavior practices as recorded by individuals in the Health in Detroit study (Verbrugge & Ascione, 1987), utilizing a diary method, revealed that persons over 18 years old had disturbed health on 16 days within a 6-week period. This means that people experienced discomfort sufficient to be considered a health problem for more than one third of the study's duration. The least commonly mentioned response to these problems was seeking medical care: Only 5% of the respondents sought medical care on the days they experienced disturbed health (e.g., by going to the physician's office, presenting themselves at hospital outpatient services, or asking for medical advice by telephone. Most individuals opted for self-treatment with prescription or nonprescribed drugs.

Self-imposed restrictions of activities (e.g., postponing errands and chores) were also common, used on nearly 24% of the days on which symptoms were noticed.

British researchers (Freund & McGuire, 1991) found that although 91% of adults studied reported symptoms during the 2 weeks prior to the interview, only 16% consulted a physician. The most frequent action in response to symptoms was taking medicine. In fact, 55% of the adults consumed some form of medication within a 24-hour period before the interview. In the Health in Detroit study, one half of the participants reported that they responded to their health problems by talking with family or friends. According to Verbrugge and Ascione (1987), this response appeared to be therapeutic in itself. Furthermore, discussing health problems with family, friends, and acquaintances often influenced a patient's decision about whether or not to seek professional help. Thus, in many cases, the patient seeks affirmation from others that the health disturbance represents a legitimization for consulting a physician.

Before an individual visits a doctor, voluntarily or not, he or she must overcome a barrier of negative feelings. As argued in chapter 2, with respect to diagnostic procedures, ill persons are often afraid of doctors, of unfavorable diagnoses and painful procedures, or are intimidated by the (overestimated) power of doctors. According to a study by Engelhardt, Wirth, and Kindermann (1973), nearly two thirds of all patients show defined fear reactions, whereas the rest show diffuse reactions. Thus, avoidance or fear-related defense strategies are quite common. Role expectations also come into play in the physician–patient relationship; that are partly contradictory in nature and increase patient anxiety. For example, the physician's knowledge, social status, and power usually lead to the situation that the physician expects the patient to assume a passive role in the relationship. That is, the doctor expects the patient to disclose all or any information requested from him or her, be cooperative during physical examinations and tests, show a willingness to accept a diagnosis, and follow directions for a proposed form of treatment. Several empirical investigations confirmed that physicians are all too aware of their authority, do not consider their patients as socially equal conversational partners, and often make unilateral decisions about the patient's welfare, whereby the patients feel dependent and helpless (Freund & McGuire, 1991).

In addition, Freund and McGuire (1991) showed that social expectations and norms pertaining to the physician–patient relationship are ambiguous. They found, for example, that most people believed that responsible persons should seek professional medical care for a serious ailment, but should not bother doctors or use medical facilities for unimportant or untreatable ailments. A British study found that 25% of the general practitioners surveyed complained that patients consulted doctors for unimportant reasons. At the same time, 56% complained that patients often did not accept a medical expert's opinions (Cartwright, 1967). The contradictory or ambiguous normative expectation is that lay persons should be able to judge correctly when the health disturbance is serious enough to warrant medical attention and which type of professional treatment should be sought, but once the person decides to seek professional advice, he or she must humbly accept the passive role of a patient.

Although patients consider the physician's role to be emotionally neutral, they expect to receive emotional support when ill, which partly explains the higher rates of seeking assistance from lay persons or semiprofessionals. In a German study, Beckmann (1984) was able to show that compared to individuals who sought medical advice from licensed physicians, those who consulted practitioners of homeopathic medicine sought and found more emotional attention. These two groups of patients did not differ with respect to the severity of illness involved. Beckmann also examined the qualities of the patient role, thereby establishing a typology of patients ranging from those who avoided doctors if at all possible to those who consulted physicians despite perfect health. From the perspective of the physician, patients' compliance is very important. However, not all patients are submissive, cooperative, and dependent; some refuse to accept the sick role. Even when the illness is very serious, these patients appear to suffer little from their bodily ailments. It is possible that they overidentify with the norms of a performance-oriented society to the point that any illness is interpreted as physical weakness. Also, the threat of losing status due to loss of income or employment are valid reasons for denying symptoms. In contrast to the patient exhibiting denial of the illness, the physician-avoiding patient is convinced that he or she is ill. Nevertheless, this patient does not expect the doctor to help, and compliance may clearly worsen. The decision to consult a physician may then be related to a cost–benefit analysis so that the subjective benefit of consulting a physician is greater than the costs involved.

## AWARENESS OF HEALTH PROBLEMS AND HEALTH CARE-SEEKING BEHAVIOR IN ADOLESCENTS

The preceding discussion focused on findings obtained in adult populations. The following section aims to examine the work that was done with respect to the behaviors of adolescents as patients, that is, how adolescents perceive physical and psychological symptoms, what they do about it, and how they react to offers of professional assistance, especially as provided by psychotherapists and counseling psychologists. In this regard, reference is made to the model proposed by Lehtinen et al. (1978) outlined earlier. In addition, special consideration is devoted to describing the developmental dynamics that play a role in characterizing adolescent health care-seeking behavior.

### Patterns of Utilization of Medical and Psychosocial Care Services

Health care professionals often find it difficult to distinguish between normal and pathological processes exhibited in adolescence; similarly, adolescents are often unable to differentiate between being *healthy* and *sick*. This results in the situation that some normal developmental changes (e.g., dramatic mood swings) are thought to be pathological, or that very serious illnesses are overlooked because the adolescents are determined to be "as normal as possible." The great discrepancies found to exist between adolescents' and physicians' perceptions and interpretations of bodily symptoms (see chap. 2, this volume) are partly a result of different normative understandings of what being sick actually means. In addition, perception of symptoms and lay diagnosis of an illness entails acceptance of the sick role, which is especially threatening for the adolescent (see chap. 1, this volume). This may explain why adolescents voluntarily seek professional medical help far less often than do adults. For example, a recent representative study of 2,000 German adolescents showed that despite frequent body complaints, 15% of the boys and 11% of the girls did not utilize any medical care service in more than 1 year (Palentien & Hurrelmann, 1995). Utilization of medical services was low even in cases of frequently occurring, acute illnesses.

Similarly, adolescents with emotional or behavioral problems rarely made use of psychological counseling services. In a representative sample of German adolescents, Remschmidt (1989) examined the prevalence of psychological disorders and the frequency with which the adolescents sought assistance from clinical psychologists or counseling services. He found that 13% of the adolescents were in need of counseling, but only 3% sought help from psychosocial care services. Research conducted on North American samples produced similar findings (see chap. 3, this volume). According to the results of the Health and Welfare Canada survey (1989), 28% of Canadian children and adolescents between 4 and 16 years old did not have any contact with a physician during a 1-year period, and only 1% were seen in mental health clinics.

There are many factors that hinder the awareness of physical or mental illness and encourage self-diagnosis and lay etiologies. First, psychological symptoms are more difficult to perceive than bodily symptoms. In his studies on illness behavior, Mechanic (1962) pointed out that mental illness itself precludes an awareness of the illness. Experimental studies of neurotic individuals revealed selective distortions in perception (Young & Martin, 1981). In particular, selective perception and recall of negative, self-related information is commonly seen in depressive patients (Lehtinen et al., 1978). Studies of adolescent coping behavior also showed that greatly troubled adolescents exhibit increased rates of defensiveness, repression, denial, or avoidance (see chaps. 6 and 7, this volume).

In contrast to clinically referred adolescents, nonclinical samples made quite accurate evaluations of psychological dysfunction. In a study on 561 adolescents, a content analysis of responses to the open question, "What does psychological disturbance mean?" revealed a basic awareness of the symptoms of emotional illness. The most frequently named symptoms were inadequate coping with reality, extreme moodiness, and rather neurotic behavior (Seiffge-Krenke, 1986). The causes of psychological dysfunction were predominantly attributed to external factors (e.g., stress at school or at work) rather than internal ones. Females' and males' depictions of symptoms did not significantly differ. Developmentally related factors have an effect on the adolescent's ability to evaluate the psychogenic cause of a disorder. For example, in describing the self, young children rely on concrete behaviors, activities, and a person's external physical characteristics; psychological and relational aspects are not included until the onset of puberty (Damon & Hart, 1982; Livesly & Bromley, 1973).

The perception of a disturbance and the ascribed internal and external causes are also illness dependent. Aarons (1970) proposed that neurotically ill adolescents are preconsciously aware of being disturbed, whereas delinquent adolescents perceive their environment to be more disturbed than they consider themselves to be. Family stressors represent further important factors that influence the adolescent's perception of an illness and the decision to seek help (see chap. 6, this volume). Many psychiatrically ill adolescents have a history of vulnerability factors such as parental divorce, parental criminal activity, parental alcoholism, or a history of being physically abused (Rutter et al., 1977). In a study of adolescents at risk of suicide, Hawton and colleagues (Hawton, Osborne, O'Grady, & Cole, 1982) found that half of the adolescents had no contact with their fathers and very poor relationships with their mothers; in addition, nearly one half of the adolescents had one parent or a sibling who required psychiatric care.

Similar observations were reported by Rutter, Quinton, and Yule (1976) in their study of British adolescents. Compared to healthy control groups, psychiatrically ill adolescents had poor relationships and communication with their parents as well as a chronic family pathology. Moreover, research on family therapy demonstrated that adolescents' symptoms, their perceptions of illness, and family dynamics are closely interwoven (Minuchin et al., 1978). An adolescent who grew up in a pathological family may be compelled to fulfill certain needs of other family members. Under these circumstances, the adolescent is hindered in seeking help from counseling services or practicing psychotherapists. For example, adolescents in pathological families become the family scapegoats; they also may be made responsible for ensuring family cohesion and conflict resolution, as Minuchin et al. (1978) described for anorexic girls. The interindividual bonding in the family thus limits the perception of symptoms and works against the adolescent's decision to seek help. This is important insofar as adolescents do not usually refer themselves to health care providers, but are encouraged to do so by concerned adults, such as teachers and parents.

In the framework of the German Health Services survey (Palentien & Hurrelmann, 1995), 800 physicians and counseling psychologists were asked to state the reasons why their adolescent patients consulted them. Most physicians (74%) stated that adolescents consulted them because of parental influence; only about 45% reported that their adolescent patients consulted them on their own initiative. Adolescents' decisions to make use of medical care were often based on their discussions with their friends and personal acquaintances. Like adults, they typically consulted individuals in the lay network and rarely sought professional health care voluntarily. A comparison with the ratings of psychologists revealed that only 42% reported that their patients were referred by parents, whereas 45% of their adolescent clients were encouraged by teachers to seek help. Self-referral was relatively uncommon; only 19% of psychologists reported that their adolescent patients consulted them on their own account.

Data from a large epidemiological survey of Canadian children between ages of 4 and 16 years old showed similar patterns of medical and psychosocial care use (Woodward et al., 1988). Seventy percent of children and adolescents with physical health problems were referred to physicians by parents, and 57% of those suffering from mental health problems were brought to counseling centers or psychiatric outpatient clinics by their parents. In this regard, it is important to note that parents are often called on to provide information that is relevant to the diagnosis and subsequent treatment. However, as detailed in chapter 2, it is questionable whether parents are the most reliable sources of information that contribute to an appropriate diagnosis and treatment of their child's disorder.

In summary, especially in adolescence, illness-specific factors (e.g., increased defensive reactions associated with certain disorders) and developmentally related factors (e.g., lack of willingness to declare oneself as needing help or to accept help from an adult, dependency on the parents' consent, or function in the family system) have an effect on an individual's awareness of or sensitivity to health problems and his or her willingness to seek help.

### Low Motivations for Seeking Health Care, or "Counseling Aversion"

As described in chapter 2, obtaining diagnostically relevant information from the adolescent can be very difficult. The adolescent may be extremely reticent or offer only vague replies about his or her health. When health care providers offer to help the adolescent or suggest a specific kind of treatment, the adolescent's response is often antagonistic (Garrison & McQuiston, 1989) and resistant (Rinsley, 1980). This led Nadler (1978) to question whether professional therapists are truly helping the adolescent by offering their assistance. Similarly, many physicians complain that their adolescent patients are uncooperative and noncompliant (see chap. 7, this volume). For example, 35% of adolescents suffering from cystic fibrosis studied by Czajkowski and Koocher (1986) were found to be noncompliant: they refused to participate in physical therapy, medical examinations, and tests, did not regularly take their prescribed medication, and did not adhere to dietary restrictions. Other authors reported that adolescents belonging to certain risk groups show especially marked tendencies to avoid doctors. For example, DuBois (1989) reported that delinquent adolescents avoided having any normal contact with doctors; their contact with the health-care-providing system was practically limited to cases when they were brought to hospital emergency rooms.

This low motivation is even more apparent in cases in which adolescents require psychotherapeutic care. Adolescent patients who require extended hospitalization or residential treatment show a strong tendency to avoid therapeutic collaboration (O'Malley, 1990). Adolescents rarely attempt to cope with their emotional problems by seeking psychological counseling or consulting a psychiatrist. In our studies of adolescent coping, it was found that only 9% of normal adolescents considered counseling to be an acceptable strategy for coping with stressors (Seiffge-Krenke, 1995). An analysis of age differences revealed that early adolescents (12–14 years old) had even lower scores than late adolescents (17–19 years old). This percentage increased to about 16% for adolescents who described themselves as being highly stressed. However, more females than males were prepared to accept institutional help in case of pressing problems.

## PRE-EXISTING KNOWLEDGE AND ATTITUDES: IS MORE INFORMATION NEEDED?

Lack of knowledge or especially negative attitudes about psychotherapy and psychological counseling do not solely account for the counseling aversion. In the already mentioned study of 561 12- to 19-year-old adolescents (Seiffge-Krenke, 1986), adolescents were not only asked to describe what they knew about the symptoms of psychological dysfunction, but also were inquired about prevalence rates, possible methods of treatment, and prognoses. The majority of respondents thought that psychological dysfunction was more common today than in the past. Eighty percent of the adolescents stated that there was more mental illness today than in the past and that mainly adolescents and adults were affected as compared to children (48%, 47%, and 5%, respectively). Adolescents learned about types of treatment predominantly from extrafamilial sources, in particular, through the mass media. They generally showed a guarded optimism about the possibilities of treating behavioral or emotional symptoms successfully. Over 70% stated that psychological disturbances could be cured. No differences were found to exist between male and female ratings with respect to sources of information and estimates about the likelihood of successful treatment. However, females were slightly better informed than males and were more interested in further information about treatment procedures. Figure 8.1 displays the different sources adolescents used for information about mental health care services.

These findings, obtained in a study of nonclinical adolescents, only slightly differ from the ratings made by 129 psychotherapists practicing in family counseling centers and psychiatric hospitals (Seiffge-Krenke, 1989). The therapists estimated the chances for successful treatment to be more positive (nearly 90% of the therapists compared to 70% of the adolescents thought that psychological dysfunction could often or very

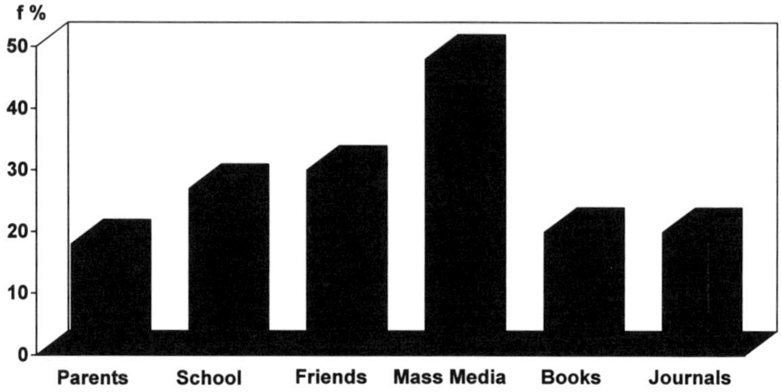


FIG. 8.1 Adolescents' sources of information about the utilization of institutionalized mental health care services ($N$ = 352).

often be treated successfully), but estimated the prevalence rates to be lower. Only 35% of the therapists thought that more adolescents exhibited psychological dysfunction today than in the past, whereas 47% of the adolescents thought this. The adolescents were thus well-informed about the prevalence rates and types of treatment for behavioral and emotional symptoms, and were also convinced that psychological disturbances can be treated successfully. However, only one half of the adolescents in this study imagined that they themselves would make use of existing forms of mental health care services; 30% said that they would do so only when parents, physicians, or teachers urged them to do so, and 19% said that they would not seek such care in any circumstances. Only 10% of adolescents in this sample actually sought professional help because of pressing problems. Obviously, there is a discrepancy between the perception of problems and the readiness to seek professional help, which can only partly be explained by a lack of information.

Although this comparably steadfast refusal to make use of professional care is surprising, it nevertheless corresponds to the finding that 48% of the therapists reported that the most typical problem involved in treating adolescents was motivating them to begin a specified form of treatment (Seiffge-Krenke, 1989). Results from the German Health survey (Palentien & Hurrelmann, 1995) mentioned earlier are helpful in clarifying the motivation problem. In this study, physicians and psychologists were asked to state what reasons their potential adolescent patients and clients have for not utilizing their services.

As is seen in Table 8.1, physicians and psychologists cited insufficient information and shame as being the main reasons behind nonutilization of medical and psychosocial care services in their adolescent patients. In general, psychologists thought that many of the reasons were more important than did the physicians (e.g., prejudices against health providers, insufficient confidence in the physician or counselor, shame, long distance to facilities, etc.). Rather striking were the comparably high numbers of physicians and psychologists who stated that the adolescent patient might not have developed a sufficient sense of suffering.

TABLE 8.1
Physicians' and Psychologists' Ratings of Possible Reasons Why Adolescents With Problems Do Not Seek Professional Help

| *Ratings* | *Physicians* f% | *Psychologists* f% |
|---|---|---|
| 1. Insufficient information about counseling or treatment. | 63.9 | 78.5 |
| 2. Shame about disclosing a problem. | 59.0 | 84.5 |
| 3. Uncertainty about the sense and effectiveness of professional counseling. | 58.2 | 85.7 |
| 4. Insufficient awareness of problems and insufficient sense of suffering. | 56.3 | 74.9 |
| 5. Fear about parents being notified. | 48.4 | 47.2 |
| 6. Parents' resistance. | 37.7 | 66.6 |
| 7. Prejudice against physicians or counselors. | 37.3 | 74.8 |
| 8. Insufficient confidence in physician or counselor. | 26.2 | 52.7 |
| 9. Long waiting or waiting lists. | 23.6 | 49.4 |
| 10. Bad experiences with physicians or counselors. | 22.0 | 54.3 |
| 11. Distances too great to competent facilities. | 20.3 | 45.0 |
| 12. Apprehension about transmission of information | 15.9 | 33.1 |
| 13. Insecurity about financing. | 14.5 | 28.8 |

*Note*. Table compiled from data appearing in "Adolescents' Health Problems and Utilization of Medical and Psychological Care Sessions in East and West Germany" by C. Palentien and K. Hurrelman (1995), in M. du Bois-Reymond, R. Diekstra, K. Hurrelmann, & E. Peters (Eds.), *Childhood and Youth in Germany and The Netherlands* (pp. 219–220). Berlin, Germany: de Gruyter.

## Gender-Specific Differences in Health Care-Seeking Behavior and Attitudes Toward Seeking Help

Several studies demonstrated that the rates of utilization of institutionalized health care services begin to differ for boys and girls around mid-adolescence. Whereas in childhood, more male patients utilize such services, around the age of 15 years, girls seek health care more often than do boys. This trend continues into adulthood (Seiffge-Krenke, 1986; Toolan, Jaffe, & Ryan, 1988). A comparison with gender differences in the use of social resources by nonclinical samples (see chap. 6, this volume) reveals some rather striking parallels. Compared with males, with increasing age, female coping behavior becomes increasingly characterized by a tendency to use informal sources of help and by a greater openness in expressing feelings and discussing problems. This, in turn, leads to corresponding gender differences in the inclination to accept institutional help. Gender differences in the acceptance of being ill and needing help thus appear to emerge already in adolescence. As adults, it was consistently found that females more frequently seek psychiatric help than do males (Dohrenwend & Dohrenwend, 1974). In fact, in a prospective study of a large sample of asymptomatic subjects, it was found that 70% of the subjects who consulted a physician were female (Andrews, 1981).

More specifically, male and female motivations for seeking care become different in adolescence. A representative study of 805 healthy adolescents' attitudes about psychotherapy showed that with increasing age, gender differences in attitudes toward psychotherapeutic help became more obvious (Seiffge-Krenke, 1986). In this study, the Psychotherapy Questionnaire designed by Schmitz (1981) was used to assess attitudes about psychotherapy.

Figure 8.2 shows the results of Scale 2 of the Psychotherapy Questionnaire, which assesses readiness to accept psychotherapy. The scale includes such items as: "I think that psychotherapy would help me if I ever had emotional problems," "It is easier to discuss emotional problems with a professional than with somebody one knows well," or "Most psychotherapists can help their patients reduce their worries and fears." Female adolescents were generally more willing to seek help from a psychotherapist when they had serious problems. Their readiness to do so increased with age, whereas male adolescents remained skeptical of psychotherapy regardless of their age. According to the majority of male adolescents in this study, most psychotherapists chose their profession because they were interested in possessing power over other individuals. Furthermore, male adolescents thought that people should learn to take care of their problems on their own instead of seeking help from others.

Females cited these reasons, as well, but with lower frequencies. Northman (1978) reported similar findings obtained in a study of 242 boys and girls in Grades 3, 6, 9, and 12. Whereas adolescents preferred to receive help from their peers, children preferred to seek help from their parents. The readiness to accept help from health care professionals in difficult circumstances increased with age, whereby females were much more willing to accept help than males were. Both males and females preferred to accept help from female health care providers.

These findings show that the counseling aversion observed in adolescents must be differentiated according to gender. In addition, the aspect of being sent to health care providers must be taken into account. Adolescents, who often are sent by parents or teachers to seek help from a therapist or counselor, may appear to be poorly motivated. However, they may in fact be basically motivated and although they do not outwardly show it, are relieved that their parents sent them to the doctor or counselor (i.e., they are happy to have an external reason for seeking treatment). For the adolescent who generally finds it difficult—especially in the phase of separation from the parents—to become attached to an adult therapist, this kind of "command from above" is a good opportunity to accept treatment and yet save face. Patients in this age group generally are openly or latently distrustful of all institutions. The last thing an adolescent wants to do is ask an adult for help. Therapists are often confronted with such statements as: "I don't need you," "You can't help me," "I can't talk about it," or "You're only helping me for the money" (Laufer & Laufer, 1984).

Adolescents are often unable to admit that they are desperate or hurt. As patients, they may present themselves as being omnipotent or

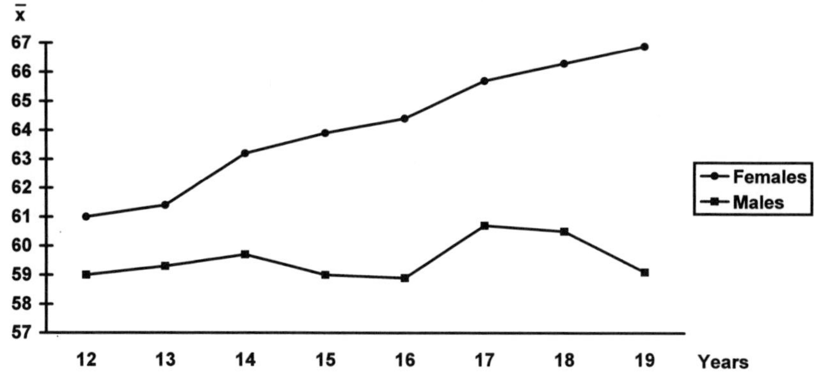


FIG. 8.2. Changes in attitudes about seeking psychotherapeutic care in 378 male and 427 female youths throughout adolescence.

superior to the therapist, considering themselves to be adults, thus needing no one's help.

Moreover, adolescents frequently discontinue their participation in treatment, usually shortly after treatment has begun (see chap. 9, this volume). However, as Rogers (1970) impressively showed, in most cases they resume participation in therapy when the therapist actively encourages them to do so. This points to the possibility that ill adolescents are latently motivated to seek treatment and thus require a situation that encourages them to accept help. This is especially true for males. In addition, some of the difficulties involved in obtaining diagnostically relevant information from adolescents and maintaining their participation in therapy are related to the adolescent's attempts to achieve independence. Yet, the majority of health care offerings imply an attachment to adults and a regression to child behavior patterns. Given the nature of the developmental tasks particular to adolescence (e.g., obtaining autonomy and independence), it is not surprising that the adolescent refuses to accept help or follow directives from health care professionals.

This also applies to physical examinations. As was detailed in chapter 4, most adolescents initiate changes in the kinds and amounts of physical contact they have with adults, and they can easily perceive such examinations to be an invasion of their privacy. Thus, before beginning treatment, it is advisable to clarify the adolescent's motivations for consulting a health care provider. Furthermore, diagnosis must be supplemented by such information about the adolescent's awareness of disturbances and perceived level of suffering. As the previous discussion showed, such information reveals that a vital interest in receiving treatment exists even in unmotivated patients.

### Factors Accounting for Adolescents' Aversion to Seeking Psychotherapeutic Care

Lack of suffering and low awareness of disturbances are not sufficient reasons in themselves for explaining why adolescents avoid consulting psychotherapists, because an increased suffering cannot be equated with increased likelihood to seek such care. Other factors play a role, for example, opinions of physicians and health care facilities or attitudes about being labeled "sick." An analysis of factors that contribute to non-utilization or delayed utilization of psychological counseling services is certainly warranted, because treatment is more likely to be successful the sooner a patient consults a health care professional.

As was seen, only a small number of adolescents seek help on their own initiative. The first contact with a psychotherapist or counseling psychologist is frequently initiated by the adolescent's parents. This situation is experienced as most threatening by those adolescents who most urgently require treatment (Rinsley, 1967). As Rogers (1970) pointed out, however, adolescents seldom passively accept their parents' directives to seek treatment. In this and other matters, they want to be active in making decisions that affect them directly. When parents do not afford the adolescent with an opportunity to make the decision to seek treatment on his or her own, the only self-determining decision left to make is to refuse any treatment. This is true of highly motivated patients as well. It should be noted, however, that depending on the applicable statutory circumstances, health care providers may not be permitted to initiate medical or psychosocial treatment without the parents' or legal guardians' informed consent. Thus, the adolescent is forced to include his or her parents in the decision-making process. In addition, the therapeutic setting, with its fixed parameters of regular visits, appears to signal renewed dependency and childlike regression (Laufer & Laufer, 1984; Redl, 1969) thus standing in the way of age-typical attempts to achieve separation from the parents and increase autonomy. This basic difficulty in accepting help from adults is certainly the most decisive factor behind an adolescent's aversion to seeking psychotherapeutic care and is responsible for a variety of latent and manifest attempts to discontinue treatment (Novick, 1980).

Furthermore, it should be recalled that the willingness to share personal information with adults dramatically decreases during adolescence. Thus, the adolescent has great difficulties in accepting a situation where he or she will be asked to disclose intimate details to an adult (see chap. 2, this volume). The importance of this was pointed out by McClure, Mitchell, and Greschuck (1982) in their study of college students. Compared to students who did not seek assistance from psychological counseling services, despite serious problems, those who sought help showed lower self-concept and a greater willingness to talk about their problems. In another study (Seiffge-Krenke, 1989), it was shown that the relation between awareness of problems and willingness to talk about them was nonlinear (see also chap. 6, this volume). This was especially obvious in the comparison of adolescents who were highly burdened with problems (see Table 8.2).

When asked about their reasons for not seeking psychotherapeutic care, the highly stressed adolescents reported significantly more often than their less-stressed peers that they were afraid that their parents might find out they were seeing a therapist or that their friends might

TABLE 8.2
Reasons for Not Consulting Psychotherapists in Highly Stressed Adolescents ($n = 43$) and Low-Stressed Adolescents ($n = 42$).

| | *Highly Stressed Adolescents* | | *Low-Stressed Adolescents* | | | |
|---|---|---|---|---|---|---|
| *Items* | *M* | *SD* | *M* | *SD* | *F* | *p* |
| 1. Adolescent afraid that parents would find out. | 3.9 | 1.0 | 3.0 | 1.1 | 3.1 | .00** |
| 2. Adolescent does not want to discuss personal matters with a stranger. | 4.2 | .76 | 3.7 | 1.1 | 2.7 | .00** |
| 3. Adolescent not well-informed about psychotherapeutic care providers. | 4.3 | .87 | 4.2 | 1.0 | .44 | .66 |
| 4. Adolescent does not know if psychotherapist or counseling service is in the vicinity. | 3.5 | 1.2 | 3.5 | 1.3 | –.56 | .96 |
| 5. Adolescent does not think psychologist can help. | 3.6 | 1.0 | 3.7 | 1.1 | –.37 | .71 |
| 6. Adolescent does not know what counseling or therapy costs. | 3.7 | 1.1 | 3.3 | 1.3 | 1.5 | .12 |
| 7. Adolescent thinks that one should try to deal with the problems alone. | 3.6 | 1.1 | 3.3 | 1.1 | 1.0 | .31 |
| 8. Adolescent is afraid that friends or acquaintances will think her or she is "crazy." | 3.9 | 1.1 | 3.3 | 1.2 | 2.3 | .02* |
| 9. Adolescent is afraid that therapist will tell others about his or her problems. | 3.0 | 1.3 | 2.1 | 1.2 | 3.0 | .00** |
| 10. Adolescent would rather try to solve problem by talking with parents or friends. | 3.5 | 1.1 | 4.0 | .90 | -2.2 | .03* |

*Note*. 5-point scale from *applies completely* (5) to *does not apply at all* (1); $^{*}p < .05$; $^{**}p < .001$.

think they were "crazy." They were distrustful of whether the therapist would uphold the confidentiality of their discussions and were generally disinclined to talk about their problems with strangers.

In fact, lack of confidentiality is a significant access barrier to health care. In a large study of 1,295 ninth through twelfth graders, Cheng,

Savagean, Sattler, and de Witt (1993) found that 58% of these adolescents had health concerns that they wished to keep private from their parents. Sixty-nine percent wanted to conceal this information from friends and classmates. Thus, a majority of adolescents have concerns they wish to keep private. It is important to note that one fourth of the adolescents reported that they would not seek health care for these concerns if they thought that their parents, friends, or teachers might find out.

According to Palentien and Hurrelmann (1995), adolescents are indeed more reluctant to seek help from psychologists and psychiatrists than from other types of health care professionals. Such reservations persist even among older adolescents, who are more likely to have been informed about the methods used to treat psychological symptoms. Parish and Kappes (1979) found, for example, that college students were very ambivalent toward psychologists and psychiatrists. Although the majority (92%) of students acknowledged the importance of receiving treatment for psychological and psychiatric disorders, more than one half of them stated that they would be reluctant to consult a psychiatrist or psychologist if they had a serious problem and would only place themselves under psychiatric care in an extreme emergency.

In interpreting such findings, it is important to consider the general issue of social acceptance of individuals afflicted with psychological disorders. Indeed, the prevailing attitude toward psychiatric patients is quite negative (Halpert, 1969). Most people are alienated by overt behavioral disturbances, and the tolerance of such behaviors varies only slightly according to SES or educational level. Similar findings were reported by Lehtinen et al. (1978). Such attitudes among the general population tend to be steadfast, despite information campaigns designed to reduce prejudices against the psychiatrically ill. In fact, sporadic reports were made that such prejudices about psychiatric patients increase the dropout rates in patients in treatment for psychiatric disorders (Malhotra, Inam Shastri, & Chopra, 1978). In his review of studies on this topic, Halpert (1969) pessimistically concluded that whereas the general population has become considerably more informed about psychiatric disorders over the past 50 years, most people remain nonaccepting of individuals suffering from psychiatric dysfunction.

Although adolescents' attitudes toward psychiatrists or psychologists are ambivalent, especially with respect to accepting help from an adult, they are, overall, more tolerant of individuals with psychiatric disorders. This may partly be related to the fact that adolescents perceive themselves to be greatly troubled or disturbed or that they are less threatened by individuals who violate socially accepted forms of behavioral conduct (see chap. 2, this volume). Nevertheless, as outlined earlier, they are afraid of being stigmatized as a psychiatric patient, which again confirms their rejection of being dependent on therapists, counseling psychologists, and psychiatrists.

### Changes in Attitudes During Treatment

In the preceding sections, we tried to illustrate the adolescent's inner conflict about seeking health care, especially with respect to the dilemma of needing help yet wanting to retain independence and protect privacy. Unfortunately, not many studies to date have dealt with those adolescents who, for whatever reasons, sought health care.

A few investigators examined adolescents' attitudes about psychiatric care directly before their admission to a psychiatric hospital and during the course of their stay. For example, Martin and Diehl (1983) studied adolescents admitted to a psychiatric hospital in the United States. Results revealed that most adolescents hardly anticipated being committed to the hospital and felt that they were not part of the decision-making process. Female adolescents, however, recognized the likelihood that they would require inpatient psychiatric care and thus were more accepting of their parents' decisions than were males. Martin and Diehl explained this finding by noting that girls tend to conform to social norms more than boys do and are used to having their parents or legal guardians make decisions about their welfare. The adolescents were generally positive about the effects of being committed to a hospital for psychiatric care, and girls were more positive than were boys.

Empirical studies focusing on the patterns of utilization of health care services, with respect to outcome and dropout rates, showed that psychotherapy is as effective for adolescents who do not discontinue treatment as it is for older age groups. In their comparison of different kinds of therapy, Gomes-Schwartz (1978) and Tramontana (1980) concluded that the percentage of adolescents who showed positive effects of psychotherapy, 75%, was only slightly below that for adult patients and above the 39% spontaneous remission rate for adolescents. Therefore, the rates for spontaneous remission were somewhat higher and treatment efficacy somewhat lower for adolescents than for adult patients. Weisz, Weiss, Alicke, and Klotz (1987) addressed the question of treatment effectiveness in their meta-analysis of 108 well-designed outcome studies with 4- to 18-year-old patients. Across various outcome measures, the average treated youngster was better adjusted after treatment than 79% of those not treated. Therapy proved to be more effective for children (mean effect size was .92) than for adolescents (mean effect size was .58). As in research on adult patients, general interactions were found between therapy type, target problem, therapist training, and effectiveness. In any case, these studies suggest that when adolescents agree to undergo treatment for psychiatric or psychological disorders, they can profit considerably.

In our studies of different referred samples (Seiffge-Krenke, 1986, 1989; Seiffge-Krenke & Wester, in prep.), we found that clinical groups expressed a more positive, less ambivalent attitude toward psychotherapy or counseling than did unselected groups of adolescents. Seventy-five percent of the adolescents who received counseling thought they would use mental health care services if they had another serious problem, as compared to 21% of the nonclinical adolescents. Thus, although adolescents show a strong aversion to counseling at first and are likely to refuse or discontinue treatment, counseling and therapy apparently seem to have a markedly positive effect on their attitudes and motivation. In one of our studies, this positive outlook was found to be a therapy outcome in itself (Seiffge-Krenke & Wester, in prep.). Forty-six adolescents receiving inpatient or outpatient care for various psychiatric disorders were studied at the beginning and end of 1 year of treatment and compared with a nontreated control group receiving the same diagnoses. Attitudes toward psychotherapy were assessed by means of the Psychotherapy questionnaire (Schmitz, 1981).

As is seen in Table 8.3, significant differences in attitudes between adolescents treated for 1 year and nontreated adolescents were found in three subscales. At the end of the year, treated adolescents were less skeptical of therapists, more prepared to accept help, and less concerned with protecting their privacy than both clinically referred but untreated subjects, and highly stressed adolescents who did not yet make contact with a counseling center (see chap. 6, this volume). The treated subjects thus had a much more positive attitude about health care than did

TABLE 8.3
Differences in Attitudes Toward Psychotherapy Between Adolescents in Treatment and Referred But Not Yet Treated Adolescents

| | *Treated* | | *Not Treated* | | | |
|---|---|---|---|---|---|---|
| *Scale* | *M* | *SD* | *M* | *SD* | *F* | *p* |
| 1. Scepticism toward psychotherapy. | 26.7 | 11.8 | 33.1 | 7.6 | 3.31 | .001 |
| 2. Readiness to accept help. | 74.1 | 15.1 | 62.4 | 11.9 | 4.58 | .001 |
| 3. Need for privacy. | 21.4 | 7.4 | 25.9 | 6.8 | 3.97 | .001 |
| 4. Attitudes toward mental illness. | 22.0 | 5.9 | 23.4 | 5.0 | 1.65 | .10 |

adolescents who had no experience with therapy or counseling. On the average, the treated adolescents expressed fewer fears about psychotherapy than did nontreated adolescents and felt that these reservations were not sufficient reasons for foregoing treatment. In particular, they placed less value on their independence and self-sufficiency and were not worried that their self-esteem or psychological stability could be damaged by therapy. They were less suspicious of the therapist and more likely to accept the therapist's help when they needed to solve an urgent problem. It should be emphasized that this generally positive attitude was characteristic of both hospitalized patients ($n$ = 20) and outpatients ($n$ = 26) in the sample.

The more positive attitude of patients receiving treatment could, of course, be due to selection. Adolescents without any motivation to try psychotherapy or with negative expectations about its efficacy will probably not contact a therapist or go to a counseling center or they will discontinue therapy. Although the treated adolescents showed conspicuous differences compared to nontreated adolescents with respect to attitudes and motivation at the end of 1 year, it is not clear whether these differences were explicitly related to treatment or nontreatment. An inspection of the scores of the Psychotherapy questionnaire at the beginning and end of the psychotherapy revealed significant changes in three scales: The skepticism toward psychotherapy, as well as the need for privacy, decreased during 1 year, whereas the readiness to accept help increased during that time. These significant changes were further substantiated by interviews. An analysis of the data obtained from interviews carried out with the 46 adolescents at the beginning of therapy and after approximately 6 months of treatment revealed that initial ambivalent or negative motivation increasingly diminished. In the initial phase, only 35% of the patients willingly consented to begin therapy or receive counseling, but this figure increased to 67% at a later time point. At the same time, fears and doubts about the efficacy of therapy were reduced. In the first few weeks, 42% of the adolescents expressed such reservations; after 6 months of treatment, only 5% reported such thoughts. This was due to the fact that within this time, 57% of the patients showed clear improvements in their symtoms. In the interviews, the majority of adolescents described therapy or counseling as a difficult but worthwhile process. This indicates that positive experiences during the course of treatment had a favorable effect on their attitudes. Other investigators reported similar findings. Martin and Diehl (1983), for example, observed that during the first few weeks of psychotherapy, adolescents were plagued with doubts and negative expectations. Similarly, according to one summary of research findings related to this topic (Feinstein, 1990), more positive attitudes toward psychotherapy emerged in the later phases of treatment.

In our study, it was important for the patients to consider the therapist as someone they could trust, someone with whom they could discuss anything that worried them (Seiffge-Krenke & Wester, in prep.). To a certain extent the therapist was seen as a model of constructive coping behavior. Given the patient's generally positive attitude once therapy was consolidated, it was assumed that although at the beginning of treatment the relationship with the therapist is overshadowed by mistrust, fear, and uncertainty, a working alliance is established and the adolescent begins to focus his or her achieving therapeutic goals.

This decidedly positive attitude about psychotherapy and counseling seems to contradict observations described in previous sections about the typical dilemma that greatly troubled adolescents have in seeking help and deciding to begin therapy. Nevertheless, it appears quite clear that the experience with therapy in both inpatient and outpatient settings helps the adolescents to be more open to receive professional care. Even adolescents with an initially ambivalent or rejecting attitude toward health care are able to change their expectations and redefine their wishes, and the relationship with the health care professional assumes the characteristics of a working alliance. This latter aspect proves to be of instrumental importance, especially because adolescents are so highly intent on achieving autonomy. In any case, our study showed that when adolescents agree to undergo treatment, they enormously profit from the experience.

### Readiness of Parents With Ill Adolescents to Accept Offers of Help

The reservations about therapy and counseling among the general population and the specific developmental changes occurring in adolescence are not the only factors that effect adolescents' utilization of mental health care services. Parents' expectations and attitudes toward such care also plays a role. In extreme circumstances, for example, in pathological families, health care-seeking behavior is discouraged. In contrast to families suffering from psychological dysfunction, most parents of chronically physically ill adolescents show a clear readiness to make use of mental health care services. However, rates of actual service use are not high either.

**Parental Stress in Families With Chronically Ill Adolescents.** As was discussed in chapter 7, the outbreak of a serious chronic illness in adolescence places the adolescent in an unfavorable situation. The ill adolescent must deal with developmentally related stressors as well as nonnormative stressors associated with the conditions of chronic illness. The management of the illness also represents a long-term burden for the parents (C. Eiser, 1985). The parents are overwhelmed with "chronic worries" (Wilker, Wasaw, & Hatfield, 1981) and suffer from a high number of stress-related symptoms (Cummings, 1976). In addition, they are confronted with new responsibilities and demands related to the care of their adolescent child. Their focus on the ill child is time-consuming and drains their emotional resources; the marriage is often jeopardized (Sabbeth & Leventhal, 1984). Many authors studying families with chronically ill adolescents explained their findings in relation to a deficit model, that is, the child's illness is perceived as a stressor that compromises the relationships among family members. This approach most likely encouraged attempts to identify signs of marital dissatisfaction in families with ill children. According to the model proposed by McCubbin et al. (1983), the family's ability or inability to adapt is not solely determined by the stressor's severity. The family's coping resources and subjective attitudes moderate their reactions to the illness. In addition, the response to the onset of a chronic illness is neither uniform nor temporally limited, as Knafl and Deatrick (1987) clearly showed. Clinical observations and research findings showed that in some families, the experience of having to deal with chronic stressors increases marital satisfaction, because the parents must cooperate closely, which often enhances intimacy (Kazak & Marvin, 1984; Silbert, Newburger, & Fyler, 1982). In addition, Ritchie (1981) showed that such families become even more competent in their decision-making abilities.

In summary, the awareness and recognition of the illness demands that the family adjust to the new situation of having a sick child. Whereas some families are successful in adapting to the imposed changes in family life and learn to accept new, more appropriate strategies in dealing with the sick adolescent's needs, others seem unable to deviate from previous patterns of interaction. The degree of cooperation in the family plays a decisive role in determining how initial reactions develop and which solutions are worked out in dealing with problems. Some families are able to organize and integrate initial reactions to the illness. Each family member assumes clearly defined tasks and recognizes his or her limits in dealing with the adolescent's illness so that the burden of the illness is shared. For example, cooperative interaction among family members was found to be an efficient coping strategy in families with children afflicted with diabetes or phenylketonuria (Hauser et al., 1988). In other cases, family members act on their own and in their own interests, often hindering other family members' attempts to care for the sick adolescent. One parent may devote most of his or her time and efforts to caring for the ill adolescent and thus become isolated from the other family members. In this case, open or latent conflicts flare up, thus undermining the chances of successful treatment of the illness as well as the adolescent's own adjustment process. In families unable to cope with the new demands placed on the family and marriage, the illness is often used to reorganize the family in a certain manner. Examples of such a dysfunctional coping style are outlined in chapter 7. One basic question is whether the chronicity (i.e., the duration of the stressor) as such promotes familial dysfunction. There are some indications that although the burden of the illness itself can be managed, its chronicity represents an additional stressor, which leads to rigidity or chaos, even in otherwise well-functioning families (Trute & Hauch, 1988).

**Desired and Actual Utilization of Psychological Counseling Services.** Although there are individual differences in dealing with the multiple stressors related to the care of a chronically ill child or adolescent, most parents show a clear readiness to make use of psychosocial care offerings. This strong wish was documented in many studies and becomes more pronounced the more serious and threatening the illness is (e.g., Cook, 1984; Slater & Rubenstein, 1987). Nevertheless, the desire or readiness to seek help cannot be equated with the actual utilization of services offering and providing such help. In our longitudinal study of chronically ill adolescents (Seiffge-Krenke et al., 1996) it was found that nearly all of the parents spoke openly about their burdens and worries and articulated a wish to obtain help (see chap. 7, this volume). However, only a small proportion of them actually sought psychological counseling for the family (16% compared to 22% of the families with healthy adolescents). The relatively high readiness of ill adolescents' parents to utilize services offering psychotherapeutic care found in most studies is related to the fact that they were responsible for supervising their children's medical care and cooperating with the attending physicians. However, this argument is one-sided, especially when one considers older adolescents. Observations made in this longitudinal study of chronically ill adolescents (see chap. 7, this volume) revealed that the adolescents assumed a great deal of responsibility for the management of their illness, even in its early stages.

Nevertheless, most of the parents remained worried about whether the adolescent was self-reliant and dependable. Hauser et al. (1988) described this kind of parental monitoring in detail as well as the far-reaching restructuring of everyday family life, leisure time, and planning of vacations. Parents reported being emotionally strained by the burdens involved in the continuous monitoring of their child's activities and bearing the responsibility for supervising the management of their child's illness. In addition, the parents' needs to seek psychological counseling were often related to their fears about the dangers of their child's illness. In fact, parents attributed more importance to the long-term effects of illness than the adolescents themselves. Moreover, the separation process in itself places an additional strain on parents of chronically ill adolescents. Indeed, many parents reported being unable to make the distinction between illness-specific and development-related problems, an observation that was made in other studies as well (Slater & Rubinstein, 1987). Thus, it is easy to imagine that the parents exhaust their emotional resources and find themselves unable to cope with the burdens in their lives. Nevertheless, despite good reasons for consulting psychotherapists or counseling psychologists, the actual rates for utilization of such services in our study were much lower than those for articulated wishes to receive professional support. This discrepancy is further discussed in the following section.

### Accepting Help in Adolescents With Psychological Dysfunction

The previous discussion is valid not only for adolescents afflicted with a chronic physical illness, but also for those suffering from severe psychiatric disorders. In a study of families with anorexic adolescents participating in family therapy programs, Minuchin et al. (1978) observed that interactions among members of such families were often very complex and mutually opposed. Coleman (1987) documented additional examples of inadequate cooperation or protest in families with adolescents undergoing inpatient or outpatient psychotherapy for compulsive neurotic, phobic, or psychosomatic disorders. During psychotherapy, adolescents often reported that they were having problems with parental cooperation and support in therapy. Such problems are explained by the fact that most treatment aims support and promote adolescent autonomy, thus requiring parents to face the difficult situation of having to redefine their relationships with their child and with one another.

Compared with the adolescent's ambivalence about accepting help from psychotherapists, which is, in part, progressive and developmentally appropriate because it hinders a reattachment to an adult, the motives of uncooperative parents are often regressive: The adolescent is fixed in a former relationship pattern. Accordingly, literature published on family research often contains reports of splitting maneuvers, in which individual family members attempt to rally the therapist to take sides (Framo, 1970; Shapiro, 1979). For example, parents or other family members attempt to make arrangements so that only certain topics are discussed during family therapy sessions, they withhold important information because of shame or guilt, or they show a regular pattern of nonattendance (Feinstein, 1990). Such examples show how difficult it is for some families to accept help as well as show regular cooperation in therapy. Often therapists complain that parents abruptly discontinue the family's or the adolescent's further participation in psychotherapy on some pretext (Sandler, Kennedy, & Tyson, 1982).

Even if parental interventions or ambivalent behavior about a child's recovery are not always obvious, it must be remembered that parents generally determine whether or not their adolescent should undergo psychotherapy. Only a small percentage of adolescents spontaneously come for treatment, and few inform their parents about their intention to do so. Many parents come without the adolescent, some without his or her knowing or consent. This affects not only the diagnostic situation, but also the adolescent's general motivation for treatment and cooperation. Health care professionals easily feel as if they must serve two parties, not being fair to either. For example, the adolescent patient may become healthier and more autonomous, but the parents will become more dysfunctional or depressed. Owing to these difficulties, many authors suggest group therapy with parents to accompany the adolescent's inpatient treatment or additional opportunities for the parents to participate in parent or marriage counseling sessions with another therapist, while the adolescent undergoes therapy alone (Coleman, 1987; Feinstein, 1990).

Psychosocial dysfunction in chronically ill adolescents is a topic of much controversy in the literature. A few authors reported that the likelihood of developing a psychiatric disorder is two to three times greater in patients with a chronic physical illness (Wilkinson, 1987). Other studies showed that the majority of adolescents afflicted with a chronic physical illness do not show manifest psychiatric symptoms (for a summary, see Roth & Seiffge-Krenke, 1996). Psychiatric dysfunction is not common, but the population of individuals suffering from a chronic physical illness is generally at increased risk of developing a psychiatric disorder, or at least, adjustment problems (Drotar & Bush, 1985; Wallander et al., 1988). For example, Cadman, Boyle, Szatmari, and Offord (1987) reported that adolescents afflicted with a chronic physical illness were more socially isolated and had more problems in school compared to those in a healthy control group. Similar observations were made in our longitudinal study of adolescents afflicted with diabetes (Seiffge-

Krenke et al., 1996; see chap. 7, this volume). Although the diabetic adolescents did not show increased rates of emotional or behavioral symptoms, they were delayed in their psychosocial development, had less autonomy, and their relationships with friends were poor. Reference was already made to the finding that the diabetic adolescents' families had relatively lower rates of health care-seeking behavior. These rates did not change when the group was differentiated according to the status of metabolic control (as measured by $HbA_1$ values) and psychological symptomatology (as measured by the YSR and the CBCL, Achenbach, 1991b, 1991d). The families of diabetic adolescents with both good or poor metabolic control did not differ with respect to the utilization of therapy and counseling; even the duration of the illness did not exert any significant influence. This result is probably related to the fact that these families used all the family resources at their disposal to cope with the illness, despite the disadvantage to some family members. The most common reactions observed in the ill adolescents ("I have to deal with this on my own") support this view.

Despite a high amount of stress and strain compared to healthy control groups, neither the parents nor the afflicted adolescents expressed a strong desire to accept professional psychological counseling. This was reflected in the already reported exceptionally low rates of utilization of psychological counseling services in families with diabetic adolescents, which was even lower than the rates for families with healthy adolescents. In coping with an illness of long duration, however, it is very likely that individual and familial resources are easily exhausted. Thus, in the presence of strong resistance and ambivalence toward seeking psychological counseling, special motivation or intervention strategies are required to make professional help acceptable for highly stressed families. The indications for and practical applications of such strategies are discussed in the final chapter.

# 9

# Some Implications for Prevention, Intervention, and Future Research

In the preceding chapter, an attempt was made to clarify which variables influence adolescents' decisions to seek health care. It became apparent that adolescents are not passive recipients of health care. They actively interpret their interactions with and critically evaluate the services provided by health care providers. Health care providers and planners should therefore include adolescents in their discussions of how to design a system that meets the needs and ultimately improves the health status of youth. Therefore, in this concluding chapter some of the research deficits that investigators in the field should be aware of in the planning of future studies are pointed out. In addition, the implications of available findings on adolescent health for the development of intervention strategies and for improving the health care of chronically ill or particularly troubled adolescents are discussed.

## FUTURE DIRECTIONS IN RESEARCH

There is currently a high level of public interest in adolescent problems and risk-taking behaviors. In this regard, more research efforts should be devoted to identifying the precursors of these behaviors and the developmental processes that accompany them. Much of the literature on variables determining adolescents' health and health care-seeking behavior was reviewed in this volume. However, the need for further research in specific areas has also become obvious. For example, additional studies are needed to clarify the links between psychological dysfunction and avoidant coping. In particular, the critical switch from the beneficial effects of avoidant coping or withdrawal to the maladaptive forms of coping must be examined. Thus, we need to broaden our assessment of coping strategies over a longer time span so that we can determine how and why coping styles change over time or situation. This argues for the use of longitudinally designed studies. This research might also help to explain observed gender differences in dealing with stress and in psychopathology. Another area of research concerns the reports of frequent body complaints found in adolescent samples. Despite reports of high rates of somatization in adolescent patients, such medically unexplained physical symptoms were not systematically investigated. The links among multiple or chronic stressors and recurrent pain, headaches, or diffuse body ailments are still poorly understood. Although studies on adult samples confirmed that minor events and everyday stressors negatively affect physical health, no study to date analyzed this relationship in adolescent samples. In fact, little work has been done to explain the relationship between major events and bodily symptoms.

The variety of explanatory variables that determine adolescents' access to health care is a further area of future research. The majority of existing studies addressing barriers to adolescent health care focused on race and gender. However, developmentally relevant variables, such as changes in disclosure behavior and in dealing with nudity, were neglected. Moreover, two key aspects of adolescents' access to health care—namely, consent and confidentiality—were not adequately addressed and remain controversial topics among health care professionals involved with adolescents. Pediatricians' and patients' views on confidentiality and consent were examined in a few empirical studies. Nevertheless, it is still unclear whether adolescents underutilize health care services because such use is only possible with parental consent or because they are wary that health care providers are unable or unwilling to keep information confidential. More work needs to be done to explain if and how adolescents' perceptions about the confidentiality of health care influence their decisions to use such services.

Much research focused on investigating the noncompliant behavior of adolescent patients. Many researchers attempted to document the extent of the problem, to describe its possible correlates and determinants, and to propose specific interventions to enhance compliance. However, our understanding of the phenomena involved in compliance and noncompliance is still very limited. This volume has addressed the enormous developmental barriers that hinder adolescent compliance. Future research efforts aimed at elucidating the variables and mechanisms of compliance and noncompliance would greatly profit from taking such developmental factors into account. It is quite likely, for example, that the developmentally related changes in parent–adolescent relationships affect physician–adolescent relationships. At any rate, such a differential likelihood for adherence in adolescent patients argues for the value of developing strategies designed to promote cooperation between the adolescent patient and physician.

Such strategies are especially appropriate for the psychotherapeutic treatment of adolescents. As was seen, adolescents tend to be unmotivated patients, who frequently discontinue their participation in therapeutic programs or abruptly stop seeing their psychotherapist on a regular basis. More work needs to be done to understand exactly which variables and contexts are necessary in order to encourage the unmotivated adolescent to continue therapy. Nevertheless, successful therapy often hinges on the therapist's ability to establish a positive and open relationship with the client. One can suspect that basically the same developmental forces that are at the roots of a difficult patient–physician relationship or noncompliant behavior are also involved in the failure of the psychotherapist to establish a therapeutic alliance with the adolescent patient.

## IMPLICATIONS FOR PREVENTION AND INTERVENTION

### Acknowledging Adolescents as "Health Seismographs"

In this volume, mortality and morbidity data were presented in order to provide the reader with rough estimates of adolescent health. Such data probably overestimate the health of the adolescent population (Millstein & Litt, 1990). In particular, measures of health-related behavior, such as utilization of physicians' or psychosocial services, appointment-keeping, or hospital discharge rates, are of marginal value. For example, adolescents tend to underutilize services even in cases of severe health problems. In addition, many surveys reveal that adolescents often report having many, often frequently occurring, bodily complaints, most of which were not serious enough to require the attention of a physician. Nevertheless, mortality and morbidity data highlight areas of adolescent health that merit concern. As detailed herein, most adolescent deaths are related to preventable social, environmental, and behavioral factors. Although there is some variation in the ranking of specific mortality causes across nations, this basic trend is observed in most Western industrialized countries. In light of other findings about the high rates of recurrent somatic complaints, adolescents are particularly sensitive to the adverse effects of social and environmental factors.

According to a WHO Regional Office for Europe (1994) memorandum on improving medical and psychological care for children and adolescents, adolescents are considered to be "health seismographs," who "show, through their social, psychological, and somatic troubles, not just where their own problems lie, but where the problems of society are as a whole" (p. 2).

Following this line of thought, one might profit from critically re-evaluating the values on which health education, prevention, and intervention are based. Some health experts complained that in Western societies, health has become a fetish, and illness a taboo. Health is associated with efficiency and achievement, youth, and attractiveness. Health care professionals may be strongly influenced by these values; for example, they may learn that to preserve or re-establish health brings about success and recognition, whereas accompanying people in their illness process does not. Perhaps our health system and our attitudes toward health are overly achievement-oriented. Too often it is proclaimed that health is an individual merit, and that health can be produced by physical exercise, not smoking, a healthy diet, and sufficient sleep. However, the alternation of health and illness are as important as tension and relaxation, effort and rest, or sleep and wakefulness.

Illness is an integral part of human development. This becomes obvious, for example, in the developmental progression many children and adolescents show during times of illness. For many adults, the lost sensitivity to physical processes indicating stress is often regained only once physical symptoms and complaints become intolerable. Similarly, the development of psychological symptoms is a signal indicating distress and conflicts. Thus, physical complaints and psychological symptoms are considered to be messages that we should listen to and use productively. Chronically ill adolescents should be supported in a way that enhances their abilities to live with the illness in a self-determined and human manner. The guiding principles for providing care should, therefore, be to respect the rights and meet the needs of the adolescent.

### Gender Differences in Adolescents' Perceptions of Health, Illness, and Health-Related Behavior

Throughout this book, a variety of research findings pertaining to strong gender differences in perceptions of physical and psychological symptoms and attitudes about health-care-seeking behavior have been presented. For example, adolescent females are much more preoccupied with aspects of physical maturation and attractiveness than are males. In addition, females view the process of physical maturation more negatively and possess a more negative body image than do males. In particular, early maturation is most negatively perceived by females; in contrast, males make positive associations with the changes brought on by early development. For example, weight gain is perceived negatively by females, whereas males consider this to be a positive change. The intense desire in young females to be attractive, coupled with the insecurity about their attractiveness, can lead to pathological outcomes such as extreme dieting or eating disorders. Female adolescents are also more concerned about nudity and more sensitive about violations of physical privacy. They generally report having more body complaints and also perceive the same stressors as being more stressful than do males. Females worry more about disagreements with parents, peer approval and acceptance, relationships with the opposite gender, and their academic performance. Also, they cope differently with these stressors than do males. In particular, they tend to brood over their problems instead of trying to seek distraction from their negative moods. Finally, the occurrence of highly stressful events increases the number or severity of somatic complaints and potentiates depressed moods in female adolescents.

Although there is a possible danger that females are oversensitive to physical ailments and stressors, health experts must acknowledge that males tend to underreport physical and psychological symptoms. Furthermore, males are far less willing than females to talk about their problems with others, including health care providers. This reluctance is strongly associated with a socially reinforced attitude that it is unmanly to talk about personal problems or to seek help. This attitude represents a serious problem, because, as demonstrated in this volume, the mortality rates and morbidity rates in many domains are much higher for males than for females. Violence as a primary cause of death and high rates of suicide are seen predominantly in adolescent male samples. Male adolescents are also less informed and less concerned about the implications of certain behaviors that are associated with increased risks to health (e.g., sex without contraception, drinking alcohol and operating a motor vehicle, etc.). Furthermore, they are less prepared to change their attitudes and behaviors. Health care experts must be aware of these differences in their assessments of adolescent health. Illness prevention and intervention strategies must also take these differences into account, for example, by helping female adolescents to view their bodies more positively or helping males to speak more openly about their problems.

### Giving Up the Splitting Between Body and Mind

The emergence of transient, unclearly defined disorders and comorbidity are two striking aspects of adolescent psychopathology. The latter is widely recognized as a diagnostic problem and has important consequences for treatment and prognosis. Comorbidity is not a new phenomenon; for example, reports of the co-occurrence of eating disorders and adolescent depression were made centuries ago. However, due to biased preconceptions among health-care professionals, as well as the tendency of many adolescents to conceal symptoms of illness, which might be socially unacceptable, this problem was generally overlooked (Habermas, 1989). Today, the increase in comorbidity is regarded as reflecting more severe psychopathology. Adolescents with co-occurring diseases are perceived as being significantly more impaired than peers with a single diagnosis and are offered help more frequently. From a developmental perspective, comorbidity reflects the amorphous, nonspecific expression of disturbances in younger age groups, in contrast to more clearly articulated clinical presentations in older adolescents and adults. Learning processes also determine how and which health problems are culturally and socially accepted and how they are expressed. Other authors, for example, Caron and Rutter (1991), explain comorbidity in terms of shared and overlapping risk factors.

It is important to recognize that the two phenomena are typical of adolescence and they do not necessarily represent negative outcomes. They are, in fact, considered to reflect the adolescent's cognitive abilities to distinguish between body and mind (Fabrega & Miller, 1995). Thus, adolescents often do not understand *psychopathology* in a manner that splits body and mind, preferring to integrate bodily and psychological aspects into their concepts of illness or well-being. In order to understand how anxiety or depression symptoms are described and explained by adolescents, more studies using open-ended interviews with adolescents, accompanied by more standardized measurement procedures, must be done. Only then can we appreciate what a certain pathology means for the adolescents in their respective cultural and ethnic settings.

### Tailoring Health Care According to the Cultural and Social Context in Which Adolescents Live

In general, demographic variables, such as age, gender, and SES, figure as important parameters that, in conjunction with prevalence rates, help to determine the causes of illness and need for treatment. However, adolescents' health problems cannot fully be understood unless they are viewed in comparison to those shown by other social groups in their society. As a rule, cultural and ethnic factors tend to be disregarded, although it is well known that ethnic minorities show high prevalence rates for certain disorders and tend to underutilize health services. Much progress was made in developing specific, operational criteria that may facilitate the diagnosis of some disorders; however, such definitions rarely acknowledge the potential contribution of cultural background. In their cultural analysis of adolescent psychopathology, Fabrega and Miller (1995) argued for recognizing the need to include cultural factors in assessments of adolescent health. Such information is obtained by asking adolescents from different cultural and ethnic backgrounds to describe their perceptions of a health problem.

Perhaps more than any other age group, adolescents are a product of a society's historical, social, and cultural circumstances. The development of individual identity during late childhood and throughout adolescence is guided by collective attitudes that prevail in a large part of community or society. The influence of culture becomes especially apparent when adolescents from different societies or different cultural backgrounds are compared. Such comparisons reveal the social and cultural differences in the importance ascribed to transition into adulthood. In addition, it becomes clear that each culture develops a unique array of attitudes and values about health. Acculturational forces also introduce conflicting goals, divergent strategies of dealing with stressors, and new kinds of challenges. The extent of parental or adult supervision and monitoring of adolescents' behavior, as well as the collective attitude toward risk-taking activities, varies among different ethnic groups.

The descriptive analysis of adolescents' life circumstances and stressors and the assessment of adolescent psychopathology must be more culturally sensitive. Although we were able to identify many universal stressors (i.e., stressors experienced by virtually all adolescents living in Western societies), research findings suggest that certain cultural groups are experiencing greater social stress and need special services. The fact that adolescents from immigrant families or ethnic minorities underutilize health care services is related to different subjective evaluations of professional health care. In addition, the characteristics of health care providers themselves might affect ethnic minorities' willingness to seek help. For example, many African Americans in the United States are socialized to conceal their true feelings, particularly when relating to Whites (Ridley, 1984). This can be problematical for the African American client who needs counseling, because most counselors in the United States are White. In an experiment designed by Poston,

Craine, and Atkinson (1991) on African American and White women, the client's gender, educational and cultural background, as well as the (fictitious) counselor's gender, ethnic background, and attitudes about racial and ethnic confrontation, served as predictor variables, and patients' willingness to disclose personal information and perceived counselor credibility served as criterion variables. These investigators found that the counselor's being White negatively affected his or her ascribed credibility. Some evidence was found that the client's willingness to disclose personal information to a white counselor increased with more education. Nevertheless, African Americans were generally unwilling to cooperate with a White counselor. These findings suggest that White counselors need to do more than simply confront racial and ethnic differences in the initial counseling session in order to increase their credibility among patients from minority groups.

### Enhancing Communication Between Adolescents and Health Experts About Sexual Behavior and Risk Prevention

As outlined in this volume, three characteristics of the communication between health care providers and patients deviate from everyday experience: asymmetric power relations, the request to disclose personal or private information, and the fact that physical privacy is not possible. Developmental changes in self-disclosure behavior and the manner in which nudity is dealt with may make communication between health care providers and adolescent patients extremely difficult. The reservations adolescents have about being examined or talking about their bodies with health care providers or other adults are seen as being related to the process of becoming separated from parents. Some parents are unable to talk about physical maturation and sexuality with their children. Consequently, many adolescents complain that they have no one with whom they can openly talk about sex. Thus, it may be easier for the adolescent to discuss these topics with an adult who is ascribed an expert status. However, although communication about sexual behaviors, such as contraceptive practices or intercourse, is expected, it is unlikely that adolescents will readily talk about other aspects of sexuality, such as masturbation, nocturnal emission, and erotic fantasies. Adolescents consider these to be private and somewhat shameful activities. Nevertheless, such information helps the health care provider determine whether an adolescent is developing normally. Health care professionals should be aware of the fact that acceptance of most sexual behaviors is greater among boys than among girls. In addition, males are more carefree and more permissive in their sexual behavior, whereas females tend to be more committed to their sexual partners. Also, male and female adolescents' knowledge about sexuality and contraceptive behavior differs. There is a strong association between physical maturity and experience with sexual intercourse, but peer pressure also influences the onset of heterosexual relations. Misjudgments of risks related to sexual relations are common during early adolescent years, when egocentrism peaks. After about 16 years old, developmental progression enables the adolescent to perceive risks more objectively. Nevertheless, health care professionals must recognize that even when young people are able to adequately perceive a behavior's potential risk, risk taking is an integral part of most adolescents' lifestyles.

Physicians represent valuable sources of information about sexual matters for this age group. They are in the position to provide accurate and nonjudgmental information about sex and risk prevention tailored to their patients' needs. Although professional medical organizations recommend that physicians discuss sexual matters and risk prevention with their adolescent patients, physicians do not always follow these recommendations. In the survey of Schuster, Bell, Petersen, and Kanouse (1996) on 2,026 students in the ninth and twelfth grades, most adolescents reported not having received these services. Thirty-nine percent of the adolescents reported discussions with physicians about how to avoid getting AIDS, 37% about using condoms, 15% about the adolescent's sex life, 13% about how to say "no" to unwanted sex, and 8% about sexual orientation. Nonvirginal females and males reported having more communication with their doctors. However, over 80% of all adolescents stated that they would find it helpful to talk with a physician about various sexual matters. One explanation of physicians' hesitance to address sexual issues is that many physicians do not feel adequately trained to do so. Furthermore, some physicians also feel too embarrassed to talk about sexual matters or they are afraid of negative parental reactions. At any rate, adolescents are clearly interested in discussing these matters with health experts. However, it is important for the adolescent to know that the contents of such discussions are kept confidential.

### Addressing Barriers to Adolescent Health Care: The Issue of Confidentiality

Recognized barriers to obtaining health care, such as inadequate health insurance or lack of transportation to a health care provider, are known to affect adolescents' utilization of health care services. Among others, social and psychological factors may also be relevant. As pointed out in the earlier discussion of developmentally related changes in self-disclosure behavior and in dealing with nudity, privacy is very important to the adolescent. Accordingly, health care-seeking behavior can be powerfully influenced by concerns about privacy. Adolescents rate "confidentiality" as being very important in their choice of health care services (Hodgson, Feldman, Corber, & Quinn, 1986). According to Cheng et al. (1993), the majority of adolescents have concerns they wish to keep confidential, and a striking percentage reported that they would not seek health services because of these concerns. However, health experts' and patients' views about confidentiality diverge, and not all health experts support confidential care. Fleming, O'Connor, and Sandeis (1994) found that the majority of pediatricians investigated were less likely to respect confidentiality in dealing with adolescents, especially early adolescents. Significantly more pediatricians believed that, should a patient under 15 years old require treatment, parental consent should be obtained or at least, that the parents should be notified. Yet most pediatricians supported the right of adolescents to seek care without parental permission for health problems related to substance abuse and sexuality. Younger pediatricians, female pediatricians, and pediatricians who were not self-employed were more likely to support adolescents' requests for confidentiality. These findings suggest that one may expect great differences in the attitudes toward confidentiality among health care providers. Nevertheless, health care professionals must be encouraged to recognize the importance of confidentiality for the adolescent patient. Admittedly, this is a difficult goal to achieve in light of parental rights and responsibilities to be informed about the health of their children.

### Toward Improving the Relationship Between the Adolescent Patient and the Physician

Previous studies suggest that confidentiality is the most important factor involved in adolescents' decisions to seek health care. However, the quality of the patient–physician relationship and perceptions of a physician's competence also play a role. One of the few studies in this area was conducted by Ginsburg et al. (1995) on 6,821 ninth graders from 39 public high schools in Philadelphia. This study was important because the sample included disproportionately high numbers of African American (65% of the sample), Hispanic (11%), and Asian (4%) adolescents; only 20% of the students were White. In this survey, adolescents were asked to describe the impact of several factors on their decisions to seek care. Factor analysis revealed three main factors. The first factor was related to the physician's competency and hygienic practices (e.g., information attesting to a physician's experience, handwashing, use of clean instruments). Most adolescents in this study said that variables relating to the physician's competence, knowledge, and carefulness were important. The second factor pertained to the provider–patient relationship. The physician's interpersonal characteristics (e.g., honesty, respect, equal treatment of the patients, confidentiality, friendliness, and the ability to relate to young people) were emphasized. Confidentiality, honesty, and respect ranked very high. Equal treatment of patients was interpreted by the students in different ways. Minority students related stories of having to wait in physicians' offices, clinics, and emergency departments while others moved ahead. The third factor was related to autonomy issues and special services offered. The adolescents thought it was important that they could go on their own to seek health care, that appointments could be easily made, that visits and test results would remain anonymous, and that crisis or counseling centers were available.

Other investigators found that adolescents who are satisfied with their providers keep appointments more consistently, and providers who are skilled in adolescent care are more likely to experience better patient compliance with treatment regimens (Litt & Cuskey, 1984). Marks, Fisher, and Lasker (1991) found that many pediatricians they surveyed continued to interact with their adolescent patients in the same manner used for younger children. Adolescent care requires a new approach, that will inevitably require extra time on the part of the pediatrician to implement care effectively. This new approach includes offering the patient a choice. Thus, pediatricians state that they are happy to provide care, but every patient has the right to seek care from another physician.

### Understanding Noncompliance and the Function of Cheating

In a review of studies on patient compliance, Cromer and Tarnowksi (1989) found that between 30% to 50% of adolescents with various types of chronic illness showed poor compliance. The problem of noncompliance cannot be separated from the central issue of the adolescent's struggle to achieve independence. Furthermore, one must not overlook the dangers associated with *hypercompliance*, for example, the risk of learned dependency.

Paradoxically, being well-informed about one's illness or disease does not always imply good compliance, as several studies have shown (see chap. 7, this volume). In one study of diabetic adolescents, good knowledge of the disease was negatively associated with diabetic control (Hamburg & Inoff, 1982). Chronically ill adolescents typically know quite a lot about their disease, but this knowledge implies being aware of having to depend on others. This dependence is all the more intolerable because it is unavoidable. According to Marcelli and Alvin (1994), adolescents frequently solve this conflict by cheating (e.g., they report false results of self-performed blood tests). By cheating they are attempting to preserve some measure of autonomy. They also are trying to forget or make others forget that they are sick. Health experts have to understand that cheating is a functional compromise between having knowledge and avoiding unbearable dependence. Physicians often maintain that poor compliance is the adolescent's fault. This negative judgment only reinforces the patient's already heightened guilt. Guilt increases anxiety and thus increases defense mechanisms. Therefore, health care providers should try to understand the chronically ill adolescent's dilemma. In this regard, it is important to be aware of the aggressive nature inherent in many noncompliant behaviors. According to Winnicott (1970), aggression is a normal part of adolescent development. It may be directed toward one's own body, as is seen, for example, in such self-destructive behaviors as delinquency, suicide, or substance abuse. Noncompliance may thus also represents the expression of aggressive tendencies.

### Searching for Alternatives: Peer Support Groups for Prevention

Without a doubt, early recognition and management of emotional distress and behavioral problems in high school students are great challenges. The magnitude of the problem is quite clear: Offer, Howard, Schonert, and Ostrov (1991) reported that 22% of 500 adolescents in high school suffered from psychosocial distress. Frymier and Gansneder (1989) evaluated the records of 22,000 students and found that one fourth to one third were at risk of developing severe disorders that might impair their future development and school performance. These and similar studies established that adolescents suffering from severe disturbances rarely seek help from professionals. In fact, the majority of those who suffer from emotional disturbances do not receive any help. It should be pointed out that adolescents frequently report that health care services are either unavailable to them or that the access to these services is low (Cheng & Klein, 1995). In general, health care is available for those with sufficient financial means or for those with severe problems, but other factors may be involved. As was outlined in this volume, compared to children, adolescents are more involved and intimate with peers and friends, turning to them for support formerly provided by the family. In addition, they are better able to formulate and evaluate possible solutions of problems and are more willing to make compromises. Also, social comparison with other peers of like gender becomes more likely. As a result, adolescent behavior becomes more strongly oriented to that of their peers. This is reflected in adolescents' preferences to seek assistance and support from their peers when they have problems.

Considering the magnitude of the problem, budgetary limitations, and adolescent patterns of seeking help, current forms of organized mental health or school counseling services are not likely to succeed in providing prevention or early intervention. In such situations of limited resources and access barriers, it is worth encouraging efforts to tap adolescents' interpersonal resources and to exploit their tendencies to reach out to peers for help.

For example, school and health systems might provide better care of adolescents with mental health problems by introducing peer counseling services. Wassef, Ingham, Collins, and Mason (1995) suggested establishing peer support groups in schools for adolescents suffering from emotional distress and behavioral problems and gave concrete guidelines for their organization. They proposed that such in-school, early intervention programs for adolescents should, for example, use available school resources (such as school student assistant programs), be designed to operate within the school budget (e.g., by having volunteers), uphold confidentiality, and aim to provide support to students who are in distress rather than represent a disciplinary body to control problem students.

In the long run, such peer support groups are not only more economical, but also more effective in helping students in distress before more serious problems develop. The peer support approach also encourages adolescents to assume an active role in evaluating and structuring services to their peers. Due to the more egalitarian structure of communication between peers, highly stressed adolescents are more likely to feel at ease about talking about their problems in the peer setting.

### Understanding the Parents' Perspectives

In some respects, the role of the health expert in helping the troubled adolescent is similar to that of the parents. Consequently, many difficulties in the treatment of adolescents emerge as a result of the health care provider's insecurity about his or her roles and functions. Although it is important for care providers to understand and acknowledge the parents' perspectives about their adolescent's difficulties, they cannot always act in the interests of two parties. This dilemma often occurs when parents insist on being physically present during their adolescent's discussions with health care providers. In this case, it is advisable to encourage separate meetings with the parents. Such an approach allows the provider to obtain information that supplements that supplied by the adolescent on an individual basis. It is also important to recognize that despite adolescents' protests and separation-oriented activities, most of them continue to maintain a close and meaningful relationship with their parents. Although adolescents are more likely to turn to peers for help, satisfaction with parental support is more strongly related to psychological well-being than satisfaction with support provided by peers. The protective function of supportive and cohesive family relations and the developmentally inhibiting influence of high parental control and low warmth were demonstrated throughout this volume. Adolescents treated in mental health facilities frequently struggle with feelings of being rejected by their families, which creates difficulties in their relationships with therapists, physicians, and nurses (Weissman & Appleton, 1995). The parents must also recognize that the separation–individuation process is a learning experience. Unfortunately, not all families are able to be flexible and make adjustments in their interactions with their adolescent children who are seeking autonomy.

As demonstrated, increasing adolescent autonomy puts an additional strain on the parents, especially if their child suffers from severe health impairments such as chronic physical illness. Many parents find it difficult to make the distinction between illness-specific and developmentally related problems. This is behind the rather unexpected finding that despite good reasons for consulting psychological services, actual rates for utilization of such services are quite low. When adolescents undergo psychotherapy or counseling, they frequently report that they were having problems with parental cooperation and support in the therapy. Such problems are explained by the fact that most treatment aims to support and promote adolescent autonomy, so that parents are often required to restructure their relationships with their child and with one another. Health care professionals must recognize the challenges involved for both parties and take the parents' worries and concerns seriously. Indeed, the parents themselves sometimes also need counseling during the process of adolescent separation. The parents of chronically ill children and adolescents especially need the support of health care providers, because they are particularly hesitant to seek and accept help.

### Developing a Therapeutic Alliance in the Treatment of Disturbed Adolescents

Some disturbed adolescent patients who undergo psychotherapy have great difficulties in developing an optimal alliance with the therapist and some never do at all. However, after an initial phase of resistance, most patients are able to show signs of genuine collaboration, which increases the likelihood that the patient will profit from psychotherapy (Rinsley, 1980). Obstacles to therapeutic collaboration are especially obvious in hospitalized adolescents. In the vast majority of cases, the parents request that their adolescent child be admitted to the hospital for treatment. Regardless of their awareness of needing hospitalization, many adolescents experience forced hospitalization as a validation of their sense of powerlessness. They are emotionally torn by the forces of a "regressive pull" (Blos, 1967) toward passivity, dependency, and the wish for autonomy and independence. It is important for therapists to look for rudimentary aspects of cooperation (often quite disguised). O'Malley (1990) noted that most adolescents progress from rudimentary to high levels of collaboration via several steps:

1. The acceptance of containment.
2. The formation of attachments.
3. The communication of symptoms.
4. The collaboration in conflict-free spheres.
5. Developmental achievement.

In order for patients to establish a sense of trust in the effectiveness of hospitalization, they must become convinced that their developmental needs will be met by staff members who will provide containment, structure, and acceptance of dependency without control for its own sake. A disturbed adolescent's engagement in normal developmental activities with members of the treatment team (such as talking about motorcycles instead of discussing his problems) signals the beginning of a tentative collaboration. Some adolescents are then willing to talk about their symptoms. Other adolescents steadfastly resist cooperating with adults; nevertheless, active collaboration in problematic areas fosters a willingness to work with team members toward success and mastery in conflict-free spheres. The adolescent thus gains competencies in other developmentally relevant areas enabling him or her to deal with the frustrating and anxiety-arousing aspects of his or her disturbances. Finally, collaboration involves both the active use of treatment for constructive change and the recognition of one's own contribution. Thus, adolescent patients may either work to alter an external situation or work to achieve personal change by accepting some degree of responsibility for their situation. Thus, therapists must be able to accept that there are different levels of collaborative behavior that facilitate treatment of adolescent patients.

### Learning From Treatment Difficulties

In this volume, we have outlined some of the most difficult problems in the health care of adolescents—e.g., the lack of adolescent motivation, which led stigmatizing adolescents to being unmotivated patients, frequent use of avoidant coping or withdrawal in highly stressed adolescents, and the strong increase in defense mechanisms exhibited by chronically ill adolescents shortly after the onset of a severe illness. However, we have learned from psychoanalysis that although an adolescent's resistance to change impedes the course of therapy, it indicates a healthy capacity to protect an established and familiar way of functioning against outside interference (Blos, 1983).

From a developmental perspective, psychotherapy of the adolescent client involves several difficulties—defensive passivity, acting out, negative therapeutic motivation, and the termination of treatment. As Rosenheim and Gaoni (1977) outlined, self-proclaimed powerlessness often cited by mid-adolescents is actually a rationalization for avoiding decision making or actively attempting to cope. As patients, these adolescents seem to be content with being recognized and treated as children. This defensive passivity causes major problems if it persists, especially if it is coupled with countertransference reactions such as rescue fantasies involving the therapist (Rodrigues-Lima, Eisenthal, & Lazare, 1981). In contrast, acting out on the part of the adolescent patient demonstrates the patient's activity and control while suppressing thoughts and feelings (Blos, 1963). In this case, the therapeutic process requires much effort to develop the patient's reality-testing skills (Feinstein, 1990). Autonomy and control in adolescence are also obvious in instances of negative therapeutic motivation and discontinuation of treatment (Novick, 1976, 1980). Negative therapeutic motivation is present when the patient goes for counseling or agrees to undergo psychotherapy with the intention of making the therapist fail.

Unlike the negative therapeutic reaction as described by Freud, negative therapeutic motivation occurs long before the patient sees the therapist or knows what therapy entails. This phenomenon is more visible in patients with certain kinds of disorders and at certain ages such as adolescence. It is interesting to note that negative therapeutic motivation is often shown by the patient and the patient's parents. In this case, it is related to their mutually shared, defensive needs to maintain an idealized image of a loving and omnipotent parent. In this situation, the therapist is perceived as a threat, hence there are conscious or unconscious efforts to undermine the therapist's efforts to establish a good relationship with the young patient or to enable transference processes to unfold. Whereas negative therapeutic motivation often occurs as a result of parental resistance, termination of treatment is more likely to be linked to the adolescent's strong drive to achieve independence. As Novick (1976) outlined, in the terminal phase of therapy, the therapist and client discuss the initial goals of treatment and the client is encouraged to recognize the fact that therapy has an end. Many adolescents have great difficulties in accepting this fact, and they drop out of therapy prematurely. This behavior represents the adolescent's wish to avoid unhappy departure scenes. It is important that therapists and other related health care professionals do not feel offended by this abrupt farewell.

# References


Aarons, A. (1970). Normality and abnormality in adolescence. *Psychoanalytic Study of the Child, 25,* 309–338.

Abholz, H.-H., Borgers, D., Karmans, W., & Korporal, J. (Eds.). (1982). *Risikofaktorenmedizin* [Risk factor medicine]. Berlin: de Gruyter.

Achenbach, T. M. (1990). "Comorbidity" in child and adolescent psychiatry: Categorical and quantitative perspectives. *Journal of Child and Adolescent Psychopharmacology, 1,* 1–8.

Achenbach, T. M. (1991a). The derivation of taxonomic constructs: A necessary stage in the development of developmental psychopathology. In D. Cicchetti (Ed.), *Rochester symposium on developmental psychopathology* (Vol. 3, pp. 120–132). Hillsdale, NJ: Lawrence Erlbaum Associates.

Achenbach, T. M. (1991b). *Manual for the Child Behavior Checklist and 1991 Child Behavior Profile.* Burlington: University of Vermont.

Achenbach, T. M. (1991c). *Manual for the Teachers Report Form and 1991 TRF profile.* Burlington: University of Vermont.

Achenbach, T. M. (1991d). *Manual for the Youth Self-Report and 1991 YSR Profile.* Burlington, VT: University of Vermont.

Achenbach, T. M., McConaughy, S. H., & Howell, C. T. (1987). Child and adolescent behavioral and emotional problems: Implications of cross-informant correlations for situational specificity. *Psychological Bulletin, 101,* 213–232.

Adams, P. F., & Hardy, A. M. (1989). Current estimates from the National Health Interview Survey: United States, 1988. *Vital and Health Statistics, Series 10,* No. 173.

Adelman, H. S., Taylor, L., Fuller, W., & Nelson, P. (1979). Discrepancies among student, parent and teacher ratings of the severity of a student's problems. *American Educational Research Journal, 16,* 38–41.

Ahmed, P. I., & Ahmed, N. (Eds.). (1985). *Coping with juvenile diabetes.* Springfield, IL: Thomas.

Allgood-Merten, B., Lewinsohn, P. M., & Hops, H. (1990). Sex differences and adolescent depression. *Journal of Abnormal Psychology, 99,* 55–63.

Amann-Gainotti, M., Di Prospero, B., & Nenci, A. M. (1989). Adolescent girls' representations of their genital inner space. *Adolescence, 94,* 473–480.

Amato, R. P., & Keith, B. (1991). Parental divorce and the well-being of children: A meta-analysis. *Psychological Bulletin, 110,* 26–46.

American Academy of Pediatrics and Center to Prevent Handgun Violence. (1994). *STOP: Steps to prevent firearm injury.* Atlanta: Author.

American Psychiatric Association. (APA). (1987). *Diagnostic and Statistical Manual of Mental Disorders* (3rd rev. ed.). Washington, DC: American Psychiatric Association.

Amir, D. (1987). Preventive behavior and health status among the elderly. *Psychology and Health, 3*, 353–378.
Anderson, B. J., Auslander, W., Jung, K. C., Miller, J. P., & Santiago, J. V. (1990). Assessing family sharing of diabetes responsibilities. *Journal of Pediatric Psychology, 15,* 477–492.
Anderson, B. J., Miller, J. P., Auslander, W. F., & Santiago, J. V. (1981). Family characteristics of diabetic adolescents: Relationship to metabolic control. *Diabetes Care, 4,* 586–594.
Anderson, P. B., & Aymami, R. (1993). Reports of female initiation of sexual contact: Male and female differences. *Archives of Sexual Behavior, 22,* 335–343.
Anderson Moore, K., Myers, D. E., Morrison, D. R., Nord, C. W., Brown, B., & Edmonston, B. (1993). Age at first childbirth and later poverty. *Journal of Research in Adolescence, 3,* 393–422.
Andrews, G. (1981). A prospective study of life events and psychological symptoms. *Psychological Medicine, 11,* 759–801.
Andrus, J. K., Fleming, D. W., Heumann, M. A., Wassell, J. T., Hopkins, D. D., & Gordon, J. (1991). Surveillance of attempted suicide among adolescents in Oregon, 1988. *American Journal of Public Health, 81,* 1067–1069.
Antonovsky, A. (1987). The salutogenic perspective: Toward a new view to health and illness. *Advances, 4,* 47–55.
Argyle, M. (1972). *Soziale Interaktion* [Social interaction]. Köln, Germany: Kiepenheuer & Witsch.
Arnett, J. (1990). Contraceptive use, sensation seeking and adolescent egocentrism. *Journal of Youth and Adolescence, 2,* 171–180.
Aseltine, R. H., & Gore, S. (1993). Mental health and social adaptation following the transition from high school. *Journal of Research on Adolescence, 3,* 247–270.
Ashworth, M. (1982). The cultural adjustment of immigrant children in English Canada. In R. C. Nann (Ed.), *Uprooting and surviving: Adaptation and resettlement of migrant families and children* (pp. 77–84). Dordrecht, Holland: Reidel.
Badura, B. (Ed.). (1971). *Soziale Unterstützung und chronische Krankheit. Zum Stand sozialepidemiologischer Forschung* [Social support and chronic illness. Findings from social epidemiological research]. Frankfurt, Germany: Suhrkamp.
Badura, B. (1983). Sozialepidemiologie in Theorie und Praxis. [Social epidemiology in theory and practice]. *Europäische Monographien zur Forschung in Gesundheitserziehung*, 5, 29–48.
Bailey, S. L. (1992). Adolescents' multisubstance use patterns: The role of heavy alcohol and cigarette use. *American Journal of Public Health, 82,* 1220–1224.
Balint, M. (1964). *The doctor, his patient and the illness.* London: Pitman.
Baltes, M. M., & Wahl, H. W. (1987). Dependency in aging. In L. L. Carstensen & B. A. Edelstein (Eds.), *Handbook of clinical gerontology* (pp. 204–221). New York: Pergamon.
Barglow, P., Edidin, E. V., Budlong-Springer, A. S., Berndt, D., Phillips, D., & Dubrow, E. (1983). Diabetic control in children and adolescents: Psychosocial factors and therapeutic efficacy. *Journal of Youth and Adolescence, 10,* 77–94.
Baron, P., & McGillivray, R. G. (1989). Depressive symptoms in adolescents as a function of perceived parental behavior. *Journal of Adolescent Research,* 4, 50–62.
Barrera, M. (1981). Social support in the adjustment of pregnant adolescents: Assessment issues. In B. H. Gottlieb (Ed.), *Social networks and social support* (pp. 69–96). Beverly Hills, CA: Sage.
Baum, A., & Grunberg, N. E. (1991). Gender, stress, and health. *Health Psychology, 10,* 80–85.
Bauman, K. E., & Ennett, S. E. (1994). Tobacco use by Black and White adolescents: The validity of self-reports. *American Journal of Public Health, 84,* 394–398.

Beardslee, W. R., & Podorefsky, D. (1988). Resilient adolescents whose parents have serious affective and other psychiatric disorders: Importance of self-understanding and relationships. *American Journal of Psychiatry, 145,* 63–69.

Beckmann, D. (1984). *Grundlagen der Medizinischen Psychologie* [Basics of medical psychology]. Göttingen, Germany: Vandenhoeck & Ruprecht, Verlag für Medizinische Psychologie.

Bell, R. (1985). *Holy anorexia.* Chicago: Chicago University Press.

Belle, D. E. (1987). Gender differences in moderators of stress. In R. D. Barnett, L. Biener, & G. K. Baruch (Eds.), *Gender and stress* (pp. 21–36). New York: The Free Press.

Ben-Sira, Z. (1984). Chronic illness, stress and coping. *Social Science and Medicine, 18,* 725–736.

Berkhan, K. (1863). Irresein bei Kindern [Mania in children]. *Korrespondenzblatt der Deutschen Gesellschaft für Psychiatrie, 10,* 65–76.

Berman, A. L., & Jobes, D. A. (1995). Suicide prevention in adolescents (age 12–18). *Suicide and Life-Threatening Behavior, 25,* 143–154.

Bernfeld, S. (1923). Über eine typische Form der männlichen Pubertät [On a typical male puberty]. *Imago, 9,* 169–188.

Bibace, R., & Walsh, M. E. (1981). Children's conceptions of illness. In R. Bibace & M. E. Walsh (Eds.), *Children's conceptions of health, illness, and body functions* (pp. 31–48). San Francisco: Jossey-Bass.

Billings, A. G., & Moos, R. H. (1981). The role of coping responses and social resources in attenuating the stress of life events. *Journal of Behavioral Medicine, 4,* 157–189.

Billings, A. G., & Moos, R. H. (1982). Family environments and adaptation: A clinically applicable typology. *American Journal of Family Therapy, 10,* 26–38.

Bingham, C. R., Miller, B. C., & Adams, G. R. (1990). Correlates of age at first sexual intercourse in a national sample of young women. *Journal of Adolescent Research, 5,* 18–33.

Bird, H. R., Gould, M. S., & Staghezza, B. M. (1993). Patterns of diagnostic comorbidity in a community sample of children aged 9 through 16 years. *Journal of the American Academy of Child and Adolescent Psychiatry, 32,* 361–368.

Blanchard-Fields, F., & Irion, J. (1988). Coping strategies from the perspective of two developmental markers: Age and social reasoning. *Journal of Genetic Psychology, 149,* 141–151.

Blaxter, M. (1983). The causes of disease: Woman talking. *Social Science and Medicine, 17,* 59–69.

Blos, P. (1954). Prolonged adolescence. *American Journal of Orthopsychiatry, 24,* 733–742.

Blos, P. (1963). The concept of acting out in relation to the adolescent process. *Journal of the American Academy of Child Psychiatry, 2,* 121–138.

Blos, P. (1967). The second individuation process of adolescence. *Psychoanalytic Study of the Child, 22,* 162–186.

Blos, P. (1973). *Adoleszenz. Eine psychoanalytische Interpretation* [Adolescence. A psychoanalytic interpretation]. Stuttgart, Germany: Klett-Cotta.

Blos, P. (1983). The contribution of psychoanalysis to the psychotherapy of adolescents. *Psychoanalytic Study of the Child, 38,* 577–599.

Blumstein, A. (1994). *Youth violence, firearms, and illicit drug markets.* Pittsburgh, PA: Carnegie Mellon University.

Blyth, D. A., Hill, J. P., & Thiel, K. S. (1982). Early adolescents' significant others: Grade and gender differences in perceived relationships with familial and nonfamilial adults and young people. *Journal of Youth and Adolescence, 11,* 425–450.

Blyth, D. A., Simmons, R. G., & Zakin, D. F. (1985). Satisfaction with body image for early adolescent females: The impact of pubertal timing within different school environments. *Journal of Youth and Adolescence, 14,* 207–225.

Bolton, F. G., & MacEachron, A. E. (1988). Adolescent male sexuality: A developmental perspective. *Journal of Adolescent Research, 3,* 259–273.

Brähler, E. (Ed.). (1988). *Body experience. The subjective dimension of psyche and soma.* New York: Springer Verlag.

Brand, A. H., Johnson, J. H., & Johnson, S. B. (1986). Life stress and diabetic control in children and adolescents with insulin-dependent diabetes. *Journal of Pediatric Psychology, 11,* 481–496.

Brooks-Gunn, J. (1987). Pubertal processes: Their relevance for developmental research. In V. B. van Hasselt & M. Hersen (Eds.), *Handbook of adolescent psychology* (pp. 111–130). New York: Pergamon.

Brooks-Gunn, J., (1988). Antecedents and consequences of variations in girls' maturational timing. *Journal of Adolescent Health Care, 9,* 365–373.

Brooks-Gunn, J., & Furstenberg, F. F. (1989). Adolescent sexual behavior. *American Psychologist, 44,* 249–257.

Brooks-Gunn, J., & Ruble, D. N. (1983). The experience of menarche from a developmental perspective. In J. Brooks-Gunn & A. C. Petersen (Eds.), *Girls at puberty. Biological and psychosocial perspectives* (pp. 155–177). New York: Plenum.

Brooks-Gunn, J., & Warren, M. P. (1985). The effects of delayed menarche in different contexts: Dance and nondance students. *Journal of Youth and Adolescence, 14,* 285–300.

Broughton, J. M. (1981). The divided self in adolescence. *Human Development, 24,* 13–32.

Bruch, H. (1982). Psychotherapy in anorexia nervosa. *International Journal of Eating Disorders, 1,* 3–14.

Bry, B. H., McKeon, P., & Pandima, R. J. (1982). Extent of drug use as a function of number of risk factors. *Journal of Abnormal Psychology, 91,* 273–279.

Buhrmester, D., & Furman, W. (1987). The development of companionship and intimacy. *Child Development, 58,* 1101–1113.

Bulcroft, R. A. (1991). The value of physical change in adolescence: Consequences for the parent–adolescent exchange relationship. *Journal of Youth and Adolescence, 20,* 89–105.

Bulman, R. J., & Wortman, C. B. (1977). Attributions of blame and coping in the real world. *Journal of Personality and Social Psychology, 35,* 351–361.

Bundesminister für Gesundheit (Ed.). (1991). *Daten des Gesundheitswesens. Ausgabe 1991* [Health data. 1991 edition] Baden Baden, Germany: Nomos.

Burke, R., & Weir, T. (1978). Benefits to adolescents of informal helping relationships with their parents and peers. *Psychological Reports, 42,* 1175–1184.

Burt, C., Cohen, L. H., & Bjorck, J. (1988). Perceived family environment as a moderator of young adolescents' life stress adjustment. *American Journal of Community Psychology, 16,* 101–122.

Byers, R. H., Lindegren, M. L., Hanson, I. C., Sweeney, P. A., & Onorato, I. M. (1992, October). *AIDS patients infected during adolescence. United States.* Paper presented at the 32nd Interscience Conference on Antimicrobial Agents and Chemotherapy, Anaheim, CA: Abstract No. 284.

Cadman, D., Boyle, M. H., Szatmari, P., & Offord, D. R. (1987). Chronic illness, disability, and mental and social well-being: Findings of the Ontario child health study. *Pediatrics, 79,* 805–813.

Calnan, M. (1987). *Health and illness: The lay perspective.* New York: Tavistock.

Campo, J. V., & Fritsch, S. L. (1994). Somatization in children and adolescents. *Journal of the American Academy of Child and Adolescent Psychiatry, 33,* 1223–1235.

Cantor, N., Acker, M., & Cook-Flannagan, C. (1992). Conflicts and preoccupation in the intimacy life task. *Journal of Personality and Social Psychology, 63*, 644–655.

Cantwell, D. P., Sturzenberger, S., Buroughs, J., Salkin, B., & Green, K. (1977). Anorexia nervosa— an affective disorder? *Archives of General Psychiatry, 34,* 1087–1093.

Carlson, G., & Kashani, J. (1988). Phenomenology of major depression from childhood through adulthood analysis of three studies. *American Journal of Psychiatry, 145,* 1222–1225.

Caron, C., & Rutter, M. (1991). Comorbidity in child psychopathology: Concepts, issues and research strategies. *Journal of Child Psychology and Psychiatry, 32,* 1063–1080.

Cartwright, A. (1967). *Patients and their doctors.* New York: Atherton.

Caspar, R. C. (1983). On the emergence of bulimia nervosa as a syndrome. *International Journal of Eating Disorders, 2,* 3–16.

Cauce, A. M., & Strebnik, D. S. (1989). Peer networks and social support: A focus for preventive efforts with youth. In L. Bond & B. E. Compas (Eds.), *Primary prevention and promotion in the schools* (pp. 235–254). Beverly Hills, CA: Sage.

Centers for Disease Control and Prevention. (1986). *Youth suicide in the United States, 1970–1980.* Atlanta: US Dept. of Health and Human Services, Public Health Service.

Centers for Disease Control and Prevention. (1990). Fatal injuries to children, United States, 1986. *Morbidity and Mortality Weekly Report, 39,* 42.

Centers for Disease Control and Prevention. (1991). Health objectives for the nation: Attempted suicide among high school students—United States, 1990. *Morbidity and Mortality Weekly Report, 40,* 633–635.

Centers for Disease Control and Prevention. (1992a). Abortion surveillance: preliminary analysis —United States, 1989. *Morbidity and Mortality Weekly Report, 40,* 817–819.

Centers for Disease Control and Prevention. (1992b). Selected behaviors that increase risk of HIV infection among high school students—United States, 1990. *Morbidity and Mortality Weekly Report, 41,* 237–240.

Centers for Disease Control and Prevention. (1992c). Tobacco, alcohol, and other drug use among high school students—United States, 1991. *Morbidity and Mortality Weekly Report, 41,* 698–703.

Centers for Disease Control and Prevention. (1994a). Homicides among 15–19-year-old males—United States, 1963–1991. *Morbidity and Mortality Weekly Report, 43,* 725–727.

Centers for Disease Control and Prevention. (1994b). Prevalence of overweight among adolescents—United States, 1988 – 1991. *Morbidity and Mortality Weekly Report, 43,* 818–821.

Centers for Disease Control and Prevention. (1994c). *Preventing tobacco use among young people: A report of the surgeon general.* Atlanta, GA: Author.

Centers for Disease Control and Prevention. (1994d). Update: Trends in AIDS diagnosis and reporting under the expanded surveillance definition for adolescents and adults—United States, 1993. *Morbidity and Mortality Weekly Report, 43,* 826–831.

Centers for Disease Control and Prevention. (1995a). Disabilities among children aged < 17 years—United States, 1991–1992. *Morbidity and Mortality Weekly Report, 44,* 609–612.

Centers for Disease Control and Prevention. (1995b). Notifiable diseases. *Morbidity and Mortality Weekly Report, 44,* 10.

Centers for Disease Control and Prevention. (1995c). Trends in sexual risk behavior among high school students—United States, 1990, 1991, and 1993. *Morbidity and Mortality Weekly Report, 44,* 124–125, 131–132.

Centers for Disease Control and Prevention. (1995d). Trends in smoking initiation among adolescents and young adults—United States, 1980–1989. *Morbidity and Mortality Weekly Report, 44,* 521–525.

Centers for Disease Control and Prevention. (1996). Asthma mortality and hospitalization among children and young adults—United States, 1980–1993. *Morbidity and Mortality Weekly Report, 45,* 350–353.

Chase, H. P., & Jackson, G. G. (1981). Stress and sugar control in children with insulin dependent diabetes mellitus. *Journal of Pediatrics, 98,* 1011–1013.

Chasseguet-Smirgel, J. (Ed.). (1979). *Psychoanalyse der weiblichen Sexualität* [Psychoanalysis of female sexuality]. Frankfurt, Germany: Suhrkamp.

Chavez, E. L., & Swaim, R. C. (1992). An epidemiological comparison of Mexican-American and White non-Hispanic 8th- and 12th-grade students' substance use. *American Journal of Public Health, 82,* 445–447.

Chelune, G. J., & Waring, E. M. (1984). Nature and assessment of intimacy. In P. McReynolds (Ed.), *Advances in psychological assessment* (pp. 23–56). San Francisco: Jossey-Bass.

Chen, K., & Kandel, D. B. (1995). The natural history of drug use from adolescence to the mid-thirties in a general population sample. *American Journal of Public Health, 85,* 41–47.

Cheng, T. L., & Klein, J. D. (1995). The adolescent viewpoint, implications for access and preventives. *Journal of the American Medical Association, 273,* 1957–1958.

Cheng, T. L., Savagean, J. A., Sattler, D. L., & de Witt, T. G. (1993). Confidentiality in health care. A survey on knowledge, perceptions, and attitudes among high school students. *Journal of the American Medical Association, 269,* 1404–1407.

Chin, M. L., Feldman, S. S., & Rosenthal, D. A. (1992). The influence of immigration on parental behavior and adolescent distress in Chinese families residing in two Western nations. *Journal of Research on Adolescence, 2,* 205–239.

Cicchetti, D. (1984). The emergence of developmental psychopathology. *Child Development, 55,* 1–7.

Claes, M. E. (1992). Friendships and personal adjustment during adolescence. *Journal of Adolescence, 15,* 39–55.

Clement, U., Schmidt, G., & Kruse, M. (1984). Changes in sex-differences in sexual behavior: A replication of a study on West German students (1966–1981). *Archives of Sexual Behavior, 13,* 99–120.

Coddington, R. D., & Troxell, J. R. (1980). The effect of emotional factors on football injury rates: A pilot study. *Journal of Human Stress, 6,* 3–5.

Codega, S. A., Pasley, B. K., & Kreutzer, J. (1990). Coping behaviors of adolescent mothers: An exploratory study and comparison of Mexican-Americans and Anglos. *Journal of Adolescent Research, 5,* 34–53.

Cohen, L. H., Burt, C. E., & Bjorck, J. P. (1987). Life stress and adjustment: Effects of life events experienced by young adolescents and their parents. *Developmental Psychology, 23,* 583–592.

Cohen, P., Cohen, J., Kasen, S., Velez, C. N., Hartmark, C., Johnson, J., Rojas, M., Brook, J., & Streuning, E. L. (1993). An epidemiological study of disorders in late childhood and adolescence - I. Age- and gender-specific prevalence. *Journal of Child Psychology and Psychiatry and Allied Disciplines, 34,* 851–867.

Cohen, S., & Wills, T. A. (1985). Stress, social support and the buffering hypothesis. *Psychological Bulletin, 98,* 310–357.

Cohn, L. D., Adler, N. E., Irwin, C. E., Jr., Millstein, S. G., Kegeles, S. M., & Stone, G. (1987). Body–figure preferences in male and female adolescents. *Journal of Abnormal Psychology, 96,* 276–279.

Cole, R., & Reiss, D. (Eds.). (1993). *How do families cope with chronic illness?* Hillsdale, NJ: Lawrence Erlbaum Associates.

Coleman, J. S. (Ed.). (1987) *Working with troubled adolescents.* London: Academic Press.

Coletta, N. D., Hadler, S., & Gregg, C. H. (1981). How adolescents cope with the problems of early motherhood. *Adolescence, 16,* 499–512.

Compas, B. E. (1987). Stress and life events during childhood and adolescence. *Clinical Psychological Review, 7,* 275–302.

Compas, B. E., Ey, S., & Grant, K. E. (1992). *Taxonomy, assessment and diagnosis of depression during adolescence.* Unpublished manuscript, University of Vermont, Burlington.

Compas, B. E., Forsythe, C. J., & Wagner, B. M. (1988). Consistency and variability in causal attributions and coping with stress. *Cognitive Therapy and Research, 12,* 305–320.

Compas, B. E., Hinden, B. R., & Gerhardt, C. A. (1995). Adolescent development: Pathways and processes of risk and resilience. *Annual Review of Psychology, 46,* 265–293.

Compas, B. E., Howell, D. C., Phares, V., Williams, R. A., & Giunta, C. T. (1989). Risk factors for emotional/behavioral problems in young adolescents: A prospective analysis of adolescent and parental stress and symptoms. *Journal of Consulting and Clinical Psychology, 57,* 732–740.

Compas, B. E., Howell, D. C., Phares, V., Williams, R. A., & Ledoux, N. (1989). Parent and child stress and symptoms: An integrative analysis. *Developmental Psychology, 25,* 550–559.

Compas, B. E., Malcarne, V. L., & Fondacaro, K. M. (1988). Coping with stressful events in older children and young adolescents. *Journal of Consulting and Clinical Psychology, 56,* 405–411.

Compas, B. E., Orosan, P. G., & Grant, K. E. (1993). Adolescent stress and coping: Implications for psychopathology during adolescence. *Journal of Adolescence, 16,* 331–349.

Compas, B. E., Slavin, L. A., Wagner, B. M., & Vanatta, K. (1986). Relationship between life events and social support with psychological dysfunction among adolescents. *Journal of Youth and Adolescence, 15,* 205–221.

Condon, S. L., Cooper, C. R., & Grotevant, H. D. (1984). Manual for the analysis of family discourse. *Psychological Documents,* No. 2616. (Unpublished manuscript, University of Santa Barbara, CA).

Cook, J. A. (1984). Influence of gender on the problems of parents of fatally ill children. *Journal of Psychosocial Oncology, 2,* 71–91.

Cotterell, J. L. (1992). School size as a factor in adolescent's adjustment to the transition to secondary school. *Journal of Early Adolescence. 12,* 28–45.

Cotterell, J. L. (1994). Analyzing the strength of supporting ties in adolescent social support. In F. Nestmann & K. Hurrelmann (Eds.), *Social networks and social support in childhood and adolescence* (pp. 257–267). New York: de Gruyter.

Cozby, P. C. (1973). Self-disclosure: A literature review. *Psychological Bulletin, 2,* 73–91.

Crain, A. J., Susman, M. B., & Weil, W.B. (1986). Effects of a diabetic child on marital integration and related measurements of family functioning. *Journal of Health Behavior, 7,* 122–127.

Cromer, B. A., & Tarnowski, K. J. (1989). Noncompliance in adolescents: A review. *Developmental Behavioral Pediatrics, 10,* 207–215.

Cummings, S. T., (1976). The impact of the child's deficiency on the father: A study of fathers of mentally retarded and of chronically ill children. *American Journal of Orthopsychiatry, 46,* 246–255.

Czajkowski, D. R., & Koocher, G. P. (1986). Predicting medical compliance among adolescents with cystic fibrosis. *Health Psychology, 5,* 297–305.

Dacey, J. (1982). *Adolescents today.* Glenview, IL: Scott, Foresman.

Damon, W., & Hart, D. (1982). The development of self-understanding from infancy through adolescence. *Child Development, 53,* 841–864.

Daniels, D., & Moos, R. H. (1990). Assessing life stressors and social resources among adolescents: Applications to depressed youth. *Journal of Adolescent Research, 5,* 268–289.

Dawson, D. (1991). Family structure and childrens' health and well-being. Data from the 1988 National Health Interview Survey on Child Health. *Journal of Marriage and the Family, 53,* 573–584.

Davies, E., & Furman, A. (1986a). Body satisfaction in adolescent girls. *British Journal of Medical Psychology, 59,* 279–287.

Davies, E., & Furman, A. (1986b). The dieting and body shape concerns of adolescent females. *Journal of Child Psychology and Psychiatry, 27,* 417–428.

Davis, S. M., & Harris, M. B. (1982). Sexual knowledge, sexual interests, and sources of sexual information of rural and urban adolescents from three cultures. *Adolescence, 17,* 471–492.

Delamater, A. M., Kurtz, S. M., Bubb, J., White, N. H., & Santiago, J. V. (1987). Stress and coping in relation to metabolic control of adolescents with type I-diabetes. *Journal of Developmental Behavior Pediatrics, 8,* 136–140.

Delbridge, L. (1975). Educational and psychological factors in the management of diabetes in childhood. *Medical Journal of Australia, 2,* 737–739.

DeLongis, A., Folkman, S., & Lazarus, R. S. (1988). The impact of daily stress on health and mood: Psychological and social resources as mediators. *Journal of Personality and Social Psychology, 54,* 486–495.

Desmond, S. M., Price, J. H., Gray, N., & O'Connell, J. K. (1986). The etiology of adolescents' perceptions of their weight. *Journal of Youth and Adolescence, 15,* 461–474.

D'Hontand, A., & Field, M. G. (1984). The image of health. *Sociology of Health and Illness, 6,* 30–60.

Diekstra, R. F. W. (1989). Suicidal behavior and depressive disorders in adolescents and young adults. *Neuropsychobiology, 22,* 194–207.

Diekstra, R. F. W. (1990). Suicide, depression and economic conditions. In D. Lester (Ed.), *Current concepts of suicide* (pp. 71–94). Philadelphia: Charles.

Dirks, J. F., Schraa, J. C., & Robinson, S. K. (1982). Patient mislabeling of symptoms: Implications for patient–physician communication and medical outcome. *International Journal of Psychiatry in Medicine, 12,* 15–27.

Dohrenwend, B. S., & Dohrenwend, P. (Eds.). (1974). *Stressful life events: Their nature and effects*. New York: Wiley.

Dohrenwend, B. S., & Dohrenwend, P. (Eds.). (1981). *Stressful life events and their contexts*. New York: Prodist.

Donovan, J. E., & Jessor, R. (1983). Problem drinking and the dimension of involvement with drugs. *American Journal of Public Health, 73,* 543–552.

Dornbusch, S. M., Carlsmith, J. M., Gross, R. T., Martin, J. A., Jennings, D., Rosenberg, A., & Duke, P. (1981). Sexual development, age, and dating: A comparison of psychological and social influences upon one set of behaviors. *Child Development, 52,* 179–185.

Drotar, D., & Bush, M. (1985). Mental health issues and services. In N. Hobbs & J. M. Perrin (Eds.), *Issues in the care of children with chronic illness* (pp. 218–230). San Francisco: Jossey-Bass.

Drotar, D., Owens, R., & Gotthold, J. (1980). Personality adjustment of children and adolescents with hypopituitarism. *Child Psychiatry and Human Development, 11,* 59–66.

D'Hontand, A., & Field, M. G. (1984). The image of health. *Sociology of Health and Illness, 6,* 30–60.

Du Bois, R. (1989). Gesundheit und Leistungsfähigkeit im Jugendalter [Health and performance in adolescence]. In M. Markefka & R. Nave-Herz (Eds.), *Handbuch der Familien-und Jugendforschung* {Handbook of research on adolescence and the family] (Vol. 2, pp. 211–328). Neuwied, Germany: Luchterhand.

Dunn, S. M., & Turtle, J. R. (1981). The myth of diabetic personality. *Diabetes Care, 4,* 640–645.

Dusek, J. B., & Flaherty, J. F. (1981). The development of the self-concept during the adolescent years. *Monographs of the Society for Research in Child Development, 46,* 1–64.

East, P. L., & Rook, K. S. (1992). Compensatory patterns of support among children's peer relationships: A test using school friends, nonschool friends, and siblings. *Developmental Psychology, 28,* 163–172.

Ebata, A. T., & Moos, R. H. (1994). Personal, situational and contextual correlates of coping in adolescence. *Journal of Research in Adolescence, 4,* 99–125.

Eisele, J., Hertsgaard, D., & Light, H. K. (1986). Factors related to eating disorders in growing adolescent girls. *Adolescence, 21,* 283–300.

Eiser, C. (1985). *The psychology of childhood illness*. New York: Springer Verlag.

Eiser, C. (1990). *Chronic childhood disease.* New York: Cambridge University Press.

Eiser, E. (1992). Psychological consequences of chronic disease in children. In S. Maes, H. Leventhal, & M. Johnston (Eds.), *International review of health psychology,* (Vol. 1, pp. 145–166). New York: Wiley.

Eissler, R. K. (1958). Notes on problems of technique in the psychoanalytic treatment of adolescents. *Psychoanalytic Study of the Child, 13*, 223–254.

Elder, G. H., Jr. (1974). *Children of the great depression.* Chicago: University of Chicago Press.

Elkind, D. (1967). Egocentrism in adolescence. *Child Development, 38*, 1025–1034.

Elkind, D., & Bowen, R. (1977). Imaginary audience behavior in children and adolescents. *Developmental Psychology, 15,* 38–44.

Emminghaus, H. (1887). *Die psychischen Störungen des Kindesalters* [Psychological disturbances in childhood]. Tübingen, Germany: Laupp.

Engelhardt, K. H., Wirth, R., & Kindermann, L. (1973). *Kranke im Krankenhaus* [Ill people in the hospital]. Stuttgart, Germany: Enke.

Erdheim, M. (1988). *Psychoanalyse und das Unbewußte in unserer Kultur* [Psychoanalysis and the unconscious in our culture]. Frankfurt, Germany: Suhrkamp.

Erlich, H. S. (1987). Denial in adolescence. *Psychoanalytic Study of the Child, 42,* 315–336.

Etzwiler, D. D., & Sines, L. K. (1962). Juvenile diabetes and its management: Family, social and academic implications. *Journal of the American Medical Association, 181,* 304–308.

Fabrega, H., & Miller, B. D. (1995). A cultural analysis of adolescent psychopathology. *Journal of Adolescent Research, 10,* 197–226.

Fagan, J., & Chin, K. (1991). Social processes of initiation into crack. *Journal of Drug Issues, 21,* 313–343.

Farber, S. S., Felner, R. D., & Primavera, I. (1985). Parental separation/divorce and adolescents: An examination of factors mediating adaption. *American Journal of Community Psychology, 13,* 71–185.

Farrington, D. P. (1989). Long-term prediction of offending and other life outcomes. In H. Wegener, F. Lösel, & J. Haisch (Eds.), *Criminal behavior and the justice system* (pp. 26–39). New York: Springer-Verlag.

Feighner, J. P., Robins, E., Guze, S. B., Woodruff, R. A., Winokur, G., & Munoz, R. (1972). Diagnostic criteria for use in psychiatric research. *Archives of General Psychiatry, 26,* 57–63.

Feinstein, S. (Ed.) (1990). Adolescent psychiatry. *Annals of the American Society for Adolescent Psychiatry: Volume 17.* Chicago: University of Chicago Press.

Feldman, S. S., Mont-Reynaud, R., & Rosenthal, D. A. (1992). When East moves West: The acculturation of values in Chinese adolescents in the U.S. and Australia. *Journal of Research in Adolescence, 2,* 147–173.

Feldman, W., Feldman, E., & Goodman, J. T. (1988). Culture versus biology. Children's attitudes towards thinness and fatness. *Pediatrics, 81*, 190–194.

Finlay-Jones, R., & Eckhardt, B. (1984). A social and psychiatric survey of unemployment among young people. *Australian and New Zealand Journal of Psychiatry, 18,* 135–143.

Fiore, M. C. (Ed.). (1992). *Cigarette smoking. A clinical guide to assessment and treatment.* Philadelphia: Saunders.

Fisher, M., Golden, N. H., Katzman, D. K., Kreipe, R. E., Rees, J., Schebendach, J., Sigman, G., Ammerman, S., & Hoberman, H. M. (1995). Eating disorders in adolescents: A background paper. *Journal of Adolescent Health, 16,* 420–437.

Fleming, G., O'Connor, K., & Sanders, J. M. (1994). Pediatricians' view of access to health services. *Journal of Adolescent Health, 15,* 473–478.

Fleming, J. E., & Offord, D. R. (1990). Epidemiology of childhood depressive disorders: A critical overview. *Journal of the American Academy of Child and Adolescent Psychiatry, 29,* 571–580.

Florenzano, R. U. (1991). Chronic mental illness in adolescence: A global overview. *Pediatrician, 18,* 142–149.

Folkman, S., & Lazarus, R. S. (1985). If it changes it must be a process: Study of emotion and coping during three stages of a college examination. *Journal of Personality and Social Psychology, 48,* 150–170.

Framo, J. L. (1970). Symptoms from a family transactional viewpoint. *International Psychiatry Clinics, 7,* 125–171.

Freedman, R. J. (1984). Reflections on beauty as it relates to health in adolescent females. *Woman and Health, 9,* 29–45.

Freedman, R. J. (1989). *Die Opfer der Venus* [The victims of Venus]. Zürich, Switzerland: Kreuz.

French, S. A., Story, M., Downes, B., Resnick, M. D., & Blum, R. W. (1995). Frequent dieting among adolescents: Psychosocial and health behavior correlates. *American Journal of Public Health, 85,* 695–701.

Freud, A. (1936). *Das Ich und die Abwehrmechanismen* [Ego and defense mechanisms]. London: Imago.

Freud, A. (1958). Adolescence. *Psychoanalytic Study of the Child, 13*, 255–278.

Freud, A. (1960). Probleme der Pubertaet [Problems of puberty]. *Psyche, 14*, 1–23.

Freud, A., & Bergmann, T. (1965). *Children in the hospital.* New York: International Universities Press.

Freud, A., & Burlingham, D. (1943). *War and children.* New York: Ernest Willard.

Freud, S. (1952a). Drei Abhandlungen zur Sexualtheorie [Three essays on the theory of sexuality]. In A. Freud, E. Bibring, W. Hoffer, E. Kris, & O. Isakower (Eds.), *Sigmund Freud, Gesammelte Werke* (Vol. 15, pp. 27–145). London: Imago. (Original work published 1905)

Freud, S. (1952). Zur Einfuehrung des Narzißmus [An introduction to narcississm]. In A. Freud, E. Bibring, W. Hoffer, E. Kris, & O. Isakower (Eds.), *Sigmund Freud, Gesammelte Werke* (Vol. 10, pp. 137–170). London: Imago. (Original work published 1914)

Freud, S. (1952). Die Weiblichkeit [Femininity]. In A. Freud, E. Bibring, W. Hoffer, E. Kris, & O. Isakower (Eds.), *Sigmund Freud, Gesammelte Werke* (Vol. 15, pp. 119–145). London: Imago. (Original work published 1933)

Freund, E. E. S., & McGuire, M. B. (1991). *Health, illness and the social body.* Englewood Cliffs, NJ: Prentice-Hall.

Frost, L. A., Moffitt, T. E., & McGee, R. (1989). Neuropsychological correlates of psychopathology in an unselected cohort of young adolescents. *Journal of Abnormal Psychology, 98,* 307–313.

Frydenberg, E., & Lewis, R. (1993). Boys play sport and girls turn to others: Age, gender and ethnicity as determinants of coping. *Journal of Adolescence, 16,* 253–266.

Frymier, J., & Gansneder, B. (1989). The Phi Delta Kappa study of adolescents at risk. *Phi Delta Kappa, 10,* 142–146.

Furman, W., & Buhrmester, D. (1985). Children's perceptions of the personal relationships in their social networks. *Developmental Psychology, 21,* 1016–1024.

Furman, W., & Epstein, L. D. (1990). *Adolescent females' relationships with friends and mothers, stressful life events, and adjustment.* Unpublished manuscript, University of Denver, CO.

Gaddis, A., & Brooks-Gunn, J. (1985). The male experience of pubertal change. *Journal of Youth and Adolescence, 14,* 61–69.

Gagnon, J., Lindenbaum, S., Martin, J., May, R. M., Menkey, J., Turner, C. F., & Zabin, L. S. (1989). Sexual behavior and AIDS. In C. F. Turner, H. G. Miller, & I. E. Moses (Eds.), *AIDS. Sexual behavior and intravenous drug use* (pp. 23–48). Washington, DC: National Academy Press.

Galambos, N. L., & Tilton-Weaver, L. (1996, March). *The adultoid adolescent. Too much, too soon.* Paper presented at the meeting of the Society for Research in Adolescence, Boston.

Garbarino, J. (1990). Youth in dangerous environments: Coping with the consequences. In K. Hurrelmann & F. Lösel, F. (Eds.), *Health hazards in adolescence* (pp. 193–218). Berlin: de Gruyter.

Garber, J. (1984). Classification of childhood psychopathology: A developmental perspective. *Child Development, 55,* 30–48.

Garfinkel, P. E. (1990). Anorexia nervosa and bulimia nervosa: What knowledge of diagnosis and pathogenesis has taught about treatment. In R. J. McMahon & R. D. Peters (Eds.), *Behavior disorders of adolescence: Research, intervention, and policy in clinical and school settings* (pp. 99–110). New York: Plenum.

Garmezy, N. (1983). Stressors of childhood. In N. Garmezy & M. Rutter (Eds.), *Stress, coping and development in children* (pp. 43–84). New York: McGraw-Hill.

Garmezy, N., & Masten, A. S. (1994). Chronic adversities. In M. Rutter, L. Herzov, & E. Taylor (Eds.), *Child and adolescent psychiatry* (pp. 191–208). Oxford, England: Blackwell.

Garmezy, N., Masten, A. S., & Tellegen, A. (1984). The study of stress and competence in children: A building block for developmental psychology. *Child Development, 55,* 97–111.

Garmezy, N., & Rutter, M. (Eds.). (1983). *Stress, coping and development in children.* New York: McGraw-Hill.

Garrison, C. Z., McKeown, R. E., Valois, R. F., & Vincent, M. L. (1993). Aggression, substance use, and suicidal behaviors in high school students. *American Journal of Public Health, 83,* 179–184.

Garrison, W. T., & McQuiston, S. (1989). Chronic illness during childhood and adolescence. *Developmental Clinical Psychology and Psychiatry, 19.*

Ge, X., Conger, R. D., Lorenz, F. O., Elder, G. H., Montague, R. B., & Simons, R. L. (1992). Linking economic hardship to adolescent distress. *Journal of Research in Adolescence, 2,* 351–377.

Gersten, J. C., Langner, T. S., Eisenberg, J. G., & Simcha-Fagan, O. (1977). An evaluation of the etiologic role of stressful life-change events in psychological disorders. *Journal of Health and Social Behavior, 18,* 228–244.

Giambra, L. (1974). Daydreaming across the life-span. Late adolescence to senior citizen. *International Journal of Aging and Human Development, 5,* 115–140.

Gilbert, B. O. (1992). Insulin-dependent diabetes control, personality and life stress in adolescents. *Personality and Individual Differences, 13,* 269–273.

Gilligan, C. (1982). *In a different voice: Psychological theory and woman's development.* Cambridge, MA: Harvard University Press.

Ginsburg, K. R., Slap, G. B., Cnaan, A., Forke, C. M., Balsley, C.-M., & Ronselle, D. M. (1995). Adolescents' perceptions of factors affecting their decisions to seek health care. *Journal of the American Medical Association, 273,* 1913–1918.

Glaser, K. (1967). Masked depression in children and adolescents. *American Journal of Psychotherapy, 21,* 565–574.

Glasner, P. D., & Kaslow, R. A. (1990). The epidemiology of human immunodeficiency virus infection. *Journal of Consulting and Clinical Psychology, 58,* 13–21.

Goldman, R. J., & Goldman, J. D. G. (1988). *Show me yours: Understanding children's sexuality.* Ringwood, Great Britain: Penguin.

Goleman, D. (1986, September 2nd). Terror's children. Mending mental wounds. *The New York Times,* p. 6.

Golombek, H. (1969). The therapeutic contract with adolescents. *Canadian Psychiatric Association Journal, 14,* 497–502.

Gomes-Schwartz, B. (1978). Effective ingredients in psychotherapy: Prediction of outcome from process variables. *Journal of Consulting and Clinical Psychology, 46,* 1023–1035.

Gorny, S. W. (1994). Inhalant abuse as an adolescent drug problem: An overview. *Child Youth Care Forum, 23,* 161–175.

Gortmaker, S. L., Perrin, J. M., Weitzman, M., Halmer, C. J., & Sobol, A. M. (1993). An unexpected success story: Transition to adulthood in youth and chronic physical health conditions. *Journal of Research in Adolescence, 3,* 317–336.

Gortmaker, S. L., Walker, D. B., Weitzman, M., & Sobol, A. M. (1990). Chronic conditions, socio-economic risks, and behavioral problems in children and adolescents. *Pediatrics, 85,* 267–276.

Gottlieb, B. H., & Sylvestre, J. C. (1994). Social support in the relationships between older adolescents and adults. In F. Nestmann & K. Hurrelmann (Eds.), *Social networks and social support in childhood and adolescence* (pp. 52–73). New York: de Gruyter.

Graham, P., & Rutter, M. (1985). Adolescent disorders. In M. Rutter & L. Hersov (Eds.), *Child and adolescent psychiatry* (pp. 351–367). Oxford, England: Blackwell.

Green, W. A. (1954). Psychological factors and reticuloendothelial disease. *Journal of Health Services, 3,* 247–261.

Greenberger, E., & Steinberg, L. D. (1981). The workplace as a context for the socialization of youth. *Journal of Youth and Adolescence, 10,* 185–210.

Greene, J. W., Walker, L. S., Hickson, G., & Thompson, J. (1985). Stressful life events and somatic complaints in adolescents. *Pediatrics, 75,* 19–22.

Greydanus, D. E., & Hofmann, A. E. (1979). Psychological factors in diabetes mellitus. A review of the literature with emphasis on adolescence. *American Journal of Diseases of Children, 133,* 1061–1066.

Gruen, R. J., Folkman, S., & Lazarus, R. S. (1988). Centrality and individual differences in the meaning of daily hassles. *Journal of Personality, 56,* 743–762.

Gull, W. (1873). Proceedings of the clinical society of London. *British Medical Journal, 1,* 527–529.

Haan, N. (1974). The adolescents' ego model of coping and defense and comparisons with Q-sorted ideal personalities. *Genetic Psychology Monographs, 89,* 273–306.

Haan, N. (1977). *Coping and defending. Processes of self-environment organization.* New York: Academic Press.

Habermas, T. (1989). The psychiatric history of anorexia nervosa and bulimia nervosa: Weight concerns and bulimic symptoms in early case reports. *International Journal of Eating Disorders, 8,* 259–273.

Hall, D. J., & Stacey, M. (Eds.). (1979). *Beyond separation: Further studies of children in hospital.* London: Routledge & Kegan Paul.

Halmi, K. (1974). Anorexia nervosa: Demographic and clinical features in 94 cases. *Psychosomatic Medicine, 36,* 18–26.

Halpert, H. P. (1969). Public acceptance of the mentally ill. An exploration of attitudes. *Public Health Reports, 84,* 59–64.

Hamburg, B. A., & Inoff, G. E. (1982). Relationships between behavioral factors and diabetic control in children and adolescents: A camp study. *Psychosomatic Medicine, 44,* 321–339.

Hamburg, B. A., & Inoff, G. E. (1985). Coping behaviors in diabetes: Relationships between knowledge of diabetes, locus of control and metabolic control. In P. I. Ahmed & N. Ahmed (Eds.), *Coping with juvenile diabetes* (pp. 61–84). Springfield, IL: Thomas.

Hammarström, A. (1990). Youth unemployment and health. Results from a five-year follow-up study. In K. Hurrelmann & F. Lösel (Eds.), *Health hazards in adolescence* (pp. 131–148). Berlin: de Gruyter.

Hanl, J. (1995). *Bewältigung chronischer Krankheiten im Jugendalter* [Coping with chronic illness in adolescence]. Unpublished master's thesis, University of Bonn, Germany.

Hansell, S., & Mechanic, D. (1990). Parent and peer effects on adolescent health behavior. In K. Hurrelmann & F. Lösel (Eds.), *Health hazards in adolescence* (pp. 43–66). Berlin: de Gruyter.

Hanson, C. L., Cigrang, J. A., Harris, M. A., & Carle, D. L. (1989). Coping styles in youths with insulin-dependent diabetes mellitus. *Journal of Consulting and Clinical Psychology, 57,* 644–651.

Hanson, C. L., De Guire, M. J., Schinkel, A. M., Henggeler, S. W., & Burghen, G. A. (1992). Comparing social learning and family systems correlates of adaptation in youths with IDDM. *Journal of Pediatric Psychology, 17,* 33–47.

Hanson, C. L., & Henggeler, S. W., (1984). Metabolic control in adolescents with diabetes: An examination of systemic variables. *Family Systems Medicine, 2,* 5–16.

Hanson, C. L., Henggeler, S. W., & Burghen, G. A. (1987). Social competence and parental support as mediators of the link between stress and metabolic control in adolescents with insulin-dependent diabetes mellitus. *Journal of Consulting and Clinical Psychology, 55,* 529–533.

Hauser, S. T. (1992). *Adolescents and their families.* New York: The Free Press.

Hauser, S. T., Borman, E. H., Jacobson, A. M., Powers, S., & Noam, G. (1991). Understanding family contexts of adolescent coping: A study of parental ego development and adolescent coping strategies. *Journal of Early Adolescence, 11,* 96–124.

Hauser, S. T., & Bowlds, M. K. (1990). Stress, coping and adaptation. In S. S. Feldman & G. R. Elliot (Eds.), *At the threshold. The developing adolescent* (pp. 388–413). Cambridge, MA: Harvard University Press.

Hauser, S. T., DiPlacido, J., Jacobson, A. M., Willett, J., & Cole, C. (1993). Family coping with an adolescent's chronic illness: An approach and three studies. *Journal of Adolescence, 16,* 305–329.

Hauser, S. T., Jacobson, A. M., Weiss-Perry, B., Vieyra, M. A., Rufo, P., Spetter, L., Wertlieb, D., Wolfsdorf, J., & Herskowitz, R. D. (1988). *Family coping strategies: A new approach to assessment.* Cambridge, MA: Massachusetts Mental Health Center and Joslin Diabetes Center.

Hauser, S. T., & Solomon, M. L. (1985). Coping with diabetes: Views from the family. In P. I. Ahmed & N. Ahmed (Eds.), *Coping with juvenile diabetes* (pp. 234–266). Springfield, IL: Thomas.

Havighurst, R. J. (1953). *Human development and education.* New York: Longman.

Havighurst, R. J. (1972). *Developmental tasks and education* (3rd ed.). New York: McKay.

Hawton, K., Osborn, M., O'Grady, J., & Cole, D. (1982). Classification of adolescents who take overdoses. *British Journal of Psychiatry, 140,* 124–131.

Health and Welfare Canada (Ed.). (1989). *The health of Canadians: Report of the Canada Health Survey (1989).* (Canada catalogue No. 82–5384) Canada.

Hendren, R. L. (1983). Depression in anorexia nervosa. *Journal of the American Academy of Child Psychiatry, 22,* 59–62.

Hendry, L. B., Shucksmith, J., Love, J. G., & Glendinning, A. (1993). *Young people's leisure and lifestyles.* London: Routledge & Kegan Paul.

Henshaw, S. K. (1994). *US teenage pregnancy statistics.* New York: The Alan Guttmacher Institute.

Herman-Stahl, M. A., Stemmler, M., & Petersen, A. C. (1995). Approach and avoidant coping: Implications for adolescents' mental health. *Journal of Youth and Adolescence, 24,* 649–665.

Herzlich, C. (1973). Health and illness. *European Monographs in Social Psychology, 5.*

Herzlich, C., & Pierret, J. (1987). *Illness and self in society.* Baltimore: John Hopkins University Press.

Hetherington, E. M. (1989). Coping with family transitions: Winners, losers, and survivors. *Child Development, 60,* 1–14.

Hill, J. P., & Holmbeck, G. N. (1986). Attachment and autonomy. *Annals of Child Development, 3,* 145–189.

Hinkle, L., & Wolf, S. (1952). Importance of life stress in the course and management of diabetes mellitus. *Journal of the American Medical Association, 148,* 513–520.

Hoberman, H. M. (1989). Completed suicide in children and adolescents: A review. *Residential Treatment for Children and Youth, 7,* 61–88.

Hodge, M. J., Dougherty, G. E., & Pless, I. B. (1995). Pediatric mortality and hospital use in Canada and the United States, 1971 through 1987. *American Journal of Public Health, 85,* 1276–1279.

Hodges, K., Kline, J. J., Barbero, G., & Flanery, R. (1984). Life events occurring in families of children with recurrent abdominal pain. *Journal of Psychosomatic Research, 28,* 185–188.

Hodgman, C. H. (1990). Modern psychiatric views of adolescent depression and suicidal behavior. *Journal of Psychology and Christianity, 9,* 15–24.

Hodgson, C., Feldman, W., Corber, S., & Quinn, A. (1986). Adolescent health needs II: Utilization of health care by adolescents. *Adolescence, 21,* 383–390.

Hoehe, M. (1988). Influence of the menstrual cycle on neuroendocrine and behavioral responses. *Psychoneuroendocrinology, 13,* 339–344.

Hoffarth, S. L., & Hayes, C. D. (Eds.). (1987). *Risking the future: Adolescent sexuality, pregnancy and childbearing.* Washington, DC: National Academy of Science.

Hoffmeyer, O. (1988). Depression bei Anorexia nervosa [Depression in anorexics]. In H.-J. Friese & G.-E. Trott (Eds.), *Depression in Kindheit und Jugend* [Depression in childhood and adolescence] (pp. 134–147). Bern, Switzerland: Huber.

Hofmann, A. D., & Becker, R. D. (1973). Psychotherapeutic approaches to the physically ill adolescent. *International Journal of Child Psychotherapy, 2,* 492–511.

Hogan, D., & Astone, N. M. (1986). The transition to adulthood. *Annual Review of Sociology, 12,* 109–129.

Holahan, C. J., & Moos, R. H. (1987). The personal and contextual determinants of coping strategies. *Journal of Personality and Social Psychology, 52,* 946–955.

Holinger, P. C., & Offer, D. (1982). Prediction of adolescent suicide: A population model. *American Journal of Psychiatry, 139*, 302–306.

Hollingshead, A. B., & Redlich, F. C. (1958). *Social class and mental illness. A community study.* New York: Wiley.

House, J. S. (1981). *Work stress and social support.* Reading, MA: Addison-Wesley.

Hudson, J. J., Pope, H. G., & Jonas, J. M. (1984). Psychosis in anorexia nervosa and bulimia. *British Journal of Psychiatry, 145,* 420–423.

Hurtig, A. L., Koepke, D., & Park, K. B. (1989). Relation between severity of chronic illness and adjustment in children and adolescents with sickle cell disease. *Journal of Pediatric Psychology, 14,* 117–132.

Igra, V., & Millstein, S. G. (1993). Current status and approaches to improving preventive services for adolescents. *Journal of the American Medical Association, 269,* 1408–1412.

Ingersoll, G. M., Orr, D. P., Vance, M. D., & Golden, M. P. (1992). Cognitive maturing, stressful events, and metabolic control. In E. J. Susman, L. V. Feagans, & W. J. Ray (Eds.), *Emotion, cognition, health and development in children and adolescents* (pp. 121–132). Hillsdale, NJ: Lawrence Erlbaum Associates.

Institut für Jugendforschung. (1990). *Die Entwicklung der Drogenaffinität Jugendlicher in der Bundesrepublik Deutschland* [The development of affinity to drugs in German youth]. Köln, Germany: Bundeszentrale für gesundheitliche Aufklärung.

Jacobson, A. M., Hauser, S. T., Wertlieb, D., Wolfsdorf, J. I., Orleans, J., & Vieyra, M. (1986). Psychological adjustment of children with recently diagnosed diabetes mellitus. *Diabetes Care, 9,* 323–329.

Jamison, R. N., Lewis, S., & Burish, T. G. (1986). Psychological impact of cancer on adolescents: Self-image, locus of control, perception of illness and knowledge of cancer. *Journal of Chronic Disease, 39,* 609–617.

Jansen, E. (1992). *Ostdeutsche Jugendliche vor und nach der Wende: Problembelastung, Coping, Familienklima und andere ausgewählte entwicklungspsychologische Fragestellungen* [East German adolescents before and after the reunion: problems, coping, family climate, and other selected topics]. Unpublished master's thesis, University of Bonn, Germany.

Jemmott, J. B., & Locke, S. E. (1984). Psychosocial factors, immunologic mediation, and human susceptibility to infectious diseases. How much do we know? *Psychological Bulletin, 95,* 78–108.

Jemmott, L., & Jemmott Ill, J. B. (1990). Sexual knowledge, attitudes, and risky sexual behavior among inner-city Black male adolescents. *Journal of Adolescent Research, 5,* 346–369.

Jerusalem, M. (1992). Akkulturationsstreß und psychosoziale Befindlichkeit jugendlicher Ausländer [Stress of acculturation and psychosocial well-being of adolescent foreigners]. *Report Psychologie, 2,* 16–23.

Jessor, R. (1986). Adolescent problem drinking: Psychosocial aspects and developmental outcomes. In R. K. Silbereisen, K. Eyferth, & G. Rudinger (Eds.), *Development as action in context. Problem behavior and normal youth development* (pp. 241–264). Berlin: Springer-Verlag.

Jessor, S. L., & Jessor, R. (1975). Transition from virginity to nonvirginity among youth: A social–psychological study over time. *Developmental Psychology, 11,* 473–484.

Jessor, R., & Jessor S. L. (1977). *Problem behavior and psychosocial development.* New York: Academic Press.

Johannsen, W. J. (1969). Attitudes towards mental patients. A review of empirical research. *Mental Hygiene Bulletin, 53,* 218–228.

Johnson, J. H. (1986). *Life events as stressors in childhood and adolescence.* Beverly Hills, CA: Sage.

Johnson, J. H., & McCutcheon, S. M. (1980). Assessing life stress in older children and adolescents. Preliminary findings with the Life Events Checklist. In O. Sarason & C. D. Spielberger (Eds.), *Stress and anxiety* (pp. 230–241). Washington, D.C.: Hemisphere.

Johnson, S. B. (1980). Psychosocial factors in juvenile diabetes: A review. *Journal of Behavioral Medicine, 3,* 95–116.

Johnson, S. B. (1984). Knowledge, attitudes and behaviors: Correlates of health in childhood diabetes. *Clinical Psychology Review, 4,* 503–524.

Johnson, T. P. (1991). Mental health, social relations, and social selection: A longitudinal analysis. *Journal of Health and Social Behavior, 32,* 408–423.

Johnston, L. D., O'Malley, P. M., & Bachman, J. G. (1987). *National trends in drug use and related factors among American high school students and young adults. 1975–1986.* Washington, DC: U.S. Government Printing Office.

Johnston, L. D., O'Malley, P. M., & Bachman, J. G. (1994). *National survey results on drug use from the Monitoring the Future study, 1975–1993.* Rockville, MD.: National Institute on Drug Abuse.

Johnston, L. D., O'Malley, P. M, & Bachman, J. G. (1995). *National survey results on drug use from the Monitoring the Future study, 1975–1994.* Rockville, MD.: National Institute on Drug Abuse.

Jouriles, E. N., Barling, J., & O'Leary, K. D. (1987). Predicting child behavior problems in maritally violent families. *Journal of Abnormal Child Psychology, 15,* 165–173.

Joy, A. E. (1987). Developmental aspects of children's strategies for coping with painful medical procedures. *Dissertation Abstracts International, 41 (01),* 284B.

Kager, V. A., & Holden, E. W. (1992). Preliminary investigation of the direct and moderating effects of family and individual variables on the adjustment of children and adolescents with diabetes. *Journal of Pediatric Psychology, 17,* 491–502.

Kalmuss, D. (1986). Contraceptive use of ever- and never-pregnant adolescents. *Journal of Adolescent Health Care, 7,* 332–337.

Kandel, D. B. (1986). Processes of peer influences in adolescence. In R. K. Silbereisen, K. Eyferth, & G. Rudinger (Eds.), *Development as action in context* (pp. 203–228). Berlin, Germany: Springer-Verlag.

Kandel, D. B., & Davies, M. (1982). Epidemiology of depressive mood in adolescents. *Archives of General Psychiatry, 39, 1205–1212.*

Kandel, D. B., & Faust, R. (1975). Sequence and stages in patterns of adolescent drug use. *Archives of Genetic Psychiatry, 32,* 923–932.

Kandel, D. B., & Yamaguchi, K. (1993). From beer to crack: Developmental patterns of drug involvement. *American Journal of Public Health, 83,* 851–855.

Kanfer, F. H., & Saslow, G. (1969). Behavioral diagnosis. In C. M. Franks (Ed.), *Behavior therapy: Appraisal and status* (pp. 417–443). New York: McGraw-Hill.

Karoly, P. (1982). Developmental pediatrics: A process-oriented approach to the analysis of health competence. In P. Karoly, J. J. Steffen, & D. J. O'Grady (Eds.), *Child health psychology* (pp. 29–56). New York: Pergamon.

Karoly, P. (1985). *Measurement strategies in health psychology.* New York: Wiley.

Karoly, P. (1988). *Handbook of child health assessment.* New York: Wiley.

Karon, J. M., Rosenberg, P. S., McQuillan, G., Khare, M., Gwinn, M., & Petersen, L. R. (1996). Prevalence of HIV infection in the United States, 1984 to 1992. *Journal of the American Medical Association, 276,* 126–131.

Kashani, J., Carlson, G., & Beck, N. (1987). Depression, depressive symptoms and depressed mood among a community sample of adolescents. *American Journal of Psychiatry, 144,* 931–934.

Katchadourian, H. (1990). Sexuality. In S. S. Feldman & R. Elliot (Eds.), *At the threshold: The developing adolescent* (pp. 120–142). Cambridge, MA: Harvard University Press.

Katz, S. J., Hofer, T. P., & Manning, W. G. (1996). Physician use in Ontario and the United States: The impact of socioeconomic status and health status. *American Journal of Public Health, 86,* 520–524.

Kavšek, M., & Seiffge-Krenke, I. (1996). The differentiation of coping traits in adolescence. *International Journal of Behavioral Development, 19,* 651–668.

Kazak, A. E., & Marvin, R. (1984). Differences, difficulties and adaptation: Stress and social networks in families with a handicapped child. *Family Relations, 3,* 67–77.

Kazak, A. E., & Meadows, A. T. (1989). Families of young adolescents who had survived cancer: Social–emotional adjustment, adaptability, and social support. *Journal of Pediatric Psychology, 14,* 175–192.

Keniston, K. (1975). Youth as a stage of life. In R. J. Havighurst & P. D. Dreyer (Eds.), *Youth* (pp. 3–26). Chicago: University of Chicago Press.

Khan, A. U. (1987). Heterogeneity of suicidal adolescents. *Journal of the American Academy of Child and Adolescent Psychiatry, 26,* 92–96.

Kielholz, P., & Adams, C. (1988). Die larvierte Depression bei Kindern, Jugendlichen und Erwachsenen [Larvate depression in children, adolescents, and adults]. In H.-J. Friese & G.-E. Trott (Eds.), *Depression in Kindheit und Jugend* [Depression in childhood and adolescence] (pp. 148–155). Bern, Switzerland: Huber.

Kieselbach, T., & Svensson, P. G. (1988). Health and social policy response to unemployment in Europe. *Journal of Social Issues, 44,* 173–191.

Klingman, A., Goldstein, Z., & Lerner, P. (1991). Adolescents' responses to nuclear threat: Before and after the Chernobyl accident. *Journal of Youth and Adolescence, 20,* 519–530.

Klink, F., & Kieselbach, T. (1990). *Jugendarbeitslosigkeit als gesundheitlicher Risikofaktor.* Bremer Beiträge zur Psychologie. Reihe C: Forschungsberichte der wissenschaftlichen Einheit "Arbeit, Arbeitslosigkeit und Persönlichkeitsentwicklung" [Adolescent unemployment. Bremen contributions to psychology. Series C: Research reports on "Work, unemployment, and personality development"] (Vol. 91). University of Bremen.

Knafl, K. A., & Deatrick, J. A. (1987). Conceptualizing family responses to a child's chronic illness or disability. *Family Relations, 36,* 300–304.

Kobasa, S. C. (1982). Commitment and coping in stress resistance among lawyers. *Journal of Personality and Social Psychology, 42,* 707–717.

Koch, S. J. (1977). The interest and concerns of adolescents, grade seven through twelve, as expressed in their written composition. *Dissertation Abstracts International, 37,* 7729–7730.

Koff, E., Rierdan, J., & Stubbs, M. L. (1990). Gender, body image, and self-concept in early adolescence. *Journal of Early Adolescence, 10,* 56–68.

Kohn, P. M., LaGreniere, K., & Gurevich, M. (1991). Hassles, health and personality. *Journal of Personality and Social Psychology, 61,* 478–482.

Kohut, H. (1977). *Die Heilung des Selbst* [Recovery of the self]. Frankfurt, Germany: Suhrkamp.

Koski, M. (1969). The coping processes in childhood diabetes. *Acta Pediatrica Scandinavica, 189,* 1–82.

Koski, M., & Kumento, A. (1975). Adolescent development and behavior: A psychosomatic follow-up study of childhood diabetes. In Z. Laron (Ed.), *Diabetes in juveniles.* Basel, Switzerland: Karger.

Kovacs, M. (1989). Affective disorders in children and adolescents. *American Psychologist, 44,* 209–215.

Kovacs, M. (1990). Comorbid anxiety disorders in childhood—onset depressions? In J. D. Maser & C. R. Cloninger (Eds.), *Comorbidity of mood and anxiety disorders* (pp. 272–281). Washington, DC: American Psychiatry Press.

Kovacs, M., & Feinberg, T. (1982). Coping with juvenile onset diabetes mellitus. In A. Baum & J. Singer (Eds.), *Handbook of psychology and health* (Vol. 2, pp. 165–212). Hillsdale: Lawrence Erlbaum Associates.

Kovacs, M., Feinberg, T., Panlanskas, S., Finkelstein, R., Pollock, M., & Crouse-Novak, M. (1985). Initial coping responses and psychosocial characteristics of children with insulin-dependent diabetes mellitus. *Journal of Pediatrics, 106,* 827–834.

Krantz, D. S., Grunberg, N. E., & Baum, A. (1985). Health psychology. *Annual Review of Psychology, 36,* 349–383.

Kruesi, M. J. P., Hibbs, E. D., Zahn, T. P., Keysor, C. S., Hamburger, S. D., & Rapoport, J. L. (1992). A two year prospective follow-up study of children and adolescents with disruptive behavior disorders: Prediction from CSF 5-HIAA, HVA and autonomic measures. *Archives of General Psychiatry, 47,* 821–833.

Kutcher, S. P. (1986). Affective disorders (depression and mania) in adolescents. *Canadian Family Physician, 32,* 2475–2479.

Kutcher, S. P., & Marton, P. (1989). Parameters of adolescent depression. A review. *Psychiatric Clinics of North America, 12,* 895–918.

LaGreca, A. M. (1988). Children with diabetes and their families: Coping and disease management. In T. Field, P. M. McCabe, & N. Schneiderman (Eds.), *Stress and coping across development* (pp.139–159). Hillsdale, NJ: Lawrence Erlbaum Associates.

LaGreca, A. M. (1992). Peer influences in pediatric chronic illness: An update. *Journal of Pediatric Psychology, 17,* 775–784.

Larson, R., & Richards, M. H. (1991). Daily companionship in late childhood and early adolescence: Changing developmental contexts. *Child Development, 62,* 284–300.

Lasègue, E. (1873). On hysteria anorexia. *Medical Times Gazette, 2,* 265–269.

Lask, B., & Fosson, A. (1989). *Childhood illness: The psychosomatic approach.* New York: Wiley.

Laufer, M. & Laufer, M. E. (1984). *Adolescence and developmental breakdown.* New Haven, CT: Yale University Press.

Laufer, R. W., & Wolfe, M. (1974). The concept of privacy in childhood and adolescence. In D. H. Larson (Ed.), *Man–environment interactions (Proceedings of EDRA) (pp. 29–54). Washington, DC: Environmental Design Research Association.*

Lavigne, J. V. (1977). The pediatric hospital staff's knowledge of normal adolescent development. *Journal of Pediatric Psychology, 2,* 98–100.

Lazarus, R. S. (1985). The trivialization of distress. In P. Ahmed & N. Ahmed (Eds.), *Coping with juvenile diabetes* (pp. 33–60). Springfield, IL: Thomas.

Lazarus, R. S., & Folkman, S. (1984). *Stress, appraisal and coping.* New York: Springer-Verlag.

Lazarus, R. S., & Folkman, S. (1991). *Stress, appraisal, and coping* (3rd ed.). New York: Springer-Verlag.

Lazarus, R. S., & Launier, R. (1978). Stress-related transactions between person and environment. In L. Pervin & M. Lewis (Eds.), *Perspectives in interactional psychology* (pp. 287–327). New York: Plenum.

Leavy, R. L. (1983). Social support and psychological disorder: A review. *Journal of Community Psychology, 11,* 3–21.

Lederer, H. D. (1967). How the sick view their world. In E. G. Jaco (Ed.), *Patients, physicians and illness* (pp. 247–256). New York: Basic Books.

Lee, L., Gilpin, E. A., & Pierce, J. P. (1993). Changes in the patterns of initiation of cigarette smoking in the United States: 1950, 1965, and 1980. *Cancer Epidemiology, Biomarkers and Prevention, 2,* 593–597.

LeGaipa, J., & Wood, H. D. (1981). Friendships in disturbed adolescents. In S. Duck & R. Gilmour (Eds.), *Personal relationships in disorder* (pp. 169–189). London: Academic Press.

Lehtinen, V., Ville, C., & Väisänen, E. (1978). Attitudes towards mental illness and utilization of psychiatric treatment. *Social Psychiatry, 13,* 63–68.

Lerner, R. M. (1982). Children and adolescents as producers of their own development. *Developmental Review, 4,* 342–370.

Lerner, R. M., & Karabenick, S. A. (1974). Physical attractiveness, body attitudes, and self-concept in late adolescents. *Journal of Youth and Adolescence, 3,* 307–316.

Levi, L. (1975). *Society, stress and disease.* New York: Oxford University Press.

Levi, L. (1981). Psychosoziale Reize, psychophysiologische Reaktionen und Krankheit [Psychosocial stimuli, psychophysiological reactions, and illness]. In J. Nitsche (Ed.), *Streß* [Stress] (pp. 18–212). Bern, Switzerland: Huber.

Lewinsohn, P. M., Klein, D. N., & Seeley, J. R. (1995). Bipolar disorders in a community sample of older adolescents: Prevalence, phenomenology, comorbidity, and course. *Journal of the American Academy of Child and Adolescent Psychiatry, 34,* 454–463.

Lief, I. H., Fullard, W., & Devlin, S. J. (1990). A new measure of adolescent sexuality: Skat-A. *Journal of Sex Education and Therapy, 16,* 79–91.

Lieu, T. A., Newacheck, P. W., & McManus, M. A. (1993). Race, ethnicity, and access to ambulatory care among US adolescents. *American Journal of Public Health, 83,* 960–965.

Litt, I. F., & Cuskey, W. R. (1984). Satisfaction with health care—a predictor of adolescents' appointment keeping. *Journal of Adolescent Health Care, 5,* 196–200.

Littrell, M. A., Damhorst, M. L., & Littrell, J. M. (1990). Clothing interest, body satisfaction, and eating behavior of adolescent females: Related or independent dimensions? *Adolescence, 25,* 77–94.

Livesley, W. J., & Bromley, D. B. (1973). *Person perception in childhood and adolescence.* New York: Wiley.

Logan, D. D. (1980). The menarche experience in twenty-three foreign countries. *Adolescence, 15,* 247–256.

Lopez, H., & Fuchs, R. (1990). Rauchen [Smoking]. In R. Schwarzer (Ed.), *Gesundheitspsychologie* [Health psychology] (pp. 185–197). Göttingen, Germany: Hogrefe.

Lösel, F., Bliesener, T., & Köferl, P. (1989). On the concept of "vulnerability": Evaluation and first results of the Bielefeld Project. In M. Bambring, F. Lösel, & H. Skowronek (Eds.), *Children at risk: Assessment, longitudinal research, and intervention* (pp. 186–221). New York: de Gruyter.

Lowry, R., Kann, L., Collins, J. L., & Kolbe, J. L. (1996). The effect of socioeconomic status on chronic disease risk behaviors among US adolescents. *Journal of American Medical Association, 276,* 792–797.

Lynd, R. S., & Lynd, H. M. (1929). *Middletown.* New York: Harcourt Brace.

Magnusson, D., Stattin, H., & Allen, V. L. (1986). Differential maturation among girls and its relevance to social adjustment: A longitudinal perspective. In D. L. Featherman & R. M. Lerner (Eds.), *Life-span development and behavior* (Vol. 7, pp. 135–172). New York: Academic Press.

Malhotra, H. K., Inam Shastri, A. S., & Chopra, H. D. (1978). Does prejudice against mentally ill increase drop out from treatment? *Indian Journal of Clinical Psychology, 5,* 17–23.

Marcelli, D., & Alvin, P. (1994). Submission or cheating in chronic illness in adolescence. The therapist's stand. *International Journal of Adolescent Medicine and Health, 7,* 65–71.

Marcia, J. E. (1980). Identity in adolescence. In J. Adelson (Ed.), *Handbook of adolescent psychology* (pp. 159–187). New York: Wiley.

Marks, A., Fisher, M., & Lasker, S. (1991). Adolescents' relationships with their pediatricians. *Journal of Adolescent Health, 12,* 5–7.

Marrero, D. G., Myers, G. L., Golden, M. P., West, D., Kershnar, A., & Lau, N. (1982). Adjustment to misfortune in the use of a social support group for adolescent diabetics. In Z. Laron & A. Galatzer (Eds.), *Psychological aspects of diabetes in children and adolescents* (pp. 141–146). Basel, Switzerland: Karger.

Marteau, T. M., Bloch, S., & Baum, J. D. (1987). Family life and diabetic control. *Journal of Child Psychology and Psychiatry, 28,* 823–833.

Martin, P., & Diehl, M. (1983). Die Einweisung in ein "Mental Health Institute" als kritisches Lebensereignis—Aspekte der kognitiven Repräsentanz [Referral to psychiatric care as critical life event: Aspects of cognitive representation]. *Praxis der Kinderpsychologie und Kinderpsychiatrie, 32,* 26–33.

Marttunen, M. J., Aro, H. M., Henriksson, M. M., & Lonnqvist, J. K. (1991). Mental disorders in adolescent suicide: DSM-III-R axes I and II diagnoses in suicides among 13- to 19-year-olds in Finland. *Archives of General Psychiatry, 48,* 834–839.

Maser, J. D., & Cloninger, C. R. (Eds.) (1990). *Comorbidity of mood and anxiety disorders.* Washington, DC: American Psychiatric Press.

Masten, A. S., Neemann, J., & Andenas, S. (1994). Life events and adjustment in adolescence: The significance of event independence, desirability, and chronicity. *Journal of Research on Adolesence, 4,* 71–97.

Matarazzo, J. D. (1980). Behavioral health and behavior medicine. Frontiers of a new health psychology. *American Psychologist, 35,* 807–817.

McCabe, M. P., & Collins, J. K. (1990). Sex role and dating orientation. *Journal of Youth and Adolescence, 8,* 407–425.

McClure, R., Mitchell, C., & Greschuck, D. (1982). Self-concept and identification of students needing a counseling center. *Psychological Reports, 50,* 487–490.

McConaughy, S. H., & Skiba, R. J. (1993). Comorbidity of externalizing and internalizing problems. *School Psychology Review, 22,* 421–436.

McCrae, R. R. (1982). Age differences in the use of coping mechanisms. *Journal of Gerontology, 37,* 454–460.

McCubbin, H. J., McCubbin, M. A., Patterson, J. M., Cauble, A. E., Wilson, L. R. & Warwick, W. (1983). CHIP—Coping Health Inventory for Parents: An assessment of parental coping patterns in the care of the chronically ill child. *Journal of Marriage and the Family, 45,* 359–370.

McCubbin, H. J., & Patterson, J. M. (1982). Family adaptation to crisis. In H. J. McCubbin, A. E. Cauble, & J. M. Patterson (Eds.), *Family stress, coping and social support* (pp. 26–48). Springfield, IL: Thomas.

McCubbin, M. A., & McCubbin, H. J. (1988). Family systems assessment. In P. Karoly (Ed.), *Handbook of child health assessment* (pp. 227–261). New York: Wiley.

McKay, M. M. (1977). Adolescent problems: An examination of the rank comparison of the latent categories of problems as defined and ordered by high school students. *Dissertation Abstracts International, 38,* 3193A.

McMahon, R. J., & Peters, R. D. (Eds.). (1990). *Behavior disorders of adolescence: Research, intervention, and policy in clinical and school settings.* New York: Plenum.

McPherson, A., & Wayne, H. (1983). Psychiatric impairment, physical health and work values among unemployed and apprenticed young men. *Australian and New Zealand Journal of Psychiatry, 17,* 335–340.

Mechanic, D. (1962). Some factors in identifying and defining mental illness. *Mental Hygiene, 46,* 66–74.

Melamed, B. G., & Siegel, L. (1980). *Behavioral medicine. Practical applications in health care.* New York: Springer-Verlag.

Millen, L., & Roll, S. (1977). Adolescent males' ratings of being understood by fathers, best friends and significant others. *Psychological Reports, 40,* 1079–1082.

Miller, B. C., McCoy, J. K., & Olson, T. D. (1986). Dating age and stage as correlates of adolescent sexual attitudes and behavior. *Journal of Adolescent Research, 1,* 361–371.

Millstein, S. G., Adler, N. E., & Irwin, L. E. (1981). Conceptions of illness in young adolescents. *Pediatrics, 68,* 834–839.

Millstein, S. G., & Irwin, L. E. (1987). Concepts of health and illness: Different constructs or variations on a theme? *Health Psychology, 6,* 515–524.

Millstein, S. G., & Litt, J. F. (1990). Adolescent health. In S. S. Feldman, & G. R. Elliott (Eds.), *At the threshold. The developing adolescent* (pp. 431–456). Cambridge, MA: Harvard University Press.

Minuchin, S., Rosman, B., & Baker, L. (1978). *Psychosomatic families: Anorexia nervosa in context.* Cambridge, MA: Harvard University Press.

Mitchell, J., McCanley, E., Buke, P. M., & Moss, S. J. (1990). Phenomenology of depression in children and adolescents. *Journal of the American Academy of Child and Adolescent Psychiatry, 27,* 12–20.

Moehr, J. R., & Hahn, K. D. (Ed.). (1977). *Verden-Studie: Strukturanalyse allgemeinärztlicher Praxen* [The Verden study: Structural analysis of general practitioners' offices]. Köln, Germany: Deutscher Ärzteverlag.

Mönks, F. J. (1968). Future time perspective in adolescence. *Human Development, 11,* 107–123.

Montemayor, R. (1986). Family variation in parent-adolescent storm and stress. *Journal of Adolescent Research, 1,* 15–31.

Moore, K., Peterson, J., & Furstenberg, F. J. (1986). Parental attitudes and the occurrence of early sexuality. *Journal of Marriage and the Family, 48,* 777–782.

Moore, S., & Rosenthal, D. (1993). *Sexuality in adolescence.* London: Routledge & Kegan Paul.

Moos, R. H., & Moos, B. S. (1981). *Family Environment Scale Manual.* Palo Alto, CA: Consulting Psychologists Press.

Moreau, D. L. (1990). Major depression in childhood and adolescence. *Psychiatric Clinics of North America, 13,* 355–368.

Morgan, H. G., & Russell, F. M. (1975). Value of family background and clinical features as predictors of long-term outcome in anorexia nervosa. Four-year study of 41 patients. *Psychological Medicine, 5,* 355–371.

Morrison, D. M. (1985). Adolescent contraceptive behavior. A review. *Psychological Bulletin, 98,* 538–568.

Mott, F. L., & Haurin, R. J. (1988). Linkages between sexual activity and alcohol and drug use among American adolescents. *Family Planning Perspectives, 20,* 128–136.

Mrazek, J. (1987a). Das Gesundheitskonzept von Jugendlichen [Adolescents' health concept]. *Brennpunkte der Sportwissenschaften, 1,* 83–103.

Mrazek, J. (1987b). Struktur und Entwicklung des Körperkonzepts im Jugendalter [Structure and development of the body concept in adolescence]. *Zeitschrift für Entwicklungspsychologie und Pädagogische Psychologie, 19,* 1–13.

Muehlenhard, C., & Cook, N. S. (1988). Men's self report of unwanted sexual activity. *Journal of Sexual Research, 24,* 58–72.

Murch, R. L., & Cohen, L. H. (1989). Relationships among life stress, perceived family environment, and the psychological distress of spina bifida adolescents. *Journal of Pediatric Psychology, 14*(2), 193–214.

Murphy, L. B., & Moriarty, A. E. (1986). *Vulnerability, coping and growth from infancy to adolescence.* New Haven, CT: Yale University Press.

Musa, K., & Roach, M. (1973). Adolescent appearance and self-concept. *Adolescence, 8,* 385–394.

Nadler, R. (1978). Are we helping? *Adolescence, 13,* 453–459.

Nannis, E., & Cowan, P. (Eds.). (1988). *Developmental psychopathology and its treatment.* San Francisco: Jossey Bass.

Natapoff, J. (1978). Children's views of health. *American Journal of Public Health, 68,* 995–1000.

Nathanson, C. A., & Becker, M. H. (1986). Family and peer influence on obtaining a method of contraception. *Journal of Marriage and the Family, 48,* 513–525.

National Adolescent Student Health Survey. (1989). *A report on the health of America's youth.* Oakland, CA: Third Party.

National Center for Health Statistics. (1988). *Vital statistics, mortality data, multiple cause of death detail.* Hyattsville, MD: U.S. Department of Health and Human Services, Public Health Service.

National Center for Health Statistics. (1993a). Advance report of final mortality statistics, 1991. *Monthly Vitality Statistics Reports, 42* (2).

National Center for Health Statistics. (1993b). Advance report of final natality statistics, 1991. *Monthly Vitality Statistics Report, 42* (3).

National Center for Health Statistics. (1995). Advance report of final mortality statistics, 1992. *Monthly Vitality Statistics Reports, 43* (6).

National Safety Council (1993). *Accident facts.* Itasca, IL.

National Survey on Drugs and Drinking. (1987). *Statistical Bulletin of Metropolitan Insurance Companies.* Oakland, CA: Third Party.

Navarro, V. (1976). *Medicine under capitalism.* New York: Prodigt.

Nelson, D. E., Giovino, G. A., Shopland, D. R., Mowery, P. D., Mills, S. L., & Eriksen, M. P. (1995). Trends in cigarette smoking among U.S. adolescents, 1974 through 1991. *American Journal of Public Health, 85,* 34–40.

Neubauer, G. (1990). *Jugend und Sexualität* [Youth and sexuality]. Stuttgart, Germany: Enke.

Neugarten, B. L. (1979). Time, age and the life cycle. *American Journal of Psychiatry, 136,* 887–894.

Newacheck, P. W. (1994). Poverty and childhood chronic illness. *Archives of Pediatric and Adolescent Medicine, 148,* 1143–1149.

Newacheck, P. W., & Taylor, W. R. (1992). Childhood chronic illness: Prevalence, severity, and impact. *American Journal of Public Health, 82,* 364–371.

Newcomb, N. D., Huba, G. J., & Bentler, P. M. (1981). A multidimensional assessment of stressful life events among adolescents. *Journal of Health and Social Behavior, 22,* 400–415.

Niemcryk, S. J., Spears, M. A., Travis, L. B., & Gray, H. E. (1990). Psychosocial correlates of Hemoglobin $A_{1C}$ in young adults with type-I-diabetes. *Journal of Psychosomatic Research, 34,* 617–627.

Nolen-Hoeksema, S. (1987). Sex differences in unipolar depression: Evidence and theory. *Psychological Bulletin, 101,* 259–282.

Nolen-Hoeksema, S. (1991). Responses to depression and their effects on the duration of depressive episodes. *Journal of Abnormal Psychology, 100,* 569–582.

Nolen-Hoeksema, S., & Girgus, J. S. (1995). Explanatory style and achievement, depression, and gender differences in childhood and early adolescence. In G. M. Buchanan & M. E. P. Seligman (Eds.), *Explanatory style* (pp. 57–70). Hillsdale, NJ: Lawrence Erlbaum Associates.

Nolen-Hoeksema, S., Girgus, J. S., & Seligman M. P. E. (1991). Sex differences in depression and explanatory style in children. *Journal of Youth and Adolescence, 20,* 233–245.

Noles, S. W., Cash, T. F., & Winstead, B. A. (1985). Body image, physical attractiveness, and depression. *Journal of Consulting and Clinical Psychology, 53,* 88–94.

Norell, J. E. (1984). Self-disclosure: Implications for the study of parent–adolescent interaction. *Journal of Youth and Adolescence, 13,* 163–177.

Northman, J. E. (1978). Developmental changes in preferences for help. *Journal of Clinical Psychology, 7,* 129–132.

Nottelmann, E. D., & Jensen, P. S. (1995). Comorbidity of disorders in children and adolescents. In T. H. Ollendick & R. J. Prin (Eds.), *Advances in clinical child psychology* (Vol. 17, pp. 109–154). New York: Plenum.

Nottelmann, E. D., Susman, E. J., Dorn, L. D., Inoff-Germain, G., Loriaux, D. L., Cutler, G. B., & Chrousos, G. P. (1987). Developmental processes in early adolescence. *Journal of Adolescent Health Care, 8,* 246–260.

Novacek, J., Raskin, R., & Hogan, R. (1991). Why do adolescents use drugs? Age, sex, and user differences. *Journal of Youth and Adolescence, 20,* 475–492.

Novick, J. (1976). Termination of treatments in adolescence. *Psychoanalytic Study of the Child, 31,* 389–413.

Novick, J. (1980). Negative therapeutic motivation and negative therapeutic alliance. *Psychoanalytic Study of the Child, 35,* 299–320.

Oetting, E. R., & Beauvais, F. (1990). Adolescent drug use: Findings of national and local surveys. *Journal of Consulting and Clinical Psychology, 58,* 385–394.

Offer, D. (1984). Das Selbstbild normaler Jugendlicher [The self-concept of normal adolescents]. In E. Olbrich & E. Todt (Eds.), *Probleme des Jugendalters* [Problems of adolescence] (pp. 111–131). Berlin: Springer-Verlag.

Offer, D., Howard, K. J., Schonert, K. A., & Ostrov, E. (1991). To whom do adolescents turn for help? Differences between disturbed and nondisturbed adolescents. *Journal of the American Academy of Child and Adolescent Psychiatry, 30,* 623–630.

Offer, D., & Offer, J. (1969). *The psychological world of the teenager.* New York: Basic Books.

Offord, D. R., Boyle, M. H., & Racine, Y. (1990a). Epidemiology of behavioral and emotional disorders of adolescence: Implications for treatment, research, and policy. In R. J. McMahon & R. D. Peters (Eds.), *Behavior disorders of adolescence: Research, intervention, and policy in clinical and school settings* (pp. 13–26). New York: Plenum.

Offord, D. R., Boyle, M. H., & Racine, Y. (1990b). Ontario Child Health Study: Correlates of disorder. *Annual Progress in Child Psychiatry and Child Development,* 194–204.

Offord, D. R., Boyle, M. H., Szatmari, P., Rae-Grant, N. I., Links, P. S., Cadman, D. T., Byles, J. A., Crawford, J. W., Munroe Blum, H., Byrne, C., Thomas, H., & Woodward, C. A. (1987). Ontario Child Health Study. II. Six-months prevalence of disorder and rates of service utilization. *Archives of General Psychiatry, 44,* 831–836.

Olweus, D. (1978). *Aggression in the schools: Bullying and whipping boys.* Washington, DC: Wiley.

Olweus, D. (1990). Bullying among school children. In K. Hurrelmann & F. Lösel (Eds.), *Health hazards in adolescence* (pp. 259–298). New York: de Gruyter.

Olweus, D., Mattson, A., Schalling, D., & Low, H. (1988). Circulating testosterone levels and aggression in adolescent males: A causal analysis. *Psychosomatic Medicine, 50,* 261–272.

O'Malley, F. (1990). Developing therapeutic alliance in the hospital treatment of disturbed adolescents. *Bulletin of the Menninger Clinic, 54,* 13–24.

O'Malley, J. E., Koocher, D., Foster, L., & Slavin, L. (1979). Psychiatric sequelae of surviving childhood cancer. *American Journal of Orthopsychiatry, 49,* 608–616.

O'Malley, P. M., Johnston, L. D., & Bachman, J. G. (1995). Adolescent substance use: Epidemiology and implications for public policy. *Pediatric Clinics of North America, 42,* 241–260.

Orleans, C. T., & Slade, J. D. (Eds.). (1993). *Nicotine addiction: Principles and management.* New York: Oxford University Press.

Orr, D. P., Weller, S. C., Satterwhite, B., & Pless, I. B. (1984). Psychosocial implications of chronic illness in adolescence. *The Journal of Pediatrics, 104,* 152–157.

Padilla, A. M., & Baird, T. L. (1991). Mexican-American sexuality and sexual knowledge: An explanatory study. *Hispanic Journal of Behavioral Sciences, 13,* 95–104.

Padilla, E. R., Rohsenow, D. J., & Bergman, A. B. (1976). Predicting accident frequency in children. *Pediatrics, 58,* 223–226.

Paikoff, R. L., & Brooks-Gunn, J. (1991). Do parent–child relationships change during puberty? *Psychological Bulletin, 110,* 47–66.

Palentien, C., & Hurrelmann, K. (1995). Adolescents' health problems and utilization of medical and psychosocial care services in East and West Germany. Findings of a study based on interviews of medical, psychological, and educational experts. In M. du Bois-Reymond, R. Diekstra, K. Hurrelmann, & E. Peters (Eds.), *Childhood and youth in Germany and the Netherlands. Transitions and coping strategies of adolescents* (pp. 209–234). New York: de Gruyter.

Papini, D. R., Farmer, F. L., Clark, S. M., & Snell, W. E. (1988). An evaluation of adolescent patterns of sexual self-disclosure to parents and friends. *Journal of Adolescent Research, 3,* 387–401.

Parish, T., & Kappes, B. M. (1979). Affective implications of seeking psychological counseling. *Journal of Counseling Psychology, 26,* 164–165.

Parrott, R., Burgoon, J. K., Burgoon, M., & Lepoire, B. A. (1989). Privacy between physicians and patients. More than a matter of confidentiality. *Social Sciences and Medicine, 29,* 1381–1385.

Patterson, J. M., Budd, J., Goetz, D., & Warwick, W. J. (1993). Family correlates of a ten-year pulmonary health trend in cystic fibrosis. *Pediatrics, 91,* 383–389.

Patterson, J. M., & McCubbin, H. J. (1987). Adolescent coping style and behaviors: Conceptualization and measurement. *Journal of Adolescence, 10,* 163–186.

Patterson, J. M., McCubbin, H. J., & Warwick, W. J. (1990). The impact of family functioning on health changes in children with cystic fibrosis. *Social Science and Medicine, 2,* 159–164.

Patton, W., & Noller, P. (1984). Unemployment and youth: A longitudinal study. *Australian Journal of Psychology, 36,* 399–413.

Paxton, S. J., Wertheim, E. H., Gibbons, K., Szmukler, G. I., Hillier, L., & Petrovich, J. L. (1991). Body image satisfaction, dieting beliefs, and weight loss behaviors in adolescent girls and boys. *Journal of Youth and Adolescence, 20,* 361–379.

Pearce, J. (1978). The recognition of depressive disorder in children. *Journal of the Royal Society of Medicine, 71,* 494–505.

Pearlin, C. J., & Schooler, C. (1978). The structure of coping. *Journal of Health and Social Behavior, 19,* 2–21.

Pearlin, L. (1987). The stress process and strategies of intervention. In K. Hurrelmann, F. Kaufmann, & F. Lösel (Eds.), *Social intervention* (pp. 53–72). Berlin: de Gruyter.

Perrin, J. M. (1985). Introduction. In H. Hobbs & J. M. Perrin (Eds.), *Issues in the care of children with chronic illness* (pp. 1–10). San Francisco: Jossey-Bass.

Petersen, A. C., (1993). Presidential address: Creating adolescents. The role of context and process in developmental trajectories. *Journal of Research on Adolescence, 3,* 1–18.

Petersen, A. C., & Crockett, L. (1985). Pubertal timing and grade effects on adjustment. *Journal of Youth and Adolescence, 14,* 191–206.

Petersen, A. C., & Crockett, L. (1986). Pubertal development and its relation to cognitive and psychosocial development in adolescent girls: Implications for parenting. In J. B. Lancaster & B. A. Hamburg (Eds.), *School-age pregnancy and parenthood. Biosocial dimensions* (pp. 147–175). New York: de Gruyter.

Petersen, A. C., & Ebata, A. T. (1987). Developmental transitions and adolescent problem behavior: Implications for prevention and intervention. In K. Hurrelmann, F. Kaufmann, & F. Lösel (Eds.), *Social intervention: Potential and constraints* (pp. 167–184). Berlin: de Gruyter.

Petersen, A. C., Kennedy, R. E., & Sullivan, P. (1991). Coping with adolescence. In M. E. Colten & S. Gore (Eds.), *Adolescent stress. Causes and consequences* (pp. 93–110). Hawthorne, NY: Aldine de Gruyter.

Petersen, A. C., & Leffert, N. (1992, November). *What is special about adolescence?* Paper presented at the Youth in the Year 2000 conference, Marbach, Germany.

Petersen, A. C., & Taylor, B. (1980). The biological approach to adolescence: Biological change and psychological adaptation. In J. Adelson (Ed.), *Handbook of adolescent psychology* (pp. 117–155). New York: Wiley.

Pfeffer, C. R. (1990). Suicidal behavior in children and adolescents: A clinical and research perspective. *The Yale Journal of Biology and Medicine, 63,* 325–332.

Phares, V., & Compas, B. E. (1992). The role of fathers in child and adolescent psychopathology: Make room for daddy. *Psychological Bulletin, 111,* 387–412.

Phinney, G. V., Jensen, L. C., Olsen, J. A., & Cundick, B. (1990). The relationship between early development and psychosexual behaviors in adolescent females. *Adolescence, 25,* 321–332.

Pierce, J. P., & Gilpin, E. (1996). How long will today's new adolescent smoker be addicted to cigarettes? *American Journal of Public Health, 86,* 253–256.

Pierce, L., & Klein, H. (1982). A comparison of parent and child perception of the child's behavior. *Behavioral Disorders, 7,* 69–74.

Pinner, R. W., Teutsch, S. M., Simonsen, L., Klug, L. A., Graber, J. M., Clarke, M. J., & Berkelman, R. L. (1996). Trends in infectious diseases mortality in the United States. *Journal of the American Medical Association, 275,* 189–193.

Poston, W. S. C., Craine, M., & Atkinson, D. R. (1991). Counselor dissimilarity, confrontation, client cultural mistrust, and willingness to self-disclosure. *Journal of Multicultural Counseling and Development, 19,* 65–73.

Potter, P. C., & Roberts, M. T. C. (1984). Children's perception of chronic illness: The role of disease symptoms, cognitive development, and information. *Journal of Pediatric Psychology, 9,* 13–28.

Powers, S. I., Dill, D., Hauser, S. T., Noam, G., & Jacobson, A. M. (1985). Coping strategies of families of seriously ill adolescents. *Journal of Early Adolescence, 5,* 101–113.

Procidano, M. E., & Heller, K. (1983). Measures of perceived social support from friends and from family: Three validation studies. *American Journal of Community Psychology, 11,* 1–24.

Punamaki, R. (1987). Psychological stress responses of Palestinian mothers and their children in conditions of military occupation and political violence. *The Quarterly Newsletter of the Laboratory of Comparative Human Cognition, 2,* 76–84.

Rauste-Von Wright, M. (1988). Body image satisfaction in adolescent girls and boys: A longitudinal study. *Journal of Youth and Adolescence, 18,* 71–83.

Redl, F. (1969). Adolescents: Just how do they react? In G. Caplan & S. Lebovici (Eds.), *Adolescence: Psychosocial perspectives* (pp. 79–99). New York: Basic Books.

Reid, W. J., & Crisafulli, A. (1990). Marital discord and child behavior problems: A meta-analysis. *Journal of Abnormal Child Psychology, 18,* 105–117.

Reiser, L. W. (1987). Denial of physical illness in adolescence. *Psychoanalytic Study of the Child, 42,* 385–402.

Reiss, A. J., & Roth, J. A. (Eds.). (1993). *Understanding and preventing violence.* Washington, DC: National Academy Press.

Remmers, H. (1962). Cross-cultural studies of teenager problems. *Journal of Educational Psychology, 53,* 254–261.

Remmers, H., & Shimberg, B. (1954). *SRA Youth Inventory, Form S.* Chicago: Science Research Associates.

Remschmidt, H. (1989). Epidemiology and classification of psychiatric disorders in childhood and adolescence. In M. Brambring, F. Lösel, & H. Skowronek (Eds.), *Children at risk: Assessment, longitudinal research, and intervention* (pp. 3–23). Berlin: de Gruyter.

Renouf, A. G., & Kovacs, M. (1994). Concordance between mothers' reports and children's self-reports of depressive symptoms: A longitudinal study. *Journal of the American Academy of Child and Adolescent Psychiatry, 33,* 208–216.

Rice, K. G., Herman, M. A., & Petersen, A. C. (1993). Coping with challenge in adolescence: A conceptual model and psycho-educational intervention. *Journal of Adolescence, 16,* 235–252.

Rich, C. L., Sherman, M., & Fowler, T. C. (1990). San Diego Suicide Study: The adolescents. *Adolescence, 25,* 855–865.

Richards, M. H., Boxer, A. M., Petersen, A. C., & Albrecht, R. (1990). Relation of weight to body image in pubertal girls and boys from two communities. *Developmental Psychology, 26,* 313–321.

Ridley, C. R. (1984). Clinical treatment of the non-disclosing black clients: A therapeutic paradox. *American Psychologist, 39,* 1234–1244.

Riegel, K. F. (1976). The dialectics of human development. *American Psychologist, 31,* 689–700.

Rierdan, J., & Koff, E. (1980). Representation of the female body in early and late adolescent girls. *Journal of Youth and Adolescence 9,* 339–347.

Rierdan, J., & Koff, E. (1985). Timing of menarche and initial menstrual experience. *Journal of Youth and Adolescence, 14,* 237–244.

Rierdan, J., Koff, E., & Stubbs, M. L. (1987). Depressive symptomatology and body image in adolescent girls. *Journal of Early Adolescence, 7,* 205–216.

Rinsley, D. B. (1967). The adolescent in residential treatment: Some critical reflections. *Adolescence, 2,* 83–95.

Rinsley, D. B. (1980). *Treatment of the severely disturbed adolescent.* New York: Aronson.

Ritchie, K. (1981). Research note: Interaction in the families of epileptic children. *Journal of Child Psychology and Psychiatry, 22,* 65–71.

Robinson, N., & Fuller, J. H. (1985). Role of life events and difficulties in the onset of diabetes mellitus. *Journal of Psychosomatic Research, 29,* 583–591.
Roche, J. P. (1986). Premarital sex: Attitudes and behavior by dating stage. *Adolescence, 21,* 106–121.
Rodin, G. M., Daneman, D., Johnson, L. E., Kenshole, A., & Garfinkel, P. (1985). Anorexia nervosa and bulimia in female adolescents with insulin dependent diabetes mellitus. A systematic study. *Journal of Psychosomatic Research, 19,* 381–384.
Rodrigues-Lima, K. R., Eisenthal, S., & Lazare, A. (1981). Perception of requests in psychotherapy: Patient and therapist. *Journal of Social Service Research, 4,* 51–68.
Rogers, P. D., & Adger, H. (1993). Alcohol and adolescents. *Adolescent Medicine State of the Art Review, 4,* 295.
Rogers, R. (1970). The "unmotivated" adolescent patient who wants psychotherapy. *American Journal of Psychotherapy, 24,* 411–418.
Rohde, P., Lewinsohn, P. M., & Seeley, J. R. (1991). Comorbidity of unipolar depression: II. Comorbidity with other mental disorders in adolescents and adults. *Journal of Abnormal Psychology, 54,* 653–660.
Rosen, B. M., Bahn, A., Shellow, R., & Bower, E. M. (1965). Adolescent patients served in outpatient psychiatric clinics. *American Journal of Public Health, 55,* 1563–1577.
Rosenbaum, M.-B. (1979). The changing body image of the adolescent girl. In M. Sugar (Ed.), *Female adolescent development* (pp. 234–252). New York: Brunner/Mazel.
Rosenberg, P. S., Biggar, R. J., & Goeddert, J. J. (1993). Declining age at HIV infection in the United States. *New England Journal of Medicine, 330,* 789.
Rosenblatt, R. (1983). *Children of war.* Garden City, NY: Doubleday.
Rosenheim, E., & Gaoni, B. (1977). Defensive passivity in adolescence. *Adolescence, 48,* 449–459.
Roth, M., & Seiffge-Krenke, I. (1996). Psychische Störungen bei chronisch kranken Jugendlichen [Psychological symptoms in chronically ill adolescents: A literature review]. *Zeitschrift für Gesundheitspsychologie, 4,* 3–21.
Roth, R., Borkenstein, M., & Otto, S. (1987). Eine teststatistische Evaluation eines Wissens- und Einstellungsfragebogen für juvenile Diabetiker [A test-statistical evaluation of a questionnaire about knowledge and attitudes of juvenile diabetics]. *Zeitschrift für Klinische Psychologie, 16,* 124–134.
Roth, R., Neuper, C., & Borkenstein, M. (1988). Erprobung eines neu entwickelten Wissens-und Einstellungsfragebogens zum juvenilen Diabetes mellitus auf einem Diabetes-Sommer camp [Application of a recently developed questionnaire about knowledge and attitudes concerning juvenile diabetes in a diabetes summer camp]. In F. Strian, R. Hölzl & M. Halsbeck (Eds.), *Verhaltensmedizin und Diabetes mellitus. Psychobiologische und verhaltenspsychologische Ansätze in Diagnostik und Therapie* [Behavioral medicine and diabetes mellitus. [Psychobiological and behavioral approaches in diagnostics and therapy] (pp. 116–130). Berlin: Springer-Verlag.
Roth, S., & Cohen, L. F. (1986). Approach, avoidance, and coping with stress. *American Psychologist, 41,* 813–819.
Rovet, J. F., Ehrlich, R., & Hoppe, M. (1988). Specific intellectual deficits in children with early onset diabetes mellitus. *Child Development, 59,* 226–234.
Roy, A., Segal, N. L., Centerwall, B. S., & Robinette, C. D. (1991). Suicide in twins. *Archives of General Psychiatry, 48,* 29–32.
Rozario, J., Kapur, M., & Kaliaperumal, D. (1990). An epidemiological survey of prevalence and pattern of psychological disturbance of school-going early adolescents. *Journal of Personality and Clinical Studies, 6,* 165–169.

Rozario, J., Kapur, M., Rao, S., & Dalal, M. (1994). A comparative study of prevalence and pattern of psychological disturbances of adolescent boys and girls. *Journal of Personality and Clinical Studies, 10,* 65–70.

Runeson, B. (1989). Mental disorder in youth suicide: *DSM–III–R* axes I and II. *Acta Psychiatric Scandinavia, 79,* 490–497.

Russell, G. F. M. (1979). Bulimia nervosa. An ominous variant of anorexia nervosa. *Psychological Medicine, 9,* 429–448.

Rutter, M. (1985a). Psychopathology and development. In M. Rutter & L. Hersov (Eds.), *Child and adolescent psychiatry* (pp. 720–739). Oxford, England: Blackwell.

Rutter, M. (1985b). Resilience in the face of adversity. Protective factors and resistance to psychiatric disorders. *The British Journal of Psychiatry, 147,* 598–611.

Rutter, M. (1986). The developmental psychopathology of depression: Issues and perspectives. In M. Rutter, C. E. Izard, & P. B. Read (Eds.), *Depression in young people* (pp. 3–30). New York: Guilford.

Rutter, M. (1987). Continuities and discontinuities from infancy. In J. D. Osofsky (Ed.), *Handbook of infant development* (pp. 1256–1296). New York: Wiley.

Rutter, M. (1988). Epidemiological approaches to developmental psychopathology. *Archives of General Psychiatry, 45,* 486–495.

Rutter, M. (1991). Age changes in depressive disorders: Some developmental considerations. In J. Garber & K. A. Dodge (Eds.), *The development of emotion regulation and dysregulation* (pp. 273–300). New York: Cambridge University Press.

Rutter, M., Graham, P., Chadwick, O. F. D., & Yule, W. (1976). Adolescent turmoil: Fact or fiction? *Journal of Child Psychology and Psychiatry, 17,* 36–56.

Rutter, M., Quinton, D., & Yule, W. (1976). *Family pathology and disorder in the children.* London: Will.

Rutter, M., Shaffer, D., & Sturge, C. (1976). *A guide to a multiaxial classification scheme of psychiatric disorders in childhood and adolescence.* London: Institute of Psychiatry.

Rutter, M., Tizard, J., Yule, W., Graham, P., & Whitmore, K. (1977). Epidemiologie in der Kinderpsychiatrie—die Isle of Wight Studien 1964–1974 [Epidemiology in child psychiatry—the Isle of Wight studies 1964–1974]. *Zeitschrift für Kinder und Jugendpsychiatrie, 5,* 238–279.

Rutter, M., Tuma, A. H., & Lann, I. S. (Eds.). (1988). *Assessment and diagnosis in child psychopathology.* New York: Guilford.

Ryan, C., Vega, A., & Drash, A. (1985). Cognitive defects in adolescents who developed diabetes early in life. *Pediatrics, 57,* 921–927.

Ryff, C. D., & Keyes, C. L. M. (1995). The structure of psychological well-being revisited. *Journal of Personality and Social Psychology, 69,* 719–727.

Ryland, D. H., & Kruesi, M. J. P. (1992). Suicide among adolescents. *International Review of Psychiatry, 4,* 185–195.

Sabbeth, B. F., & Leventhal, J. M. (1984). Marital adjustment to chronic childhood illness: A critique of the literature. *Pediatrics, 73,* 762–768.

Safyer, A. W., Hauser, S. T., Jacobson, A. M., & Bliss, R. (1993). The impact of the family on diabetes adjustment: A developmental perspective. *Child and Adolescent Social Work Journal, 10,* 123–140.

Salt, R. E. (1991). Affectionate touch between fathers and preadolescent sons. *Journal of Marriage and the Family, 53,* 545–555.

Sandler, J., Kennedy, H., & Tyson, R. L. (1982). *Kinderanalyse. Gespräche mit Anna Freud* [Analysis of children. Talking with Anna Freud]. Frankfurt, Germany: Fischer.

Sanger, M. S., Copeland, D. R., & Davidson, E. R. (1991). Psychosocial adjustment among pediatric cancer patients: A multidimensional assessment. *Journal of Pediatric Psychology, 26,* 463–474.

Sanok, R. J. (1975). *Egocentric conceptualizations among adolescents and adults.* Unpublished manuscript, Pennsylvania State University, Pittsburgh.

Savin-Williams, R. C., & Berndt, T. J. (1990). Friendship and peer relations. In S. S. Feldman & G. R. Elliott (Eds.), *At the threshold: The developing adolescent* (pp. 99–119). Cambridge, MA: Harvard University Press.

Scheidt, P. C., Harel, Y., Trumble, A. C., Jones, D. H., Overpeck, M. D., & Bijur, P. E. (1995). The epidemiology of nonfatal injuries among US children and youth. *American Journal of Public Health, 85,* 932–938.

Schmid-Tannwald, I., & Urdze, A. (1983). *Sexualität und Kontrazeption aus der Sicht der Jugendlichen und ihrer Eltern* [Sexuality and contraception in the view of adolescents and their parents]. Stuttgart, Germany: Kohlhammer.

Schmidt, G., Klusmann, D., Zeitzschel, U., & Lange, C. (1994). Changes in adolescents' sexuality between 1970 and 1990 in West Germany. *Archives of Sexual Behavior, 23,* 489–513.

Schmitz, K. (1981). *Einstellungen zur Inanspruchnahme therapeutischer Hilfe.* [Attitudes towards psychotherapeutic services]. Unpublished paper, University of Gießen, Germany.

Schonfield, W. A. (1969). The body image in adolescents. In G. Caplan & S. Lebovici (Eds.), *Adolescence* (pp. 27–53). New York: Basic Books.

Schulz, A. (1991). *Das Körperbild weiblicher Jugendlicher und seine Auswirkungen auf Erleben und Verhalten* [Body image of female adolescents and its impact on perception and behavior]. Unpublished master's thesis, University of Bonn, Germany.

Schuster, M. A., Bell, R. M., Petersen, L. P., & Kanouse, D. E. (1996). Communication between adolescents and physicians about sexual behavior and risk prevention. *Archives of Pediatric and Adolescent Medicine, 150,* 906–913.

Schwefel, D., Svensson, P. G., & Zöllner, H. (1987). *Unemployment, social vulnerability and health in Europe.* Berlin: Springer-Verlag.

Scott-Jones, D., & Turner, S. L. (1988). Sex education, contraceptive and reproductive knowled ge, and contraceptive use among Black adolescent females. *Journal of Adolescent Research, 3,* 171–187.

Scott-Jones, D., & White, A. B. (1990). Correlates of sexual activity in early adolescence. *Journal of Early Adolescence, 10,* 221–238.

Seiffge-Krenke, I. (1986). *Psychoanalytische Therapie Jugendlicher* [Psychoanalytic therapy of adolescents]. Stuttgart, Germany: Kohlhammer.

Seiffge-Krenke, I. (1989). Problem intensity and the disposition of adolescents to take therapeutic advice. In M. Brambring, F. Lösel, & H. Skowronek (Eds.), *Children at risk: Assessment and longitudinal research* (pp. 457–477). New York: de Gruyter.

Seiffge-Krenke, I. (1990). Coping and health-related behavior: A cross-cultural perspective. In K. Hurrelmann & F. Lösel (Eds.), *Health hazards in adolescence* (pp. 339–360). New York: de Gruyter.

Seiffge-Krenke, I. (1992). Coping behavior of Finnish adolescents: Remarks on a cross-cultural comparison. *Scandinavian Journal of Psychology, 33,* 301–314.

Seiffge-Krenke, I. (1993a). Close friendships and imaginary companions in adolescence. In B. Laurssen (Ed.), *Close friendship in adolescence* (pp. 73–88). San Francisco: Jossey-Bass.

Seiffge-Krenke, I. (1993b). Coping behavior in normal and clinical samples: More similarities than differences? *Journal of Adolescence, 16,* 285–304.

Seiffge-Krenke, I. (1995). *Stress, coping and relationships.* Hillsdale, NJ: Lawrence Erlbaum Associates.

Seiffge-Krenke, I. (1997a). The capacity to balance intimacy and conflict: Differences in romantic relationships between healthy and diabetic adolescents. In S. Shulman & A.

Collins (Eds.), *Romantic relationships in adolescence. New directions for child development* (pp. 73–88). San Francisco: Jossey-Bass.
Seiffge-Krenke, I. (1997b). Chronic disease and its impact on perceived developmental progression: A delicate balance. *Developmental Psychology* (in press).
Seiffge-Krenke, I. (1997c). "One body for two": The problem of boundaries between chronically ill adolescents and their mothers. *Psychoanalytic Study of the Child,* 52, 340–358.
Seiffge-Krenke, I., & Brath, K. (1990). Krankheitsverarbeitung bei Kindern und Jugendlichen. Forschungstrends und Ergebnisse [Coping with illness in children and adolescents. Research trends and results]. In I. Seiffge-Krenke (Ed.), *Krankheitsverarbeitung bei Kindern und Jugendlichen* [Coping with illness in children and adolescents] (Vol. 4, pp. 3–22). Berlin: Springer-Verlag.
Seiffge-Krenke, I., & Kollmar, F. (1997). Discrepancies between mothers' and fathers' perceptions of sons' and daughters' problem behavior: A longitudinal analysis of parent–adolescent agreement on internalizing and externalizing problem behavior. *Journal of Child Psychology and Psychiatry* (in press).
Seiffge-Krenke, I., Moormann, D., Nilles, D., & Suckow, A. (1991). *Fragebogen zur Krankheitsverarbeitung für jugendliche Diabetiker* [Questionnaire on coping with illness in juvenile diabetics]. Unpublished manuscript, University of Bonn, Germany.
Seiffge-Krenke, I., Schmidt, C., Kollmar, F., Floss, A., & Roth, M. (1996). *Chronisch kranke Jugendliche und ihre Familien: Belastung, Bewältigung und psychosoziale Folgen* [Chronically ill adolescents and their families: Stress, coping, and psychosocial consequences]. Stuttgart, Germany: Kohlhammer.
Seiffge-Krenke, I., & Shulman, S. (1990). Coping style in adolescence: A cross-cultural study. *Journal of Cross-Cultural Psychology, 21,* 351–377.
Seiffge-Krenke, I., & Wester, U. (In preparation). *Changing attitudes towards psychotherapy and counseling: A treatment outcome.*
Sells, C. W., & Blum, R. M. (1996). Morbidity and Mortality among U.S. adolescents: An overview of data and trends. *American Journal of Public Health, 86,* 513–519.
Selye, H. (1946). The general adaptation syndrome and the diseases of adaptation. *Journal of Clinical Endocrinology, 6,* 117–230.
Shaffer, D., Garland, A., Gould, M., Fisher, P., & Trautman, P. (1988). Preventing teenage suicide: A critical review. *Journal of the American Academy of Child and Adolescent Psychiatry, 27,* 675–687.
Shafii, M., Carrigan, S., Whittinghill, J. R., & Derrick, A. (1985). Psychological autopsy of completed suicide attempters: Response to suicide-prevention programs. *Journal of the American Medical Association, 264,* 3151–3155.
Shapiro, R. L. (1979). Family dynamics and object-relations theory: An analytic, group-interpretative approach to family therapy. *Adolescent Psychiatry, 7,* 118–135.
Shouval, R., Ber, R., & Galatzer, A. (1982). Family social climate and the health status and social adaptation of diabetic youth. In Z. Laron & A. Galatzer (Eds.), *Psychological aspects of diabetes in children and adolescents* (pp. 89–93). Basel, Switzerland: Karger.
Shulman, S., & Seiffge-Krenke, I. (1997). *Fathers and adolescents. Developmental and clinical perspectives.* London: Routledge & Kegan Paul.
Siddique, C. M., & D'Arcy, C. (1984). Adolescence, stress, and psychological well-being. *Journal of Youth and Adolescence, 13,* 459–473.
Siegel, J. M., & Brown, J. D. (1988). A prospective study of stressful circumstances, illness symptoms, and depressed mood among adolescents. *Developmental Psychology, 24,* 715–721.
Siegel, L. J. (1992). Somatic disorders of childhood and adolescence. In W. M. Reynolds (Ed.), *Internalizing disorders in children and adolescents* (pp. 283–310). New York: Wiley.

Sigusch, V. & Schmidt, G. (1973). *Jugendlichensexualität* [Adolescent sexuality]. Stuttgart, Germany: Enke.

Silber, I. J. (1982). The differential diagnosis of functional symptoms in adolescence. *Adolescence, 17,* 769–778.

Silbert, A., Newburger, J., & Fyler, D. (1982). Marital instability and congenital heart disease. *Pediatrics, 69,* 747–750.

Simmons, R. G., & Blyth, D. A. (1987). *Moving into adolescence: The impact of pubertal change and school context.* New York: de Gruyter.

Simmons, R. G., Blyth, D. A., & McKinney, K. L. (1983). The social and psychological effects of puberty on White females. In J. Brooks-Gunn & A. C. Petersen (Eds.), *Girls at puberty: Biological and psychosocial perspectives* (pp. 229–271). New York: Plenum.

Simmons, R. G., Burgeson, R., & Carlton-Ford, S. (1987). The impact of cumulative change in early adolescence. *Child Development, 58,* 1220–1234.

Simmons, R. G., & Rosenberg, F. (1975). Sex, sex roles, and self-image. *Journal of Youth and Adolescence, 4,* 229–258.

Simonds, J. E. (1977). Psychiatric status of diabetic children in good and poor control. In Z. Laron & A. Galatzer (Eds.), *Psychological aspects of balance of diabetes in juveniles* (pp. 8–16). Basel, Switzerland: Karger.

Singh, G. K., & Stella, M. Y. (1996). Trends and differentials in adolescent and young adult mortality in the United States, 1950 through 1993. *American Journal of Public Health, 86,* 560–564.

Slater, E. J., & Rubenstein, E. (1987). Family coping with trauma in adolescents. *Psychiatric Annals, 17,* 786–794.

Slavin, L. A., & Compas, B. E. (1989). The problem of confounding social support and depressive symptoms: A brief report on a college sample. *American Journal of Community Psychology, 17,* 57–65.

Smetana, J. G., Yau, J., & Hanson, S. (1991). Conflict resolution in families with adolescents. *Journal of Research on Adolescence, 1,* 109–134.

Smith, M. S., Mauseth, R., Palmer, J. P., Pecoraro, R., & Wenet, G. (1991). Glycosylated hemoglobin and psychological adjustment in adolescents with diabetes. *Adolescence, 26,* 31–40.

Snyder, C. R., Handelsman, M. M., & Endelman, J. R. (1978). Can clients provide valuable feedback to clinicians about their personality interpretations? A reply to Greene. *Journal of Consulting and Clinical Psychology, 46,* 1493–1495.

Society for Adolescent Medicine (Ed.) (1992). Medical screening. *Journal of Adolescent Health, 13,* 7S–51S.

Soff, M. (1989). *Jugend im Tagebuch* [Youth in diaries]. München, Germany: Juventa.

Spatz Widom, C. (1989). Does violence beget violence? *Psychological Bulletin, 106,* 3–28.

Sroufe, L. A., & Fleeson, J. (1986). Attachment and the construction of relationships. In W. W. Hartup & Z. Rubin (Eds.), *Relationships and development* (pp. 51–72). Hillsdale, NJ: Lawrence Erlbaum Associates.

Sroufe, L. A., & Rutter, M. (1984). The domain of developmental psychopathology. *Child Development, 54,* 173–189.

Stabler, B., Surwit, R. S., Lane, J. D., Morris, M. A., Litton, J., & Feinglos, M. N. (1987). Type A behavior patterns and blood glucose control in diabetic children. *Psychosomatic Medicine, 49,* 313–316.

Stark, L. J., Spirito, A., Williams, L. A., & Guevremont, D. C. (1989). Common problems and coping strategies: I. Findings with normal adolescents. *Journal of Abnormal Child Psychology, 17,* 203–212.

Statistisches Bundesamt. (1991). *Fachserie Gesundheitswesen, 12, Reihe 3* [Health Series 12, Vol. 3]. Wiesbaden, Germany: Statistisches Bundesamt.

Statistisches Bundesamt. (1992). *Statistisches Jahrbuch 1992* [Statistical yearbook of 1992]. Wiesbaden, Germany: Statistisches Bundesamt.

Stattin, H., & Magnusson, D. (1990). *Pubertal maturation in female development.* Hillsdale, NJ: Lawrence Erlbaum Associates.

Stavrakaki, C., & Ellis, J. (1989). The relationship of anxiety to depression in children and adolescents. *Psychiatric Clinics of North America, 12,* 777–789.

Stein, D. M., & Reichert, P. (1990). Extreme dieting behaviors in early adolescence. *Journal of Early Adolescence, 10,* 108–121.

Stein, J. H., & Reiser, L. W. (1994). A study of white middle-class adolescent boys' responses to "semenarche" (the first ejaculation). *Journal of Youth and Adolescence, 23,* 373–384.

Stein, S., & Charles, E. (1975). Emotional factors in juvenile diabetes mellitus: A study of early life experience of eight diabetic children. *Psychosomatic Medicine, 37,* 237–244.

Stern, M., & Zevon, M. A. (1990). Stress, coping, and family environment. *Journal of Adolescent Research, 5,* 290–305.

Stiffman, A. R., Earls, F., Dore, P., & Cunningham, R. (1992). Changes in acquired immunodeficiency syndrome-related risk behavior after adolescence: Relationships to knowledge and experience concerning human immunodeficiency virus infection. *Pediatrics, 89,* 950–956.

Stocker, C. M. (1994). Children's perceptions of relationships with siblings, friends, and mothers: Compensatory processes and links with adjustment. *Journal of Child Psychology and Psychiatry, 35,* 1447–1459.

Stone, A. A., & Neale, J. M. (1984). New measure of daily coping: Development and preliminary results. *Journal of Personality and Social Psychology, 46,* 892–906.

Storz, N. S., & Greene, W. H. (1983). Body weight, body image, and perception of diets in adolescent girls. *Journal of Nutrition and Education, 15,* 15–18.

Straus, M. A., Gelles, R. J., & Steinmetz, S. K. (1980). *Behind closed doors: Violence in the American family.* New York: Anchor.

Strouse, J. S., & Fabes, R. A. (1987). A conceptualization of transition to nonvirginity in adolescent females. *Journal of Adolescent Research, 2,* 331–348.

Strupp, H. H. (1989). Can the practitioner learn from the researcher? *American Psychologist, 44,* 717–724.

Sullivan, B. J. (1978). Self-esteem and depression in adolescent diabetic girls. *Diabetes Care, 1,* 18–22.

Sullivan, B. J. (1979). Adjustment in diabetic adolescent girls: I. Development of the Diabetic Adjustment Scale. *Psychosomatic Medicine, 41,* 119–126.

Suls, J., & Fletcher, B. (1985). The relative efficacy of avoidant and non-avoidant coping strategies. A meta-analysis. *Health Psychology, 4,* 249–288.

Susman, E. J., Nottelman, E. D., Inoff-Germain, G. E., Dorn, L. D., Cutler, G. B., Jr., Loriaux, D. L., & Chrousos, G. P. (1985). The relation of relative hormonal levels and physical development and social–emotional behavior in young adolescents. *Journal of Youth and Adolescence, 14,* 245–264.

Swearingen, E. M., & Cohen, L. H. (1985). Life events and psychological distress: A prospective study of young adolescents. *Developmental Psychology, 21,* 1045–1054.

Sweeney, P., Lindegren, M. L., Buehler, J. W., Onorato, M., & Janssen, R. S. (1995). Teenagers at risk of human immunodeficiency virus type 1 infection. Results from seroprevalence surveys in the United States. *Archives of Pediatric and Adolescent Medicine, 149,* 521–528.

Swift, C. R., Seidman, F., & Stein, H. (1967). Adjustment problems in juvenile diabetes. *Psychsomatic Medicine, 29,* 555–571.

Tanner, J. M. (1972). Sequence, tempo, and individual variation in growth and development of boys and girls aged 12 to 16. In J. Kagan & R. Coles (Eds.), *12 to 16: Early adolescence* (pp. 1–24). New York: Norton.

Thoits, P. A. (1982). Life stress, social support, and psychological vulnerability: Epidemiological considerations. *Journal of Community Psychology, 10,* 341–362.

Thoits, P. A. (1983). Dimensions of life events that influence psychological distress: An evaluation and synthesis of literature. In H. B. Kaplan (Ed.), *Psychosocial stress: Trends in theory and research* (pp. 33–103). New York: Academic Press.

Tobin-Richards, M. H., Boxer, A. M., & Petersen, A. C. (1983). The psychological significance of pubertal change. Sex differences in perceptions of self during early adolescence. In J. Brooks-Gunn & A. C. Petersen (Eds.), *Girls at puberty: Biological and psychological perspectives* (pp. 127–154). New York: Plenum.

Tolor, A., & Fehon, D. (1987). Coping with stress: A study of male adolescents' coping strategies as related to adjustment. *Journal of Adolescent Research, 2,*(1), 33–42.

Toolan, J. M. (1969). Depression in children and adolescents. In G. Caplan & S. Lebovici (Eds.), *Adolescence: Psychosocial perspectives* (pp. 263–270). New York: Basic Books.

Toolan, P., Jaffe, S., & Ryan, P. (1988). *Gender pattern in adolescent clinical service use.* Unpublished manuscript, University of Chicago, Chicago, IL.

Touliatos, J., & Lindholm, B. W. (1980). Behavioral disturbances in children of native-born and immigrant parents. *Journal of Community Psychology, 8,* 28–33.

Tramontana, M. G. (1980). Critical review of research on psychotherapy outcome with adolescents. *Psychological Bulletin, 88,* 429–450.

Treboux, D., & Busch-Rossnagel, N. (1990). Social network influences on adolescent sexual attitudes and behaviors. *Journal of Adolescent Research, 5,* 175–189.

Troiano, R. P., Flegal, K. M., Kuczmarski, R. J., Campbell, S. M., & Johnson, C. L. (1995). Overweight prevalence and trends for children and adolescents. The National Health and Nutrition Examination Surveys, 1963 to 1991. *Archives of Pediatric and Adolescent Medicine, 149,* 1085–1091.

Trute, B., & Hauch, C. (1988). Building on family strength: A study of families with positive adjustment to the birth of a developmentally disabled child. *Journal of Marriage and Family Therapy, 14,* 185–193.

Udry, J. R., & Billy, J. O. (1987). Initiation of coitus in early adolescence. *American Sociological Review, 52,* 841–855.

U.S. Department of Health and Human Services. (1990). *Seventh special report to the U.S. congress on alcohol and health.* Rockville, MD: U.S. Department of Health and Human Services, National Institute on Alcohol Abuse and Alcoholism.

U.S. Department of Health and Human Services (1994a). *HIV/AIDS Surveillance Report, year-end edition.* Atlanta, GA: U.S. Department of Health and Human Services.

U.S. Department of Health and Human Services (1994b). *Preventing tobacco use among young people: A report of the surgeon general.* Atlanta, GA: U.S. Department of Health and Human Services.

Urberg, K. A., & Rosen, R. A. (1987). Age differences in adolescent decision-making: Pregnancy resolution. *Journal of Adolescent Research, 2,* 447–454.

Vaillant, G. E. (1977). *Adaptation to life.* Boston: Little, Brown.

van Goor-Lambo, G., Orley, J., Poustka, F., & Rutter, M. (1994). Abnormal psychosocial situations: Preliminary results of a WHO and a German multicenter study. *European Child and Adolescent Psychiatry, 3,* 229–241.

Varni, J. W., Rubenfeld, L. A., Talbot, D., & Setoguchi, Y. (1989). Stress, social support, and depressive symptomatology in children with congenital/acquired limb deficiencies. *Journal of Pediatric Psychology, 14,* 515–530.

Vaugham, S., Stabler, J., & Clance, P. (1981). Children's monetary evaluation of body parts as a function of sex, race and school grade. *Journal of Psychology, 107,* 203–209.

Vega, W. A., Zimmerman, R. S., Warheit, G. J., Apospori, E., & Gil, A. G. (1993). Risk factors for early adolescent drug use in four ethnic and racial groups. *American Journal of Public Health, 83,* 185–189.

Verbrugge, L. M., & Ascione, F. J. (1987). Exploring the iceberg: Common symptoms and how people care for them. *Medical Care, 25,* 539–569.

Verhulst, F. C., & van der Ende, J. (1993). "Comorbidity" in an epidemiological sample: A longitudinal perspective. *Journal of Child Psychology and Psychiatry and Allied Disciplines, 34,* 767–783.

Vernberg, E. M. (1990). Psychological adjustment and experiences with peers during early adolescence: Reciprocal, incidental, or unidirectional relationships? *Journal of Abnormal Child Psychology, 18,* 187–198.

Versteegen, U. (1988). *Zur Bedeutung des Konzepts der "Lebensweisen" für die Gesundheitspsychologie* [The significance of the "lifestyle" concept in health psychology]. Unpublished doctoral dissertation, University of Freiburg, Germany.

Vizard, E., Monck, E., & Misch, P. (1995). Child and adolescent sex abuse perpetrators: A review of the research literature. *Journal of Child Psychology and Psychiatry, 36,* 731–756.

Vonderach, G. (1989). Arbeitslosigkeit (Berufsnot) junger Menschen [Unemployment in young people]. In M. Markefka & R. Nave-Herz (Eds.), *Handbuch der Familien- und Jugendforschung* [Handbook of research on adolescence and the family] (Vol. 2, pp. 699–716). Neuwied, Germany: Luchterhand.

Wagner, B. M., Compas, B. E., & Howell, D. C. (1988). Daily and major life events: A test of an integrative model of psychosocial stress. *American Journal of Community Psychology, 16,* 189–205.

Wallander, J. L., Varni, J. W., Babani, L., Banis, H. T., & Wilcox, K. T. (1988). Children with chronic physical disorders: Maternal reports of their psychological adjustment. *Journal of Pediatric Psychology, 13,* 197–212.

Warren-Boulton, E., Anderson, B. J., Schwartz, N. L., & Drexler, A. J. (1981). A group approach to the management of diabetes in adolescents and young adults. *Diabetes Care, 4,* 620–623.

Wassef, A., Ingham, D., Collins, M. L., & Mason, G. (1995). In search of effective programmes to address students' emotional distress and behavioral problems. Part I: Defining the problem. *Adolescence, 30,* 523–538.

Watzlawick, P., Weakland, J. H., & Fish, R. (1974). *Lösungen* [Solutions]. Bern, Switzerland: Huber.

Webster-Stratton, C. (1988). Mothers' and fathers' perceptions of child deviance: Roles of parent and child behaviors and parent adjustment. *Journal of Consulting and Clinical Psychology, 56,* 908–915.

Weddle, K. D., McKenry, P., & Leigh, G. K. (1988). Adolescent sexual behavior: Trends and issues in research. *Journal of Adolescent Research, 3,* 245–257.

Weiner, I. B. (1970). *Psychological disturbances in adolescence.* New York: Wiley.

Weiner, I. B., & Del Gaudio, A. L. (1976). Psychopathology in adolescence: An epidemiological study. *Archives of General Psychiatry, 33,* 187–193.

Weinman, J. (1990). Health psychology in the 1990's. In P. J. D. Drenth, J. A. Sergeant, & R. J. Takens (Eds.), *European perspectives in psychology* (Vol. 2, pp. 169–191). Chichester, England: Wiley.

Weis, P. A. (1961). Deformities as cues to understanding development of form. *Perspectives in Biology and Medicine, 4,* 133–151.

Weissman, J., & Appleton, C. (1995). The therapeutic aspects of acceptance. *Perspectives in Psychiatric Care, 31,* 19–23.

Weisz, J. R., Weiss, B., Alicke, M. D., & Klotz, M. L. (1987). Effectiveness of psychotherapy with children and adolescents: Meta-analytic findings for clinicians. *Journal of Consulting and Clinical Psychology, 55,* 542–549.

Werner, E. E., & Smith, R. S. (1982). *Vulnerable but invincible. A study of resilient children.* New York: McGraw-Hill.

Werner, M. J., & Adger, H. (1995). Early identification, screening, and brief intervention for adolescent alcohol use. *Archives of Pediatric and Adolescent Medicine, 149,* 1241–1248.

Wertlieb, D., Hauser, S. T., & Jacobson, A. M. (1986). Adaptation to diabetes: Behavior symptoms and family context. *Journal of Pediatric Psychology, 11,* 463–479.

Westbrook, L. E., & Stein, R. E. K. (1994). Epidemiology of chronic health conditions in adolescents. *Adolescent Medicine: State of the Art Reviews, 5,* 197–209.

Wetzel, R. D., Reich, T., Murphy, G. E., Province, M., & Miller, J. P. (1987). The changing relationship between age and suicide rates. Cohort effect, period effect or both? *Psychiatric Development, 3,* 179–218.

Whitaker, B. (1987). *The global connection: The crisis of drug addiction.* London: Ebenezer Baylis & Son, Ltd.

White, K., Kolman, M. L., Wexler, P., Polin, G., & Winter, R. J. (1984). Unstable diabetes and unstable families: A psychosocial evaluation of diabetic children with recurrent ketoacidosis. *Pediatrics, 73,* 749–755.

Wilker, L., Wasaw, M., & Hatfield, E. (1981). Chronic sorrows revisited. Parent versus professional depiction of the adjustment of parents of mentally retarded children. *American Journal of Orthopsychiatry, 51,* 63–70.

Wilkinson, G. (1987). Invited review. The influence of psychiatric, psychological and social factors on the control of insulin-dependent diabetes mellitus. *Journal of Psychosomatic Research, 31,* 277–286.

Williams, R. (1983). Concepts of health: An analysis of lay logic. *Sociology, 17,* 185–205.

Winnicott, D. W. (1969). *Kind, Familie und Umwelt* [Child, family, and environment]. München, Germany: Reinhardt.

Winnicott, D. W. (1970). *The maturational processes and the facilitating environment.* London: Hogarth.

Winokur, A., March, V., & Mendels, J. (1980). Primary affective disorder in relatives of patients with anorexia nervosa. *American Journal of Psychiatry, 17,* 695–698.

Woodward, C. A., Boyle, M. H., Offord, D. R., Cadman, D. F., Links, P. S., Munroe-Blum, H., Byrne, C., & Thomas, H. (1988). Ontario Child Health study: Patterns of ambulatory medical care utilization and their correlates. *Pediatrics, 82,* 425–434.

World Health Organization. (1946). *Constitution.* Geneva: World Health Organization.

World Health Organization. (1992). *International classification of diseases, injuries, and causes of death* (10th ed.). Geneva: World Health Organization.

WHO Regional Office for Europe (1994, January). *Memorandum on improving medical and psychological care for children and adolescents.* Report of the 2nd Health Sciences Colloquium of Bielefeld, Germany.

Wright, L. (1979). Health care psychology. Prospects for the well-being of children. *American Psychologist, 34,* 1001–1006.

Wysocki, T. (1993). Associations among teenager–parent relationships, metabolic control, and adjustment to diabetes in adolescents. *Journal of Pediatric Psychology, 18,* 441–452.

Young, C. D., & Martin, M. (1981). Processing information about self by neurotics. *British Journal of Clinical Psychology, 20,* 205–212.

Zabin, L. S., Astone, N. M., & Emerson, M. R. (1993). Do adolescents want babies? The relationship between attitudes and behavior. *Journal of Research on Adolescence, 3,* 67–86.

Zelnik, M., & Kantner, J. F. (1979). Reasons for non-use of contraception by sexually active women aged 15–19. *Family Planning Perspectives, 12,* 230–237.

Zelnik, M., & Kantner, J. F. (1980). Sexual activity, contraceptive use, and pregnancy among metro-area teenagers. *Family Planning Perspectives, 12,* 30–36.

Zelnik, M., Kantner, J. F., & Ford, K. (1981). *Sex and pregnancy in adolescence.* Beverly Hills, CA: Sage.

Zeltzer, L., Kellerman, J., Ellenberg, L., Dash, L., & Rigler, D. (1980). Psychological effects of illness in adolescence. II. Impact of illness in adolescents—crucial issues and coping styles. *Journal of Pediatrics, 97,* 132–138.

Zeltzer, L., LeBaron, S., & Zeltzer, P. (1984). The adolescent with cancer. In R. Blum (Ed.), *Chronic illness and disabilities in childhood and adolescence* (pp. 168–179). New York: Grune & Stratton.

Zola, J. K. (1966). Culture and symptoms—analysis of patients presenting complaints. *American Sociological Review, 31,* 615–630.

Zola, J. K. (1983). *Socio-medical inquiries: Recollections, reflections, and reconsiderations.* Philadelphia: Temple University Press.

Zubin, J. (1967). Classification of the behavior disorders. *Annual Review of Psychology, 18,* 373–406.

# Author Index

## A


Aarons, A., 188
Abholz, H. H., 7
Achenbach, T. M., 31, 34, 36, 37, 144, 178, 208
Acker, M., 104
Adams, C., 41
Adams, G. R., 94
Adams, P. F., 47, 50, 69
Adelman, H. S., 30
Adger, H., 62, 63
Adler, N. E., 5
Ahmed, N., 161
Ahmed, P. I., 161
Albrecht, R., 79
Alicke, M., 200
Allen, V. L., 74
Allgood-Merten, B., 120
Alvin, P., 220
Amann-Gainotti, M., 76
Amato, R. P., 104
Amir, D., 27
Andenas, S., 105
Anderson, B. J., 155, 170, 173
Anderson, P. B., 95
Anderson Moore, K., 118
Andrews, G., 194
Andrus, J. K., 56
Antonovsky, A., 7
Apospori, E., 68
Appelton, C., 222
Argyle, M., 20
Arnett, J., 97
Aro, H. M., 56
Ascione, F. J., 184, 185
Aseltine, R. H.,104, 106
Ashworth, M., 116
Astone, N. M., 97, 107
Atkinson, D. R., 216
Auslander, W. F., 155, 170
Aymami, R., 95


## B


Babani, L., 155
Bachman, J. G., 62, 62, 66,
Badura, B., 9, 167
Bahn, A., 35
Bailey, S. L., 68
Baird, T. L., 96
Baker, L., 17
Balint, M. T., 21
Baltes, M. M., 17
Banis, H. T., 155
Barbero, G., 108
Barglow, P., 159
Barling, J., 119
Baron, P., 150
Barrera, M., 129
Baum, A., 101, 102, 106, 127

Baum, J. D., 155
Bauman, K. E., 64
Beardslee, W. R., 146
Beauvais, F., 62, 64, 65, 66, 67
Beck, N., 52
Becker, M. H., 98
Becker, R. D., 154
Beckmann, D., 186
Bell, R., 40
Bell, R. M., 217
Belle, D. E., 134
Ben-Sira, Z., 152
Bentler, P. M., 106
Ber, R., 170
Bergman, A. B., 108
Bergmann, T., 5
Berkhan, K., 41
Berman, A. L:, 55
Berndt, T. J., 95
Bernfeld, S., 88
Bibace, R., 3
Biggar, R. J., 59
Billings, A. G., 134, 171
Billy, J. O., 89
Bingham, C. R., 94
Bird, H. R., 39
Bjorck, J., 110, 130
Blanchard-Fields, F., 133
Blaxter, M., 3
Bliesener, T., 142
Bliss, R., 154
Bloch, S.,155
Blos, P., 35, 71, 114, 223, 224
Blum, R. M., 44, 61, 64, 69
Blum, R. W., 58
Blumstein, A., 54
Blyth, D. A., 71, 78, 89, 106, 146
Bolton, F. G., 94
Borgers, D., 7
Borkenstein, M., 164, 165
Borman, E. H., 178
Bowen, R., 27
Bower, E. M., 35
Bowlds, M. K., 105, 142
Boxer, A. M., 77, 79
Boyle, M. H., 52. 53, 207
Brähler, E., 76, 99
Brand, A. H., 109, 155, 159
Brath, K., 152, 153
Bromley, D. B., 188
Brooks-Gunn, J., 71, 72, 72, 79, 81, 82, 96, 97, 101, 103, 106
Broughton, J. M., 23, 27
Brown, J. D., 110
Bruch, H., 17
Bry, B. H., 69
Bubb, J., 155
Budd, J., 155
Buehler, J. W., 59
Buhrmester, D., 24, 174
Buke, P. M., 41
Bulcroft, R. A., 82, 86, 91
Bulman, R. J., 167
Burgeson, R., 106
Burghen, G. A., 155
Burgoon, J. K., 21
Burgoon, M., 21
Burish, T. G., 152
Burke, R., 121, 128
Burlingham, D., 115
Buroughs, J., 40
Burt, C., 110, 130
Busch-Rossnagel, N., 94
Bush, M., 207
Byers, R. H., 59

## C

Cadman, D., 207
Calnan, M., 2
Campbell, S. M., 58
Campo, J. V., 36, 100
Cantor, N., 104
Cantwell, D. P., 40
Carle, D. L., 133
Carlson, G., 52, 54
Carlton-Ford, S., 106
Caron, C., 34, 37, 214
Carrigan, S., 56
Cartwright, A., 185
Cash, T. F., 79
Caspar, R. C., 39
Cauce, A. M., 121, 125
Centerwall, B. S., 56
Chadwick, O. F. D., 52
Charles, E., 159
Chase, H., 79, 185
Chasseguet-Smirgel, J., 88
Chavez, E. L., 66
Chelune, G. J., 22, 24
Chen, K., 65, 66
Cheng, T. L., 198, 218, 220
Chin, K., 69, 117
Chopra, H. D., 199
Cicchetti, D., 13
Cigrang, J. A., 133
Claes, M. E., 126
Clance, P., 75
Clark, S. M., 24
Clement, U., 92
Cloninger, C. R., 36
Coddington, R. D., 108
Codega, S. A., 143
Cohen, J., 53
Cohen, L. H., 110, 112, 130, 142

Cohen, P., 53
Cohen, S., 52, 126, 127, 128, 129
Cohn, L. D., 79
Cole, C., 161
Cole, D., 188
Cole, R., 161
Coleman, J. S., 206, 207
Coletta, N. D., 143
Collins, J. K., 91, 95
Collins, J. L., 50
Collins, M. L., 221
Compas, B. E., 42, 53, 102, 105, 110, 111, 112, 121, 127, 129, 133, 134, 135, 136, 139, 144
Condon, S. L., 173
Cook, J. A., 161, 205
Cook, N. S., 95
Cook-Flannagan, C., 104
Cooper, C. R., 173
Copeland, D. R., 154
Corber, S., 218
Cotterell,J. L., 118, 125, 145
Cowan, P., 13
Cozby, P. C., 25
Crain, A., 170
Craine, M., 216
Crisafulli, A., 31
Crockett, L., 72, 73, 74, 77
Cromer, B. A., 219
Cummings, S. T., 204
Cundick, B., 92
Cunningham, R., 59
Cuskey, W. R., 219
Czajkowski, D. R., 190

D

Dacey, J., 77
D'Arcy, C., 112, 121
Dalal, M., 53
Damhorst, M. L., 80
Damon, W., 188
Daneman, D., 154
Daniels, D., 129
Dash, L., 154
Davidson, E. R., 154
Davies, E., 54, 78, 80
Davis, S. M., 97, 98
Dawson, D., 104
Deatrick, J. A., 204
DeGuire, M. J., 155
Delamater, A. M., 15, 159, 160
Delbridge, L., 170
Del Gaudio, A. L., 35, 52
DeLongis, A., 102
Derrick, A., 56
Desmond, S. M., 79
Devlin, S. J., 89
de Witt, T. G., 199
Del Gaudio, A. L., 35, 52
Diehl, M., 200, 201
Diekstra, R. F. W., 55, 57, 120
Dill, D., 174
Di Placido, J., 161
di Prospero, B., 76
Dirks, J. F., 29, 30
D'Hontand, A., 2
Dohrenwend, B. S., 102, 194
Dohrenwend, P., 102, 194
Donovan, J. E., 68
Dore, P., 59
Dornbusch, S. M., 91
Dougherty, G. E., 46
Downes, B., 58
Drash, A., 177
Drexler, A. J., 174
Drotar, D., 165, 207
Dubois, R., 190
Dunn, S. M., 166
Dusek, J. B. 167

E

Earls, F., 59, 149
East, P. L., 150
Ebata, A. T., 106, 132, 138, 139
Eckhardt, B., 119
Eisele, J., 78
Eisenberg, J. G., 110
Eisenthal, S., 224
Eiser, C., 5, 16, 108, 154, 155, 204
Eiser, E., 143, 151
Eissler, R. K., 88
Elder, G. H. Jr., 117
Elkind, D., 27, 97
Ellenberg, L., 154
Ellis, J., 54
Emerson, M. R., 97
Emminghaus, H., 41
Endelman, J. R., 30
Engelhardt, K. H., 185
Ennett, S. E., 64
Epstein, L. D.,128
Erdheim, M., 88
Erlich, H. S., 156, 179
Etzwiler, D. D., 173
Ey, S., 42

F

Fabes, R. A., 92, 94
Fabrega, H., 214, 215
Fagan, J.,68
Faber, S. S., 143, 146

Farmer, F. L., 24
Farrington, D. P., 149
Faust, R., 68
Fehon, D., 131, 133
Feighner, J. P., 39
Feinberg, T., 161
Feinstein, S., 203, 207, 224
Feldman, E., 76
Feldman, S. S., 117
Feldman, W., 76, 218
Felner, R. D., 143
Field, M. G., 2
Finlay-Jones, R., 119
Fiore, M. C., 63, 148
Fish, R., 17
Fisher, M., 57, 219
Fisher, P., 56
Flaherty, J. F., 167
Flanery, R., 108
Fleeson, J., 145
Flegal, K. M., 58
Fleming, D. W., 37
Fleming, J. E., 41, 54
Fletcher, B., 142
Florenzano, R. U., 52
Floss, A., 80
Folkman, S., 102, 103, 105, 125, 131, 133
Fondacaro, K. M., 103, 133, 139
Ford, K., 93
Forsythe, C. J., 134
Fosson, A., 102
Foster, L., 156
Fowler, T. C., 56
Framo, J. L., 207
Freedman, R. J., 77, 78, 79
French, S. A., 58
Freud, A., 5, 35, 40, 71, 115
Freud, S., 88
Freund, E. E., 3, 8, 20, 101, 117, 175, 183, 184, 185
Fritsch, S. L., 36, 100
Frost, L. A., 39
Frydenberg, E., 121, 135
Frymier, J., 220
Fuchs, R., 64
Fullard, W., 89
Fuller, J. H., 159
Fuller, W., 30
Furman, A., 79, 80
Furman, W., 24, 128, 174
Furstenberg, F. F., 96, 97, 98
Fyler, D., 204

## G

Gaddis, A., 71
Gagnon, J., 93, 95
Galambos, N. L., 71, 144
Galatzer, A., 170
Gansneder, B., 220
Gaoni, B., 224
Garbarino, J., 116
Garber, J., 31
Garfinkel, P. E., 57, 58, 154
Garland, A., 56
Garmezy, N., 10, 14, 15, 105, 135, 145,
Garrison, C. Z., 63, 152, 181, 190
Ge, X., 117
Gelles, R. J., 119
Gerhardt, C. A., 136
Gersten, J. C., 110
Giambra, L., 27
Gil, A. G., 68
Gilbert, B. O., 155
Gilligan, C., 169
Gilpin, E. A., 64, 65
Ginsburg, K. R., 218
Girgus, J. S., 141
Giunta, C. T., 110, 111
Glaser, K., 41
Glasner, P. D., 60
Glendinning, A., 91
Goeddert, J. J., 59
Goetz, D., 155
Golden, M. P., 109
Goldman, J. D. G., 93
Goldman, R. J., 93
Goleman, D., 116
Golombek, H., 181
Gomes-Schwartz, B., 200
Goodman, J. T., 76
Gorny, S. W., 67
Gore, S., 104, 106
Gortmaker, S. L., 151, 152
Gotthold, J., 156
Gottlieb, B. H., 146
Gould, M., 56
Gould, M. S., 39
Graham, P., 36, 52, 53, 105, 135
Grant, K. E., 42, 111
Gray, H. E., 154
Gray, N., 79
Green, W. A., 40, 108
Greenberg, N. E., 101, 102
Geenberger, E., 146
Greene, J. W., 100, 107
Greene, W. H., 79
Gregg, C. H., 143
Greschuck, D., 197
Greydanus, D. E., 177
Grotevant, H. D., 173
Gruen, R. J., 102
Grunberg, N. E., 106, 127
Guevremont, D. C., 133
Gull, W., 39

Gurevich, M., 109

## H

Haan, N., 134, 135
Habermas, T., 214
Hadler, S., 143
Hahn, K. D., 20
Hall, D. J., 16
Halmer, C. J., 152
Halmi, K., 40
Halpert, H. P., 199
Hamburg, B. A., 161, 219
Hammarström, A., 120, 143
Handelsman, M. M., 30
Hanl, J.,153
Hansell, S., 148
Hanson, C. L., 133, 155, 159, 170
Hanson, I. C., 59
Hanson, S., 104
Hardy, A. M., 47, 50
Harris, M. A., 133
Harris, M. B., 97, 98
Hart, D., 188
Hatfield, E., 204
Hauch, C., 205
Haurin, R. J., 63
Hauser, S. T., 105, 142, 154, 155, 161, 170, 173, 174, 178, 204, 205
Havighurst, R. J., 113, 169
Hawton, K., 188
Hayes, C.D., 93
Heller, K., 125
Hendren, R. L., 40
Hendry, L. B., 91
Henggeler, S. W., 155, 170
Henriksson, M. M., 56
Henshaw, S. K., 61, 97
Herman, M. A., 106
Herman-Stahl, M. A., 133, 139, 141
Hertsgaard, D., 79
Herzlich, C., 2
Hickson, G., 100
Hill, J. P., 104, 123, 146
Hinden, B. R., 136
Hinkle, L., 159
Hoberman, H. M., 56
Hodge, M. J., 46
Hodges, K., 108
Hodgman, C. H., 55
Hodgson, C., 218
Hoehe, M., 101
Hofer, T. P., 47
Hoffmeyer, O., 41
Hoffarth, S. L., 93
Hofman, A. E., 154, 177
Hogan, D., 107
Hogan, R., 120
Holahan, C. J., 138
Holden, E. W., 154
Holinger, P. C., 120
Hollingshead, A. B., 184
Holmbeck, G. N., 104, 123
Hoppe, M., 154
Hops, H., 120
House, J. S., 128
Howard, K. J., 220
Howell, C. T., 31
Howell, D. C., 110, 111, 112
Huba, G. J., 106
Hudson, J. J., 40
Hurrelmann, K., 100, 187, 189, 190, 199
Hurtig, A. L., 154

## I

Inam-Shastri, A. S., 199
Igra, V., 47
Ingersoll, G. M., 109
Ingham, D., 221
Inoff, G. E., 165, 219
Irion, J., 133
Irwin, L. E., 5

## J

Jackson, G. G., 159
Jacobson, A. M., 154, 155, 156, 161, 174, 178, 179
Jaffe, B., 194
Jamison, R. N., 152, 166
Jansen, E., 121
Janssen, R. S., 59
Jemmott, J. B., 127
Jemmott, L., 93
Jemmott Ill, J. B ., 93
Jensen, L. C., 92
Jensen, P. S., 34, 35, 39
Jerusalem, M., 116
Jessor, R., 28, 68, 92, 94
Jessor, S. L., 92, 94
Jobes, D. A., 55
Johnson, J. H., 107, 108, 109, 110, 149
Johnson, L. E., 154
Johnson, S. B., 109, 164
Johnson. T. P., 144
Johnston, L. D., 62, 63, 64, 65, 66, 67
Jonas, J. M., 40
Jouriles, E. N., 119
Joy, A. E., 154
Jung, K. C., 155

## K

Kager, V. A., 154
Kaliapenemal, D., 53
Kalmuss, D., 97
Kandel, D. B., 28, 54, 65, 66, 68, 147, 148
Kanfer, F. H., 21
Kann, L., 50
Kanouse, D. E., 217
Kantner, J. F., 93, 97
Kappes, B. M., 199
Kapur, M., 53
Karabenick, S. A., 76
Karmans, W., 7
Karoly, P., 15, 18
Karon, J. M., 59, 60
Kashani, J., 25, 53, 54
Kaslow, R. A., 60
Katchadourian, H., 90
Katz, S. J., 47
Kavsek. M., 134
Kazak, A. E., 143, 204
Keith, B., 104
Kellerman, J., 154
Keniston, K., 114
Kennedy, H., 207
Kennedy, R. E., 107
Kenshole, A., 154
Keyes, C. L. M., 19
Khan, A. U., 56
Kielholz, P., 41
Kieselbach, T., 119
Kindermann, L.,185
Kinsey, A. C., 89
Klein, D. N., 53
Klein, H., 30
Klein, J. D., 220
Kline, J. J., 108
Klingman, A., 115
Klink, F., 119
Klotz, M. C., 200
Klusmann, D., 92
Knafl, K. A., 204
Kobasa, S. C., 131
Koch, S. J., 23
Köferl, P., 142
Koff, E., 72, 74, 76, 78
Kohn, P. M., 109
Koepke, D., 154
Kohut, H., 38
Kolbe, J. L., 50
Kollmar, F., 31, 80
Kolman, M. L., 170
Koocher, D., 156
Koocher, G. P., 190
Korporal, J., 7
Koski, M., 170
Kovacs, M., 31, 37, 41, 161
Kreutzer, J., 143
Kruesi, M. J. P., 55, 56, 57
Kruse, M., 92
Kuczmarski, R. J., 58
Kurtz, S. M., 155
Kumento, A., 170
Kutcher, S. P., 54

## L

La Greca, A. M., 157, 174
LaGreniere, K., 109
Lange, C., 92
Langner, T. S., 110
Lann, J. S., 34
Larson, R., 104, 126
Lasègue, E., 39, 40
Lask, B., 102
Lasker, S., 219
Laufer, M.,34, 87, 88, 90, 195, 197
Laufer, M. E., 34, 87, 88, 90, 197
Laufer, R. W., 23
Launier, R., 131, 142
Lavigne, J. V.,36
Lazare, A., 224
Lazarus, R. S., 102, 103, 105, 131, 133, 142, 143
Leavy, R. L., 127
LeBaron, S., 178
Lederer, H. D., 183, 184
Ledoux, N., 112
Lee, L., 64
Leffert, N., 104
LeGaipa, J., 144
Lehtinen, V., 182, 183, 187, 188, 199
Leigh, G. K., 87
Lepoire, B. A., 21
Lerner, R. M., 12, 76, 77
Leventhal, J. M., 204
Levi, L., 7, 102
Lewinsohn, P. M., 41, 53, 120
Lewis, R., 121, 135, 152
Lief, I. H., 89
Lieu, T. A., 47
Light, H. K., 79
Lindegren, M. L., 59
Lindholm, B. W., 117
Litt, J. F., 6, 211, 219
Littrell. M. A., 80
Littrell, J. M., 80
Livesley, W. J., 188
Locke, S. E., 127
Lösel, F., 142
Logan, D. D., 73
Lonnqvist, J. K., 56
Lopez, H., 64
Love, J. G., 91
Low, H., 74

Lowry, R., 50
Lynd, H. M., 123
Lynd, R. S., 123

## M

MacEachron, A. E., 94
Magnusson, D., 71, 74
Malcarne, V. L., 103, 133, 139
Malhorta, H. K., 199
Manning, W. G., 47
Marcelli, D., 220
March, V., 40
Marcia, J. E., 113
Marks, A., 219
Marrero, D. G., 126, 160, 174
Marteau, T. M., 155, 170
Martin, M., 188
Martin, P., 200, 201
Marton, P., 54
Marttunen, M. J., 56
Marvin, R., 204
Maser, J. D., 36
Mason, G., 221
Masten, A. S., 15, 105, 112
Matarazzo, J. D., 18
Mattson, A., 74
Mauseth, R., 154
McCabe, M. P., 91, 95
McCanley, E., 41
McClure, R., 197
McConaughy, S. H., 31. 38
McCoy, J. K., 91
McCrae, R. R., 133
McCubbin, H. J., 19, 134, 171, 172, 204
McCubbin, M. A., 19
McCutcheon, S. M., 107, 109
McGee, R., 39
McGillivray, R. G., 150
McGuire, M. B., 3, 8, 20, 101, 117, 175, 183, 184, 185
McKay, M. M., 122
McKenry, P., 87
McKeon, P., 68
McKeown, R. E., 63
McKinney, K. L., 71
McMahon, R. J., 35
McManus, M. A., 47
McPherson, A., 120
McQuiston, S., 152, 181, 190
Meadows, H. T., 143
Mechanic, D., 148, 188
Melamed, B. G., 15
Mendels, J., 40
Millen, L., 24
Miller, B. C., 91
Miller, B. D., 214, 215
Miller, J. P., 57, 155, 170
Millstein, S. G., 5, 6, 47, 211
Minuchin, S., 17, 154, 189, 206
Misch, P., 119
Mitchell, C., 197
Mitchell, J., 41
Moehr, J. R., 20
Moffitt, T. E., 39
Monck, E., 119
Mönks, F. J., 122
Montemayor, R., 122
Mont-Reynaud, R., 117
Moore, K., 98
Moore, S., 90, 91, 92, 93, 94, 95, 122
Moormann, D., 160
Moos, B. S., 170
Moos, R. H., 129, 132, 134, 138, 139, 170,171
Moreau, D. L., 54
Morgan, H. G., 40, 41
Moriarty, A. E., 135
Morrison, D. M., 97
Moss, S. J., 41
Mott, F. L., 63
Mrazek, J., 46, 75
Muehlenhard, C., 95
Murch, R. L., 130
Murphy, G. E., 57
Murphy, L. B., 135
Musa, K., 77

## N

Nadler, R., 190
Nannis, E., 13
Natapoff, J., 16
Nathanson, C. A., 98
Navarro, V., 8
Neale, J. M., 134
Neemann, J., 105
Nelson, D. E., 65
Nelson, P., 30
Nenci, A. M., 76
Neubauer, G., 95
Neugarten, B. L., 71
Neuper, C., 165
Newacheck, P. W., 44, 47, 50
Newburger, J., 204
Newcomb, N. D., 106, 112
Niemcryk, S. J., 154
Nilles, D., 160
Noam, G., 174, 178
Nolen-Hoeksema, S., 101, 135, 138, 141
Noles, S. W., 79
Noller, P., 119
Norell, J. E., 26
Northman, J. E., 195

Nottelmann, E. D., 34, 35, 39, 71
Novacek, J., 120
Novick, J.,197, 224, 225

## O

O'Connell, J. K., 79
Oetting, E. R., 62, 64, 65, 66, 67
Offer, D., 30, 120, 140, 167, 220
Offer, J., 140
Offord, D. R., 37, 41, 52, 53, 54, 207
O'Grady, J., 188
O'Leary, K. D., 119
Olson, T. D., 91, 92
Olweus, D., 74, 118
O'Malley, F., 181, 190, 223
O'Malley, J. E., 156
O'Malley, P. M., 62, 66
Onorato, I. M., 59
Orleans, C. T., 63, 64
Orley, J., 34
Orosan, J., 111
Orr, D. P., 109, 156
Osborn, M., 188
Ostrov, E., 220
Otto, S., 164
Owens, R., 156

## P

Padilla, A. M., 96
Padilla. E. R., 108
Paikoff, R. L., 71, 72, 103
Palentien, C., 100, 187, 189, 190, 199
Palmer, J. P., 154
Pandima, R. J., 68
Papini, D. R., 24
Parish, T., 199
Park, K. B., 154
Parrott, R., 21, 22, 25, 26
Pasley, B. K., 143
Patterson, J. M., 134, 155, 171, 172
Patton, W., 119
Paxton, S. J., 79, 80
Pearce, J., 54
Pearlin, C. J., 131, 156
Pearlin, L., 8
Pecoraro, R., 154
Perrin, J. M., 152, 156
Peters, R. D., 35
Petersen, A. C., 54, 61, 69, 72, 73, 74, 77, 79, 104, 106, 107, 133, 139
Petersen, L. P., 217
Peterson, J., 98
Pfeffer, C. R., 56
Phares, V., 105, 110, 111, 112
Phinney, G. V., 92
Pierce, J. P., 64, 65
Pierce, L., 30
Pierret, J., 2
Pinner, R. W., 48
Pless, J. B., 46, 156
Podorefsky, D., 146
Polin, G., 170
Pope, H. G., 40
Poston, W. S. C., 215
Potter, P. C., 16
Poustka, F., 34
Powers, S. I., 174, 178
Price, G., 79
Primavera, I., 143
Procidano, M. E., 125
Province, M., 57
Punamaki, R., 116

## Q

Quinn, A., 218
Quinton, D., 189

## R

Racine, Y., 52, 53
Rao, S., 53
Raskin, R., 120
Rauste-von-Wright, M., 77
Redl, F.,197
Redlich, F. C,. 184
Reich, T, 57
Reichert, P., 74, 79
Reid, W. J., 31
Reiser, L. W., 71, 74, 83, 84, 86, 156
Reiss, A. J., 45
Reiss, D., 161
Remmers, H., 122
Remschmidt, H., 187
Renouf, A. G., 31
Resnick, M. D., 58
Rice, K. G., 106, 131, 135, 136
Rich, C. L., 56
Richards, M. H., 79, 104, 126
Ridley, C. R., 215
Rierdan, J., 72, 74, 76, 79
Riegel, K. F., 159
Rigler, D., 154
Rinsley, D. B., 181, 190, 197, 223
Ritchie, K., 204
Roach, M., 77
Roberts, M. T. C., 16
Robinette, C. D., 56
Robinson, N., 159
Robinson, S. K., 29

Roche, J. P., 92
Rodin, G. M., 154
Rodrigues-Lima, K. R., 224
Rogers, P. D., 63
Rogers, R., 175, 196, 197
Rohde, P., 41
Rohsenow, D. J., 108
Roll, S., 24
Rook, K. S., 150
Rosen, B. M., 35
Rosen, R. A., 27
Rosenbaum, M. B., 77
Rosenberg, F., 77
Rosenberg, P. S., 59
Rosenblatt, R., 116
Rosenheim, E., 224
Rosenthal, D., 90, 91, 92, 93, 94, 95, 122
Rosenthal, D. A., 117
Rosman, B., 17
Roth, J. A., 45
Roth, M., 80, 207
Roth, R., 164, 177
Roth, S., 142
Rovet, J. F., 154, 177
Roy, A., 56
Rozario, J., 53
Rubenfeld, L. A., 129
Rubenstein, E., 205, 206
Ruble, D. N., 81
Runeson, B., 56
Russell, F. M., 40, 41
Russell, G. F. M., 39
Rutter, M., 10, 11, 13, 14, 34, 36, 38, 41, 52, 74, 105, 135, 136, 188, 189, 214
Ryan, C., 177
Ryan, P., 194
Ryff, C. D., 19
Ryland, D. H., 55, 56, 57

## S

Sabbeth, B. F., 204
Safyer, A. W., 154
Salkin, B., 40
Salt, R. E., 26, 84
Sandler, J., 207
Sanger, M .S., 154
Sanok, R. J., 27
Santiago, J. V., 155, 170
Sattler, D. L., 199
Satterwhite, B., 156
Saslow, G., 21
Savagean, J. A., 199
Schalling, D., 74
Scheidt, P. C., 47
Schinkel, A. M., 155
Schmidt, G., 89, 92, 95, 96, 97
Schmidt-Tannwald, I., 92, 98
Schmitz, K., 194, 201
Schonert, K. A., 220
Schonfield, W. A., 75
Schooler, C., 131, 167
Schraa, J. C., 29
Schulz, A., 25, 72, 80, 81, 82, 83, 84, 85
Schuster, M. A., 217
Schwartz, N. L., 174
Schwefel, D., 102
Scott-Jones, D., 87, 93, 96, 97, 98
Seeley, J. R., 53
Seidman, F., 178
Seiffge-Krenke, I., 16, 17, 24, 31, 32, 35, 80, 85, 91, 104, 121, 122, 128, 130, 132, 133, 134, 135, 137, 139, 140, 142, 144, 151, 152, 156, 157, 160, 169, 172, 175, 176, 179, 188, 191, 192, 194, 197, 201, 203, 205, 207
Seligman, M. P. E., 141
Sells, C. W., 44, 64, 69
Selye, H., 102
Setoguchi, Y., 129
Shaffer, D., 36
Shafii, M., 56
Shapiro, R., 207
Shellow, R., 35
Sherman, M., 56
Shimberg, B., 122
Shovral, R., 170
Shucksmith, J., 91
Shulman, S., 132, 134
Siddique, C. M., 121, 123
Siegel, J. M., 110
Siegel, L., 15
Siegel, L. J., 57
Sigusch, V., 89, 92, 96
Silber, I. J., 29
Silbert, A., 204
Simcha-Fagan, O., 110
Simmons, R. G., 71, 77, 78, 106
Simonds, J. E., 174, 178
Sines, L. K., 173
Singh, G. K., 44, 45
Skiba, R. J., 38
Slade, J. D., 63, 64
Slater, E. J., 205, 206
Slavin, L., 156
Slavin, L. A., 129
Smetana, J. G., 104, 106
Smith, R. S., 10, 14, 135
Smith, M. S., 154, 155
Snell, W. E., 24
Snyder, C. R., 30
Sobol, A. M., 151, 152
Soff, M., 86
Solomon, M. L., 170
Spatz Widom, C., 119, 150

Spears, M. A., 154
Spirito, A., 133
Sroufe, L. A., 13, 145
Stabler, B., 159
Stabler, J., 75
Stacey, M., 16
Staghezza, B. M., 39
Stark, L. J., 133, 134
Stattin, H., 71, 74
Stavrakaki, C., 54
Stein, D. M., 74, 79
Stein, H., 178
Stein, J. H., 71, 83, 84, 85
Stein, R. E. K., 49, 74
Stein, S., 159
Steinberg, L. D., 146
Steinmetz, S. K., 119
Stella, M. Y., 44, 45
Stemmler, M., 133
Stern, M., 121, 133
Stiffman, A. R., 59
Stocker, C. M., 150
Stone, A. A., 134
Story, M., 58
Storz, N. S., 79
Strouse, J. S., 92, 94
Strebnik, D. S., 125
Strupp, H. H., 19
Stubbs, M. L., 74, 76
Sturge, C., 36
Sturzenberger, S., 40
Suckow, A., 160
Sullivan, B. J., 165, 178
Sullivan, P., 107
Suls, J., 142
Susman, E. J., 74, 86
Susman, M. B., 170
Svensson, P. G., 102, 119
Swaim, R. C., 66
Swearingen, E. M., 110
Sweeney, P. A., 59
Swift, C. R., 178
Sylvestre, J. C., 146
Szatman, P., 207

## T

Talbot, D., 129
Tanner, J. M., 71
Tarnowski, K. J., 219
Taylor, B., 73
Taylor, W. R., 50
Tellegen, A., 15
Thiel, K. S., 146
Thoits, P. A., 110, 125, 127
Thompson, J., 100
Tilton-Weaver, L., 71, 144
Tizard, J., 36
Tobin-Richards, M. H., 77, 78
Tolor, A., 131, 133
Toolan, P., 41, 194
Touliatos, J., 117
Tramontana, M. G., 200
Trautman, P., 56
Travis, L. B., 154
Treboux, D., 94
Troiano, R. P., 58
Troxell, J. R., 108
Tuma, A. H., 34
Turner, S. L., 93, 96, 97, 98
Turtle, J. R,. 166
Tyson, R. L., 207

## U

Udry, J. R., 89
Urberg, K. A., 27
Urdze, A., 92, 98

## V

Väisänen, E., 182
Vaillant, G. E., 131
Valois, R. F., 63
van der Ende, J., 39
van Goor-Lambo, G., 34
Vanatta, K., 129
Vance, M. D., 109
Varni, J. W., 129, 155
Vaugham, S., 75
Vega, A., 177
Vega, W. A., 68
Verbrugge, L. M., 184, 185
Verhulst, F. C., 39
Vernberg, E. M., 130
Versteegen, U., 2
Ville, C., 182
Vincent, M. L., 63
Vizard, E., 119
Vonderach, G., 119

## W

Wagner, B. M., 112, 129, 134
Wahl, H. W., 17
Walker, D. B., 151
Walker, L. S., 100
Wallander, J. L., 155
Walsh, M. E., 3
Warheit, G. J., 68
Waring, E. M., 22, 24
Warren, M. P., 72, 73, 106
Warren-Boulton, E., 174
Warwick, W. J., 155, 171
Wasaw, M., 204

Wassef, A., 221
Watzlawik, P., 17
Wayne, H., 120
Weakland, J. H., 17
Webster-Statton, C., 31
Weddle, K. D., 87, 89, 94
Weil, W. B., 170
Weiner, I. B., 32, 35, 52
Weinman, J., 16
Weir, T., 128
Weiss, P. A., 13
Weiss, B., 200
Weissman, J.,
Weisz, J. R., 200
Weitzman, M., 151
Weller, J. M., 156
Werner, E. E., 10, 14, 135
Werner, M. J., 62
Wertlieb, D., 155, 170
Westbrook, L. E., 49
Wester, U., 201, 203
Wetzel, R. D., 57
Wexler, P., 170
Whitaker, B., 67
White, A. B., 87
White, K., 170
White, N. H., 155
Whitmore, K., 36
Wilcox, K. T., 155
Wilker, L., 204
Wilkinson, G., 178, 207
Williams, L. A., 133
Williams, R., 2
Williams, R. A., 110, 111, 112
Willett, J., 161
Wills, T. A., 126, 127, 128, 129
Winefield, C., 20
Winnicott, D. W., 23, 220
Winokur, A., 40
Winstead, B. A., 79
Winter, R. J., 170
Wirth, R., 185
Wolf, S., 159
Wolfe, M., 23
Wood, H. D., 144
Woodward, C. A., 189
Wortman, C. B., 167
Wright, L., 15

## Y

Yamaguchi, K., 68
Yau, J., 104
Young, C. D., 188
Yule, W., 36, 189

## Z

Zabin, L. S., 97
Zakin, D. F., 78
Zeitzschel, U., 92
Zelnik, M., 93, 96
Zeltzer, L., 154, 178
Zeltzer, P., 178
Zevon, M. A., 121, 133
Zöllner, H., 102
Zola, J. K., 183, 184
Zubin, J., 32

# Subject Index

## A


Abortion, 61
Accidents, 44, 46, 47, 63, 108
Adaptation, 15, 73, 74
familial, 204, 205
impact of self-concept, 167
to illness, 155
Adjustment, *see* Adaptation
Adolescence, definition of, 152
AIDS, 45, 46, 48, 59-61, 92, 114, 115, 217
age differences in infection, 59
gender differences in infection, 59
risk awareness, 60
Alcohol, 44, 62, 63
age of first drinking, 62
cultural differences in alcohol abuse, 62, 63
gender differences in alcohol abuse, 62, 63
Allergies, 50
Anorexia nervosa, *see* Eating disorders
Anxiety, 37-39, 41, 129, 110, 214
Attractiveness, 76-78, 80, 156
perception of, 77, 78
Autonomy, 221-224
Avoidance, *see* Defense mechanisms


## B


Behavior
health-related, *see* Health care-seeking behavior
problem behavior, 74
risk-taking, 6, 9, 26, 28,1 47, 209
sexual, *see* Sexuality
Birth control, *see* Contraception
Body complaints, 99-101, 107, 167, 168, 179, 213
age differences, 100
gender differences, 100,101,106
Body concept, 70
Body contact, 26
Body image, 70, 75-80, 106, 167, 168, 178, 213
definition of, 75
development of, 75
gender differences, 76, 77
negative body image, 58, 78-81
Body perception, 168
Body satisfaction, 76-81
Body weight 57, 58, 80
attitudes toward, 58
overweight, 58
impact on health, 58
Breast development, 72
Buffer model, *see* Models
Bulimia nervosa, *see* Eating disorders
Bullying, 118, 119


## C


Cancer, 143

Changes
developmental, 28, 133, 136
in living conditions, 148
physical, 41, 70-73,
Cheating, 219
Chronic illness, 9, 38, 49-52, 109, 152, 212, 219, 222-224
age differences, 49, 51
attitudes toward, 165
cultural differences, 50, 51
definition of, 49, 50
impact on development, 151, 152
impact on peer relationships, 155
incidence, 49
knowledge about, 164, 165
parental stress, 203, 204
parental monitoring, 205, 206
phases in dealing with, 162-164
prevalence, 49, 50, 51
socioeconomic differences, 50-52
Closeness, 83, 175
Cognitive complexity, 133
Coitus, *see* Sexual intercourse
Comorbidity, 34, 36-41, 154, 207, 208, 214
Compliance, 16, 154, 157, 165, 182, 190, 210, 219, 220
age differences, 154
changes over time, 165, 166,
hypercompliance, 219
Conduct disorders, *see* Disorders, conduct
Contact
avoidance of, 26, 83
body contact, *see* Body contact
changes in, 82, 83
physical, 5, 20, 25, 82-85, 127
Contraception, 60, 89, 93-98, 216
attitudes toward, 94, 95
cultural differences, 97
gender differences, 97, 98
knowledge about, 93, 96,
use of, 94-98
Coping, 124, 131, 132, 148, 151-156
active, 132, 148, 149, 242
adaptive, 137, 138
age differences, 133, 153, 154
anticipatory, 132, 133
avoidant, 133, 137-142, 149, 209, 224
conceptualization of, 131, 132, 153
developmental factors, 154, 156,
familial, 154, 155, 171, 172, 204, 205
family factors, 154, 155, 169-172
gender differences in, 134, 141, 142, 154
impact of body image, 166, 167
impact of severity of illness, 155
impact of visibility of illness, 156
impact of physician-patient relationship, 175
peers as a coping resource, 155
process, 7, 8
strategies, 155, 164
styles, 9, 12, 130, 134, 136, 141, 143, 210
cognitive strategies, 155, 156,
emotion-focused, 133, 139
problem-focused, 133, 136, 139, 149, 155, 156, 160
illness-specific strategies, 16, 151-153, 155, 156, 160
maladaptive strategies, 136, 137, 142, 150, 209, 210
Counseling aversion, *see* Health care-seeking behavior
Critical life events, *see* Stressors

## D

Dating, 91-93, 104
Daydreaming, 26, 27, 156,
Death, causes of, 44, 69, 211
Defense mechanisms, 179
asceticism, 40,
avoidance, 161, 188
denial, 156, 161, 162-164, 188
rationalization, 156
regression, 35, 184,
repression, 188,
secrecy, 161-164
Depression, 31, 52-54, 74, 79, 110-112, 126, 139-141, 214
age differences, 52-54
comorbidity, 36-41
etiology of, 54
gender differences, 54, 79, 141,
larvate depression, 41
symptoms, 53, 54, 128-130, 133, 135, 138, 141, 150, 214
syndromes, 52
prevalence of, 41, 54
Development
cognitive, 3, 70
physical, 72
Developmental breakdown, 87, 152
Developmental pediatrics, 13, 15
Developmental progression, 36, 212, 217
Developmental psychopathology, 13, 14, 135
Developmental tasks, 113, 114, 155, 158, 169, 173
Deviance hypothesis, *see* Timing, hypothesis about
Diabetes, 157-164, 219

coping with, 158-164
impact of stressors, 159-161
metabolic control, 157, 160
perception of, 161, 162
prevalence, 157
psychosocial consequences, 177-179
psychosocial factors, 157
role of the family, 159
symptoms of, 157
Diagnostics
assessment, 23
Diagnostic information, 18,21
health diagnostics, 19, 22
Diary, 85, 86
Dieting behavior, 58, 74, 78, 79, 213, *see also* Eating disorders
gender differences, 78
Disclosure, 157, 197, 198, *see also* Self-disclosure
Disease, *see also* Illness, Chronic illness, AIDS,
infectious, 48
Disorders
conduct disorders, 138
physical disorders, 127
psychological disorders, *see* Psychological disorders
transitory disorders, 35
Distress
emotional, 220,221
psychosocial, 220
Divorce *see also* Stressors, familial
Doctor-patient communication, *see* Relationships, physician-patient
Drugs, 43, 45, 52, 60, 65, 66, 68, 140, 147, 148, 218, 220 *see also* Substance abuse
cultural differences, 66
developmental patterns, 67, 68
prevalence, 66
DSM, *see* Psychiatric classification systems

## E

Eating disorders, 39-41, 57-59, 86, 213, 214
age differences, 58
anorexia nervosa, 36, 39, 40
bulimia nervosa, 39, 40
cultural differences, 58
gender differences, 57, 58
prevalence, 58
Egocentrism, 6, 26-28, 217
Erotic fantasies, 89, 90, 216
Ethnic minorities, 215

## F

Factors
protective, 9, 11-14, 124, 130, 135, 145, 148, 149
risk, 10-14, 27, 38, 124, 130, 135, 148, 149
Family
achievement-orientation, 171
cohesion, 130, 135, 145, 146, 222
communication patterns, 173
disengagement from, 146
dynamics, 17
climate, 130, 171, 172
familial coping, *see* Coping, familial
familial dysfunction, 205
familial perception of illness, 189
impact on coping 169-172
pathological, 179, 180, 189
stressors, *see* Stressors, familial
Fantasizing, *see* Daydreaming, Erotic fantasies
Friends, *see* Relationships, with peers
Future, fears about, 114, 115, 121, 178

## G

Germ theory, 4
Gender role intensification hypothesis, 172

## H

Health, 129, 212
attitudes toward, 17, 212
awareness of health problems, 187, 188, 190
care, 15, 182, 183, 209, 210, 215, 217, 218, 224
care providers, 15, 16, 32, 36, 209, 210, 212, 214-218, 221, 222
care-seeking behavior, 47, 181, 182, 184, 185, 189
age differences, 191
counseling aversion, 190, 195
gender differences, 187, 191, 194
motivation, 190, 195, 196-199
parents' readiness to accept help, 203
socioeconomic differences, 184
definition of, 1, 5, 6
development of health concepts, 3, 5

disclosure, 43, 151
lay conceptions of, 2, 3, 6, 12, 16, 19
mental health, 139, 221
models
compensation model, 15
medical model, 7, 12
pathogenic-curative model, 12
pathology-oriented model, 15
psychological model, 9, 12
risk factor model, 7, 8
salutogenetic model, 7, 12
sociological model, 8, 12
parental perception of adolescents' health, 221, 222
physical, 99
problems, 43, 144, 148, 149, 211, 214
psychological, 99
public health, 45
risk behavior, 43, 158
seismographs, 211
status, 1, 43, 99, 166, 167, 210
impact on body image, 80
unconscious attitudes toward, 2
unreliability of adolescents' perception, 35, 36
Heterosexual relationships, *see* Relationships, heterosexual
HIV, *see* AIDS
Homicide, 43, 44
age differences, 44, 45
cultural differences, 45
Hospitalization, 46, 223
Hysteria, 40

## I

ICD, *see* Psychiatric classification systems
Illness, 45, 46, 102, 212, *see also* Morbidity, Chronic illness
causes, 3
immunity to, 6
medical prevention, 46
mental, 9
perception of, 154,187
psychosomatic, 100
reaction to, 5
socioeconomic differences, 183
types of patients, 184
visibility of, 156,
Imaginary audience, 27
Immigration, 116
Inhalants, *see* Substance abuse
Injuries, 46,47
In-time, *see,* Timing
Intervention, 212,221
Intimacy, 175
Intoxication, *see* Alcohol
Invulnerability, *see* Vulnerability

## L

Life-span developmental perspective, 16
Lifestyles, 8, 21
risky, 9

## M

Maladaptation, 52, 73, 74, 104, 110, 111, 151, 152, 178
age differences, 154
emotional, 155
psychological, 73, 74, 178
Malnutrition *see* Poverty
Marijuana, 65, 66, *see also* Substance abuse, Drugs
Masturbation, 89, 90, 216
acceptance of, 89
central masturbation fantasy, 87
disclosure about, 89
frequency, 89
gender differences, 89
Maturity
assessment of, 71
cognitive, 134,213
early, 72
impact on peer relationships, 85
late, 72
perception of, 80
physical, 25, 70-74, 213, 216, 217
social, 24, 134
Menarche, 25, 71–73, 80, 101
attitudes towards, 80
cultural differences, 73
disclosure about, 82,83
perception of, 73
Mental health, *see* Health
Models, *see also* Health, models of
approach-avoidance model, 132, 134
buffer model, 127–129
main effect model, 127–129
Morbidity, 27, 47, 48, 211
age differences, 45, 46, 47
cultural differences, 47, 48
gender differences, 50, 100, 213
multimorbidity, 17
socioeconomic differences, 50–52
Moratorium, 113
Mortality, 27, 43, 44, 46, 48, 69, 211
age differences, 44, 45, 48
cultural differences, 44, 46

gender differences, 213
socioeconomic differences, 50, 51
Motivation, 224
therapeutic, 224, 225

## N

Nocturnal emission, *see* Semenarche
Nudity, 84
dealing with, 25, 26, 30, 210, 216, 218

## O

Oedipal identification, 87
Obesity, *see* Eating disorders

## P

Parents
monitoring of chronic illness, *see* Chronic illness
perception of adolescents health, *see* Health
readiness to accept help, *see* Health
relationship to adolescents, *see* Relationships, with parents
Peers, *see* Relationships, with peers
Personal fable phenomenon, 27, 97
Physical appearance, *see* Attractiveness
Physical changes, 14, 70–73
Physical contact, 82–85, *see also* Contact
Physical maturity, *see* Maturity, physical
Physical well-being, *see* Well-being
Physician–patient relationship, *see* Relationships, physician–patient
Poverty, 117,118 *see also* Stressors, macrosocial
Pregnancy, 59, 61, 69, 98, 118
cultural differences, 61
prevalence, 38–40
Prevention, 212
Privacy, 82, 84
informational, 22
physical, 22, 23, 25
psychological, 22, 25, 26
violation of, 26
Psychiatric classification systems
deficits, 32
DSM, 33, 34, 39
ICD, 33, 34, 39
utility of, 35
Psychological disorders, 52, 53, 127, 129, 178, 187
acceptance, 199, 200
age differences, 36, 52
gender differences, 36, 52, 53
perception of, 188
prevalence, 52
psychological care seeking, 187
Psychological immune system, 9
Psychosomatic medicine, 7
Psychotherapy, 224
attitudes toward, 191–193, 194, 199–203
aversion to, 196–199
effectiveness, 200–203
gender differences, 194, 195
parents' attitudes, 203–205, 206, 207
Psychopathology, 34, 37, 39, 109–111
Psychosomatic illness, *see* Illness, pychosomatic
Pubertal status, 70,71

## R

Rationalization, *see* Defense mechanisms
Regression, *see* Defense mechanisms
Relationships
compensatory relationships, 9,10
deficits in, 144–146, 150
heterosexual, 91–96, 104, 113, 114, 173, 175, *see also* Sexuality
physician–patient, 20–22, 175, 176, 181, 182, 185, 186, 211, 216–218, 222–224
improvement of, 218, 219
role expectations, 186
social, 16, 143
supportive, 128, 129
with family members, 82, 83
with parents, 17, 30, 31, 82 104, 106, 118, 128, 130, 133, 135, 136, 211
with peers, 85, 86, 104, 128–130, 133, 173–175, 220, 221
gender differences, 85, 86
Repression, *see* Defense mechanisms
Resilience, 10, 14, 135, 136, 145
Risk behavior, *see* Behavior, risk-taking
Risk factors, *see* Factors
Roles
sick person's role, 4

## S

Secrecy, *see* Defense mechanisms
Seismographs, *see* Health
Self-concept, 74, 77, 167
Self-disclosure, 22–25, *see also* Disclosure

changes in, 28, 210, 216–218
low disclosure, 31, 36
self-disclose partners, 23, 24
willingness to disclose, 146, 216
Self-esteem, 78, 79, 161, 167
Self-representation
styles of, 23, 25
Semenarche, 71, 74, 80, 82, 89, 216
disclosure about, 83
Sex-typing, 89
Sexuality, 216, 218
development of, 87–89
psychoanalytic theory, 87, 88
psychological theory, 89
diseases, 60, 61, *see also* AIDS
gender differences, 87
homosexuality, 56, 59, 60
initiation, 87, 91, 92, 94
motives, 95
risk behavior, 43, 59, 61, 89
sexual intercourse, 89, 92–95, 216
gender differences, 93
cultural differences, 93
Sickness, *see* Chronic Illness, Illness
Smoking, 63–65
age of initiation, 63,64
cultural differences, 64
gender differences, 64
prevalence, 64
Social networks, 125, 126, 134, 143, 145, 146
misperception of social networks, 145
Social resources, 12
Social support, *see* Support, social
Socioeconomic status, 2, 8
Somatization, 36, 129, 210
Stress, 7, 9, 15, 38, 101–103, 130, 131, 135, 209, 213
buffers, 128
chronic, 130, 143, 144
effects of, 138
general adaptation syndrome, 102
impact on accidents, 108
impact on chronic illness, 109
impact on development, 107
impact on health, 99
impact on psychopathology, 109–111
impact on somatic complaints, 107
perception of, 121
physical symptoms of stress, 107
psychological symptoms of stress, 107
resistance to, 10
stress illnesses, 102, 103,
Stressors, 103, 129, 215
accumulation of, 11, 105–107, 109, 128, 135
change of, 123
control of, 103
critical life events, 103, 109, 155
definition of, 9
development-related, 105, 112
everyday hassles, 103
family stressors, 104, 105, 108, 112, 143, 146
gender differences, 104
illness-related stressors, 151, 160, 161
interpersonal stress, 20
macrosocial stressors, 113, 116, 143, 148
major stressors, 143, 149
minor stressors, 131–133, 137
non-normative stressors, 103–105, 148, 149, 151
normative stressors, 103, 104, 137, 148, 149
predictability of, 103
self-related stressors, 139
Substance abuse, 41, 66, 67, *see also* Drugs
Suicide, 43, 44, 52, 55–57, 120
age differences, 55
gender differences, 55
cultural differences, 55
methods, 56
suicidal thoughts, 55, 56
risk factors for, 56, 57
Support, 151, 154, 157, 158, 167
emotional, 20,125,128
from friends, 174,221
informational, 128
instrumental, 125,128
social, 9, 124–128, 134, 135, 145, 149, 154, 157, 167
availibility of, 127
deficits in, 143, 149
perceived, 125, 127, 145, 146
influence on symptomatology, 128, 129
risk factors, *see also* Factors, risk
Symptoms
externalizing, 31, 36–38, 41, 42
internalizing, 31, 36–38, 41
evaluation by different sources, 30, 31
mislabeling of, 29
gender differences in perception of, 212
Syndromes
externalizing, 140,142
internalizing, 140

## T

Thinness, 57, 78, 80, *see also* Body weight
Timing, 12, 70–75
gender differences, 74
impact on adjustment, 74
"in-time," 71
"off-time," 71
hypotheses
stage termination stage hypothesis, 73
deviance hypothesis, 73
goodness-of-fit hypothesis, 73
perception of pubertal timing, 72
gender differences, 72

## U

Unemployment, 119, 120, *see also* Stressors, macrosocial

## V

Violence, 118, 213, *see also* Stressors, macrosocial
in family, 118
in school, 119
Virology, 7
Vulnerability, 9, 10, 14

## W

War conditions, 116, *see also* Stressors, macrosocial
Weight gain, 213, *see also* Body weight
Well-being, 17
emotional, 19
physical, 19, 125
psychological, 2, 125, 126, 222
Withdrawal, *see* Coping, avoidant